Occupational Therapy in Practice

A Collection of Articles From the
Special Interest Section Newsletters

Volume 1
1978, No. 1–1983, No. 2

The American Occupational Therapy Association, Inc.
Rockville, Maryland

Foreword

Volume 1 of *Occupational Therapy in Practice* is a collection of articles from the AOTA Special Interest Section (SIS) newsletters published from 1978 to mid-1983. The Special Interest Sections were formed in 1976 to facilitate the exchange of ideas between therapists and to encourage the development of occupational therapy in specialty practice areas. At that time, five sections were formed: developmental disabilities, gerontology, mental health, physical disabilities, and sensory integration. In 1978, each section began producing a quarterly newsletter to address the practice/communication needs of its membership. The Administration and Management SIS was formed in 1985 and therefore is not included in this volume.

After the first year of publication, it became apparent that the newsletter format fulfilled a major communication need for AOTA. The newsletters contained original high-quality practice articles. Because of the short, informal nature of the articles therapists felt encouraged to write and share clinical experiences that most likely would not have been developed into a formal journal article.

Inevitably, requests were made to preserve these articles so that their content could be referenced and retrieved. Thus, the idea for this collection was born.

In determining the content of this collection, the five members of the 1984 SIS Steering Committee reviewed the newsletters of their respective sections and selected articles that "contributed to the knowledge base of occupational therapy." The articles are presented in reverse chronological order, that is, from the most recent to the earliest. To guide the reader to a particular subject area, an index is included at the back of the book. Readers should also note that to facilitate referencing these articles have been reproduced in their original form. No further editing or correcting has been attempted.

Many people have contributed to the publication of *Occupational Therapy in Practice;* most notably, Carol Gwin, OTR, AOTA liaison to the Special Interest Sections, who served as coordinator for the project; the members of the 1984 SIS Steering Committee, Ann Conway, past chair of the Mental Health SIS, Nancy Ellis, chair of the Gerontology SIS, Gretchen Reeves, past chair of the Sensory Integration SIS, and Lana Warren, chair of the Developmental Disability SIS, who determined which articles were to be included in the collection; and Linda Tomasini, Practice Division secretary, who compiled the articles that had been selected.

From AOTA's Publications Division, Sabine J. Beisler, production editor, oversaw the production of the book, and Patsy Carpenter, managing editor, provided technical assistance.

Jeanne Melvin, OTR, MEd, FAOTA
Editor and
Past Chair (1982-1985)
Physical Disabilities SIS

CONTENTS

2 Gerontology Special Interest Section

3   Mental Health Special Interest Section

4 Physical Disabilities Special Interest Section

5   Sensory Integration Special Interest Section

Index *page* 237

1
Developmental Disabilities
Special Interest Section

Developmental Disabilities
Special Interest Section Newsletter; Vol. 6, No. 2, 1983

The Dual Diagnosis Client—A Need for Special Programming

By Shawn Miyake, MA, OTR, and Toni Quintana, Oxnard, CA

Within the last few years, clinicians have begun to deal with a newly identified group of individuals who present clinical problems that are difficult to treat. These individuals have been labeled "dual diagnosis" clients, and they possess the "dual diagnosis" of developmental disability and mental illness. The literature appears to support the high rate of psychiatric disturbance in retarded individuals. One study[1] of a population of 798 retarded individuals identified 14% as having a mental illness. Other authors[2] have begun to investigate the relationship between mental retardation and chronic mental illness.

One possible reason for the increased visibility of this client population is that cuts have forced many agencies to more accurately define those they are mandated to serve. With shrinking funds, agencies must be more selective in delineating populations that will receive services. Funding cuts frequently force agencies to combine several programs into one. This results in clients with many different problems being included in a single treatment program. These factors are frustrating to the clinician who is trying to provide the best treatment for individuals with multiple problems. These individuals are not easily handled with available resources, and they make up the therapists' "I throw up my hands in helplessness—what do I do with them?" category.

Although a definitive dual diagnosis incidence rate is not available in the literature, the public agencies of a California city of approximately 100,000 have estimated that in 1982-83 there were about 50 dual diagnosis cases living there. These individuals were visible because their acting out behaviors in the community brought them into contact with police, emergency rooms or inpatient units. Still unknown are the individuals who remain invisible in the community because they neither seek or receive services.

No policy regarding the handling of these cases exists in this city. A verbal agreement between agencies (mental health and an agency serving the developmentally disabled) has been made to handle such individuals on a case by case basis. Those clients who are clearly defined as developmentally disabled by the state's standards and clearly defined as mentally ill by DSM-III do not appear to have difficulty acquiring services from either agency. Only the primary diagnosis appears to differ (DD/MI or MI/DD) depending on the agency from which services are currently being received.

The clients who had the greatest difficulty receiving necessary and appropriate services were those individuals who were labeled mentally ill and who had "functional" retardation. In a retrospective study by Russell and Tanguay[2], the relationship between mental illness and mental retardation was investigated. The authors recognized that psychiatric disturbances that occurred in adulthood could temporarily disrupt general intellectual functioning. They then questioned whether or not a psychotic process that occurred during the developmental period could lead to a chronic depression of intellectual performance, and whether or not a person with such a condition could actually be labeled "retarded." The results of their study appeared to support the idea that persons suffering from chronic psychiatric conditions, especially psychoses, may have a prolonged or permanent depression of intelligence. Because these clients do not fit the legal definition of developmental disability, receiving specialized services for problems related to such a disability is difficult. Consequently, these clients receive only mental health services. Although such services deal effectively with acute and chronic psychiatric conditions, the clients they are not able to deal with the problems caused by depressed intellectual function or behavioral disturbances.

Behavioral disturbance is the single most important reason (next to intellectual loss) for institutionalizing mentally retarded persons[2]. Many mental health clinicians comment on the difficulties of working with dual diagnosis clients and they cite the clients' behavioral disturbances as a day-to-day frustration. Poor treatment compliance, such as with medication schedules, is another difficulty acknowledged by some mental health clinicians. Therapists often report that they have not been trained to deal with these types of problems.

In an effort to deal with these complex problems, the aforementioned city shuffles clients back and forth between agencies. Some get lost in the shuffle and receive no services. Others go to sheltered workshops for the developmentally disabled and stay as long as they remain symptomatic. During periods of stress, their psychiatric conditions often get worse, and clients then are bounced over to mental health clinics. After such episodes are brought under control, the clients then go back to the workshop. Clinicians in both settings agree that it is difficult to handle such clients and, depending upon the setting, they are able to deal with only certain aspects of their client's disabilities.

After interviewing clinicians who worked with this difficult population, ideas representing an ideal program were combined. A program was proposed that had a behavioral control component (such as behavior modification), medication for control of psychotic symptoms, social and recreational rehabilitation, vocational education and daily living skills training. Ideally, the program should be provided within the clients' living situation (e.g., board and care).

A group program for dual diagnosis clients in a community mental health facility is being developed. These clients' lowered intellectual performance, coupled with their psychotic symptoms result in such problems as behavioral acting out, impulsive behavior, inability to sit still and inability to participate in group discussions. These multiple problems render most mental-health oriented rehabilitation programs ineffective. Programs that have combined behavior modification, habit training (regarding time use, dressing and grooming skills, social

(continued)

The Dual Diagnosis Client

skills, goal attainment), and structured activities that have a low stress/demand component (including activities with clearly defined limits/rules and boundaries, low expectations for performance and constant feedback regarding behavior) have proved successful. In the near future more programs should be designed to recognize and treat the the special multiplicity of needs of this client population.

References:
1. Eaton, L. and Menolascino, F., Psychiatric disorders in the mentally retarded: types, problems and challenges, *Amer. J. of Psychiatry* Vol. 139, No. 10, Oct. 1982, pp 1297-1303.
2. Russell, A. and Tanguay, P., Mental illness and mental retardation: cause or coincidence? *Amer. J. of Mental Deficiency*, Vol. 85, No. 6, 1981, pp 570-574.

The authors wish to thank Thomas McGee, MSW, William Wakelee, MSW, and Tracy Luchetta, for their comments and observations regarding this client population.

Developmental Disabilities
Special Interest Section Newsletter; Vol. 6, No. 2, 1983

Some Coping Mechanisms of Retarded School-Age Children

By Judith Schouten, OTR, Milwaukee, WI

Charlie, a developmentally disabled boy, did not have the fine motor hand skills or muscle strength necessary to button his shirt or button and zip his pants until he was a pre-adolescent. Mom took the time to do these tasks. Charlie got his fasteners done and he got a loved one's close, warm, individual attention. Now, his environmental situation has changed. Mom has a job, a new baby, or has lost interest. Her son is older and has developed the motor skills and strength to do his own fasteners. However, Charlie still takes 20 minutes to do five shirt buttons. He frequently goes to Mom or another adult, fumbles and whines, and then waits for intervention. Independence in dressing is not achieved. Why?

Common coping mechanisms such as denial, acting out, or projection are frequently used by elementary school children when responding to a conflict situation. Students in the trainable mentally retarded range tend to manipulate their environment when confronted with obstacles that interfere with their needs. The environment then adapts to them. Classroom teachers often describe this type of coping behavior as uncooperative or noncompliant. Parents also are puzzled by such behavior. As a school-based therapist in daily contact with this population, I found two features characteristic of these coping behaviors. First, once they are learned, they are very difficult to circumvent. Second,

they are easily reinforced by ordinary adult/peer interaction or environmental demands. In Charlie's case, unless Mom buttons his shirt and pants, he will miss his school bus.

External demands to adjust (such as Charlie's learning to button) require some adaptive action on the part of the child, whether it is constructive or nonconstructive. By fumbling and waiting, Charlie fulfills all of his perceived needs. In an individual with a limited repertoire of social skills, and in some cases, little or no appropriate expressive language, adaptation of this sort can be interpreted as resistance.

Such adaptive actions frequently occur during specific task requests, the performance of which a trainable mentally retarded (TMR) child perceives as too difficult or not desirable. Charlie saw buttoning as something his mother did for him, so he put forth no effort to learn to do it himself.

The following adaptive actions have been observed in a school setting:

1. Verbal ability is used to distract the teacher/requestor from the requested task. For example, "Where did you buy this?" or, "Why?"
2. A child *actively* refuses to do a task by throwing a temper tantrum, doing a sit-down strike in the middle of class, saying "no" without trying, or by crying.
3. A child *passively* refuses by making his whole body go limp, by ignoring or gazing pathetically at the requestor,

or by waiting for outside intervention after a few nonproductive "tries."

4. Some TMR students rely on compensatory acts like saying or nodding "yes" and then doing nothing. Watching the requestor's face for a correct response or seeking frequent reassurance reflects students' inability to perform even though they want to please the requestor.
5. Destructive frustration is exhibited by biting one's own hand, throwing a requested object and kicking or pushing others.
6. Children may also use physiological responses like crying, gagging, (with no food in the mouth) during feeding training, or soiling their pants.

Charlie used a typical physiological adaptive behavior to change a situation he didn't like. Mom picked Charlie up early from school one day to take him to the dentist. She came early another day for a parent-teacher conference. Charlie wanted to go home, because lately he didn't like school. While waiting in the office for Mom, Charlie had an "accident," and soiled his pants. Mom was embarrassed. She cut the meeting short and left with Charlie.

Often these adaptive behaviors are taken at face value and the underlying cause is not addressed. We, who are supposed to help students grow and develop, can unknowingly reinforce manipulative behavior by stopping a requested task and then not resuming it after the child's action. The result is

(continued)

Coping Mechanisms

that the child's evasive maneuver is positively reinforced.

Interpreting these behaviors as learned responses to stress can give further insight into effective intervention. One can then see uncooperative behavior as a developmentally delayed child's method of coping rather than as a reflection on the ability of a teacher or a parent.

What can be done to curb this stress response? First, consider that the requested task may have a strong emotional element. The task may be so frustrating for the child that the mere sight of it provokes feelings of failure. At first, Charlie was not happy about buttoning because he had never been successful in this activity. However, when he was presented with a game that had the same motor components,

Charlie changed his attitude and eventually learned to button. In the second example, if Charlie had been changed into fresh clothes after his "accident" and the parent-teacher conference resumed, the message would have been that Charlie's evasive maneuver did not work.

A positive reward system can be used by the requestor to reinforce appropriate behavior and appropriate methods of self-expression. Acknowledging the task's difficulty while rewarding the student's efforts is one method of increasing productive use of therapy time. The therapist can reinforce appropriate elements of a multi-step task such as shoe tying by placing two shoe strings on a cardboard, calling one a "cat," the other a "mouse," and making up a story with

the student. Old jogging shoes—maybe one of Dad's—can also be used.

Another way to create a positive reward is to drop a marble into a jar whenever an appropriate behavior during "practice time" is seen. A simple agreement such as, "If you get 10 marbles in the jar, you can do this . . .", can be made. After the student reaches the predetermined number of marbles, the agreed-upon reward can be given. The child will be able to see when the requested task will end.

These are just a few ways to change the emphasis of a requested task from a threatening situation into a cooperative, pleasant experience. Charlie gets attention and warm support from his environment and learns to be more confident in his abilities. In the end, Charlie is pleased with his independence in dressing and so is Mom.

Developmental Disabilities
Special Interest Section Newsletter; Vol. 5, No. 4, 1982

Provision of Services for the Developmentally Disabled: "When Is Enough Enough?"

By Olivia Ann Unger, OTR, Los Angeles, California

The decision to terminate an independent living skills group for developmentally disabled adults forces occupational therapists to take a good hard look at what they do. What you believe you have accomplished and what really has happened may be very different. A more provocative question may be asked in terms of serving a population that is faced with a life-long disability: "When is enough, enough?" A group for emotionally disturbed developmentally disabled young adults, co-led by this writer, will be used as the spring board from which to raise questions regarding the decision to terminate services.

The group began two years ago with five clients at the Neuropsychiatric Institute of UCLA. They included both men and women who were emotionally disturbed and developmentally disabled young adults. Clients ranged from borderline to mildly retarded in intellectual functioning with moderate

to severe limitations in self-care, self-direction, learning and capacity for independent living. Four of the five members went to school or worked in sheltered environments.

Presenting problems were divergent and included: noncompliance, physical and verbal angry outbursts, lack of investment in current work program and low self-esteem. The needs, however, for all clients were similar and were primarily related to basic daily survival skills. For example, changes in routine or schedule presented serious difficulties for these individuals. Simple obstacles such as breaking a shoe lace or locking oneself out of the house posed larger than life difficulties. The major adjustment problem for our clients was in the sphere of interpersonal relationships. Whether it be in the workshop, on the bus, in the home or in the group, communication skills were the area of greatest strife.

Broadly, the focus of the group was

on interpersonal problem solving, social skill development and emotional support. The methods included a broad range of activities both within and outside the hospital setting, which included: bowling, parties, snack preparation, arts and crafts, group discussions, and role playing. Thus, a central focus of the group was not only coping with daily hassles but coping while demonstrating appropriateness in behavior.

Conscious of the limitation posed by dealing with social problems frequently out of context (i.e., out of the setting these issues normally arise), we began to explore in greater depth how and where members spent their time and the purposes and goals of other groups that they attended. Members were all well entrenched in a support network for the developmentally disabled whether it be through social clubs or other daily living skills pro-

(continued)

Provision of Services

grams. Six months ago it became clear that our group as well as these other community groups were part of a web of services offered to the developmentally disabled. By virtue of their participation in this network, they were integrated into an externally controlled system of socialization which may have excluded them from the mainstream of society. Although not our intent, our group was "the place to meet" on Thursdays whereas other programs were for Monday, Tuesday or Wednesday. Because our services no longer appeared to provide a unique function, the group leaders decided to terminate the group. This is where critical questions began to be raised, not only in regard to this specific group, but more broadly to services being provided for the developmentally disabled. The questions are not mutually exclusive but all focus on issues pertaining to

working with a population that have longstanding problems interfering with entering mainstream society. 1) What are appropriate entry and terminating goals for a daily living skills group? We as professionals perceive we have treatment goals. Are the goals of the professional consistent with those receiving the services? 2) There appears to be an informal social support network for the developmentally disabled by virtue of the number of programs being offered. If the group or program becomes the thing to do on Thursday, what function is it fulfilling? Are the groups or programs indistinguishable to the group members other than as a place to go on a given day of the week? Is this an appropriate function for occupational therapy, that is, purely a social group? 3) Occupational therapy as a profession is committed and knowledgeable in the area

of chronic disabilities. Should we be leaders in establishing models for programs for the developmentally disabled? If so, what would such a model look like? 4) How are services being coordinated within various communities for the developmentally disabled? What more specialized services do we see as needed by the dual diagnosis client? 5) Who are setting the standards for community living for the adult developmentally disabled? When do these adults no longer require our professional services?

In this article, a group co-led by this writer was used to exemplify issues related both to the initiation and the termination of services for the developmentally disabled. Questions such as these will encourage occupational therapists to scrutinize their role in the provision of effective and responsible services for this client population.

Developmental Disabilities
Special Interest Section Newsletter; Vol. 5, No. 4, 1982

Adapted Table for Multiply Handicapped Adult

By Cindy Hughes, COTA Student, Worcester, MA

This table was designed to improve the function of a multiplyhandicapped, retarded adult. He has cerebral palsy, marked by spastic quadriplegia and severe scoliosis. To attain functional use of his right arm, he needs to be in a side-lying position, supported by a bean bag. The table is used to raise activities to his level (Figure 1).

The table top can be placed at any angle to promote maximum range of motion or to fit various activities (e.g., vertical for drawing, slanted for reading or flat for table-top activities). The front is left open so that the table can be brought as close to the user as possible, fitting the bean bag underneath. Three slits are made in the top to attach an A.S.P. holder.

(continued)

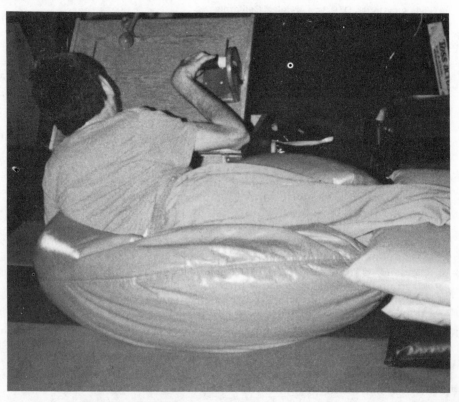

Figure 1

Adapted Table

TOP: 1/2" plywood with 1/2" pine strip edges (2-18" and 1-24"). 1/4" slits are cut 2 1/2" in from the edge for the A.S.P. holder. Underneath top a piece of wood is needed for support sticks.

SIDES: (2) 3/4" pine board 10" wide x 24" long

BACK: (1) 3/4" pine board 10" wide x 24" long

STORAGE: (1) 3" wide x 22 1/2" long (side) notch cut wide enough to clear support sticks
(1) 10" pine board 22 1/2" long (bottom) (see elevation at side)

SUPPORTS: Three-3/4" wide sticks of any length depending on angle of table top wanted. Pivot all on 4" dowel with 2 blocks on either side to hold the dowel. (See Plan at Table Base.)

FINISHED TABLE MEASUREMENTS

Total height:	10"
Total length:	24"
Total width:	15"
Raised edge:	1/2" high

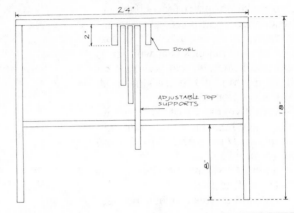

**Figure 2—
Plan at Table Base**

Developmental Disabilities
Special Interest Section Newsletter; Vol. 5, No. 3, 1982

Adaptive Equipment Construction With Tri-Wall Cardboard

By Catriona Binder-Macleod, OTR, and Gloria Walden, both of Jonesboro, Georgia

Tri-Wall

A material called Tri-Wall has revolutionized our adaptive equipment department. Adrienne Bergen of Blythedale Children's Hospital introduced us (the therapists at Clayton County Board of Education) to this material. Although this material is not new, very few therapists seem to use it. We would like to share information about Tri-Wall because we think tremendous savings can be realized in terms of cost, time, and energy by using Tri-Wall instead of the conventional plywood for building adaptive equipment.

Materials needed:
1) Tri-Wall—one-inch thick corrugated cardboard used commercially to make large heavy-duty boxes. It can be bought in sheets of square footage.

2) 1/4" dowels—used for "nails." Cut dowels in 3-1/2" to 4" lengths and sharpen in pencil sharpener.
3) Elmer's glue.
4) 1" foam for padding.
5) Terry cloth or vinyl for upholstering equipment.
6) Contact paper to "waterproof" surfaces.

Construction:
Construction is basically similar to construction with wood, except that it

(continued)

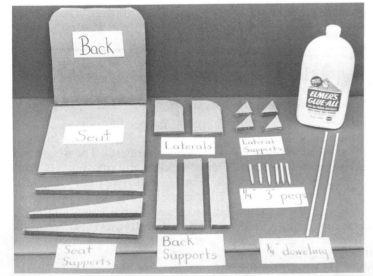

Figure 1

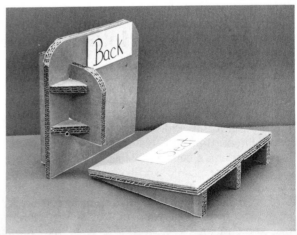

Figure 2

Adaptive Equipment Construction

is much easier and faster!

1) Cut out pattern pieces of cardboard for piece of equipment desired, e.g., to make an insert for a chair: cut out back piece, seat piece, and laterals. (Figure 1).

2) Cut out triangles that will act as supports for laterals, seat, and back.

3) Apply lots of Elmer's glue to all joint intersections.

4) Join two pieces of Tri-Wall by putting glued surfaces together and hammering 1/4″ dowel "nails" into joint. (Figure 2)

5) Support weight bearing pieces with Tri-Wall triangles.

6) Pad and upholster where needed. (Figure 3)

7) Apply contact paper to surfaces that need to be water resistant.

Uses:

We have used Tri-Wall to construct:
1) Wheelchair-adapted seat inserts
2) Classroom-adapted seat inserts
3) Footrests
4) Side-lyers
5) Small tables
6) Bench seats
7) Small prone standers
8) Flap switch for battery operated toys (March '81 issue *AJOT*).

Advantages:

1) Low cost—cheaper than plywood. A 4′x8′ piece of Tri-Wall is $9.60.

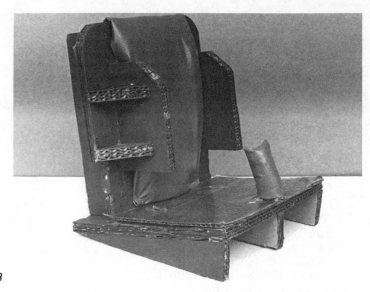

Figure 3

2) Energy and time expenditure. Easier to work with than wood. Not as time consuming to make projects.

3) Lightweight—for increased portability in classroom and home and ease of storage.

4) Because of above advantages, Tri-Wall is good to use for equipment for young children who quickly outgrow their equipment. Average life of equipment in daily use is two to three years.

Disadvantages:

1) Will not take very heavy use—i.e., will not stand up under force of extreme spasticity or excessive weight.

2) Cannot be water proofed as well as wood. Contact paper can be used to

waterproof surfaces such as table tops or seat inserts that may have liquids spilled on them and need to be wiped down (obviously not good for adapted toilet seats).

Tri-Wall Suppliers:

1. The Workshop for Learning Things; 5 Bridge Street, Watertown, MA 02172.

2. Medco, 2077 New York Avenue; Huntington Station, NY 11746.

3. Kane Paper Company, Bldg. 413, Wilson Airport Industrial Park, Macon, GA 31297.

For further information contact: Catriona Binder-Macleod, OTR, Clayton County Board of Education, 5870 Maddox Rd., Morrow, GA 30260.

Developmental Disabilities

Special Interest Section Newsletter; Vol. 5, No. 3, 1982

Weighted Cup Holder for the Severely Disabled

By Marguerite S. Emshoff, MA, OTR, Philadelphia, PA, and Robin A. Juckem, BS, Philadelphia, PA

A simple solution has been developed to enable severely disabled individuals to drink independently. It has been found useful for individuals whose gross incoordination or spasticity make handling a cup impossible. It is also an aid for people who have poor head and torso control and are therefore unable to bend over and drink from a conventional cup and straw placed on a table.

A young man with these problems

was recently treated in occupational therapy at the Community Organization for Mental Health and Retardation. He has severe spastic cerebral palsy with wrist contractures and had never been able to drink independently. He had always required someone to hold a cup for him. The adapted cup holder described below gives him freedom from this dependency. When the cup and holder are placed on his lapboard, he can push them into posi-

tion and sip when he desires. The extra height puts the straw within his head and body control area. The weight prevents sudden arm movements from tipping the cup. The plastic cup with lid is used to keep the straw in place and to prevent spills (Figure 1).

This simple device is also useful for patients with severe upper extremity weakness, particularly those whose

(continued)

Weighted Cup Holder

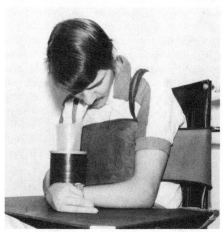

Figure 1

movement is restricted by neck collars or torso supports.

The cup holder is inexpensive and easy to construct. The cup is easily removed from the holder for filling and washing.

Materials

Materials needed are: an empty one-pound coffee can with plastic lid; convalescent feeding cup;[1] plastic flex straw; 3 two-pound diving weights or a five-pound ankle weight;[2] 14 inches Con-tact® paper.

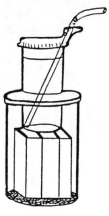

Figure 2

Fabrication

Trace the circumference of the bottom of the cup in the center of the plastic coffee can lid. Cut this out carefully, making sure the hole is not too large. Put the weights upright in the can so they support the cup (Figure 2). If necessary, wedge in cardboard to hold them upright. Cover the can with Con-tact® paper.

[1] Convalescent Feeding Cup is available from Fred Sammons Be OK.

[2] Diving weights are available in sporting goods stores and are inexpensive. Five-pound ankle weights are available from Preston.

Developmental Disabilities
Special Interest Section Newsletter; Vol. 5, No. 2, 1982

Inexpensive Adaptive Positioning Equipment for a Multiply Handicapped Child

By: June Houston, COTA, Jonesboro, Tennessee

Multiply handicapped children often need several different types of adaptive equipment for use throughout the day. This is especially true for severely involved children who have no volitional movement and are unable to change position. The unique needs of each child often make commercially constructed products unsuitable and, in addition, their cost is often prohibitive. This article describes two inexpensive positioning devices that can be made quickly and easily from objects and materials often found in the home.

The child shown in Figures 1 and 2 is 6 1/2 year old girl with severe, spastic quadriplegic cerebral palsy. Spasticity is present in all her extremities, with flexor tone dominating in the upper extremities and extensor tone in the lower extremities. This child is totally reflex dominated, with no functional gross or fine motor abilities. She lacks head and trunk control, has severe oral dysfunctions, is visually impaired and is developing scoliosis and a dislocation of her left hip. The child is totally dependent on her caretakers to provide for her basic needs. Her interaction with the environment is minimal. Wheelchair, stroller, carseat or sidelying positioner do not adquately meet her needs for postural support and reflex inhibition. Neither are sandbags able to position her in supine, prone or sidelying positions due to her strong extensor thrust pattern.

To position the child in an upright position, a plastic 13 gallon (49.21 L) kitchen garbage container (oblong rather than round) was adapted by cutting away a portion of three sides, and padding the inside and edges of the container with 1 1/2" (3.81 cm) and 1"

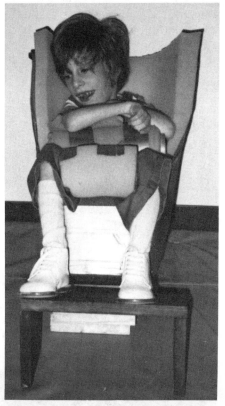

Figure 1

(continued)

9

Adaptive Positioning Equipment

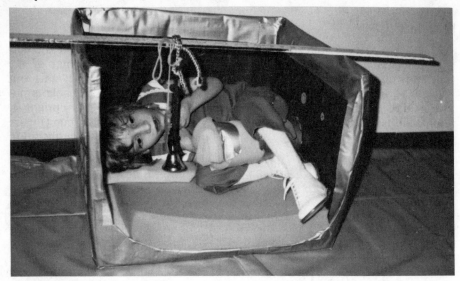

Figure 2

(2.54 cm) foam. (See Figures 3 and 4). Duct tape was used to hold the foam padding in place. The child sits in the chair and is propped against the wall at the angle which best encourages active head control. Two 1 1/2'' (3.81 cm) scraps of wood were placed under the chair to stabilize it and a footrest constructed of scrap wood was placed at the front of the chair to support the child's feet in a neutral position. Two-inch thicknesses of foam were cut in lengths varying from 6''-10'' (15.24-25.4 cm), and were taped with duct tape; these were used to provide additional support and positioning (e.g. placed between knees to maintain abduction of the hips, placed under the arms to discourage habitual flexion of the upper extremities).

To position the child in sidelying, a large, sturdy cardboard box (16''x18''x22'') (40.64x45.72x58.88 cm) was used. (Boxes of other sizes may be chosen to accommodate children of various sizes). This child's extensor thrust was so strong that she could not be positioned in sidelying unless her hips were completely flexed. The box chosen was strong enough to keep her in a flexed position and to prevent the extensor thrust pattern. The front of the box was cut away to allow contact with environmental stimuli. The floor of the box was padded with 3'' (76.2 cm) foam, the box was covered with contact paper inside and outside, and the edges were taped with duct tape. A pillow of 1'' (2.54 cm) foam was used for the child's head and could be moved to either side of the box to position the child on either the right or left side. The same foam shapes that were used to provide additional support in the upright positioner were used as needed in the sidelying positioner.

In both these positioners, a yardstick was used to hang various toys at the child's eye and hand level.

Advantages of these positioners:

1. The child can be positioned with good body alignment in both upright and in sidelying positions on both right and left sides. This will prevent worsening of orthopedic deformities, and will inhibit abnormal reflexes.

2. The upright position will encourage head control and awareness of the environment.

3. Both positioners are inexpensive, can be easily constructed by parents for use at home and can be discarded or modified when the child outgrows them.

4. Toys can be suspended from the positioners to encourage the child to reach.

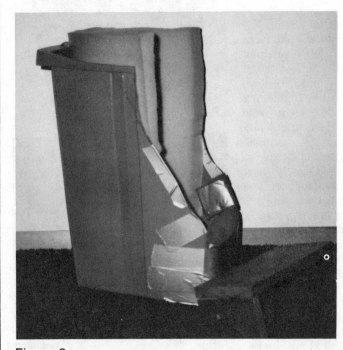

Figure 3

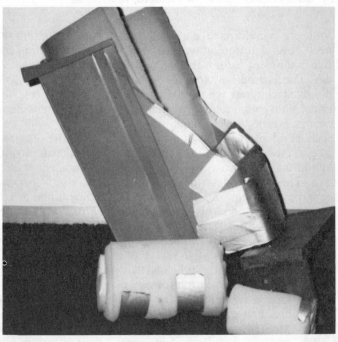

Figure 4

The Confusion in the Definition of Developmental Disabilities— Implications for Occupational Therapy Practice

The confusion that exists in the definition of developmental disabilities in general and in the practice of OT with developmentally disabled individuals in particular continues to be discussed. Recently, these issues received attention in *Mental Retardation,* December 1981, "The Definition of Developmental Disabilities: A Concept in Transition," by Jean Summers and in *AJOT,* February 1982, "Developmental Disabilities, An Ambiguous Term," by Martha Moersch. The DDSIS standing committee would like to provide a forum for the expression of the views of the members of the special interest section on these subjects. Some thoughts, opinions and questions regarding developmental disabilities and OT practice within this special interest area have been compiled here. We are sharing some of our concerns and would like to invite those of you who wish to respond to do so.

First, let us review the most commonly used current definition of developmental disabilities, from the 1978 extension of the DD Act, PL 95-602. As usually printed, it reads, "A developmental disability is a severe, chronic disability of a person which (A) is attributable to a mental or physical impairment, or combination of mental and physical impairments; (B) is manifested before the person attains age twenty-two; (C) is likely to continue indefinitely; (D) results in substantial functional limitations in three or more of the following areas of major life activity; (i) self-care, (ii) receptive and expressive language, (iii) learning, (iv) mobility, (v) self-direction, (vi) capacity for independent living, and (vii) economic self-sufficiency; and (E) reflects the person's need for a combination and sequence of special, interdisciplinary, or generic care, treatment, or other services which are individually planned and coordinated (42 USC 6102(7))." Some people have expressed the belief that this functional definition is excessively general, that it is inconsistent in purpose, creates difficulty in implementation and that too much emphasis is placed on severity of involvement.

The standing committee believes that the definition's emphasis on the functional aspects of developmental disabilities is properly palced, and that, furthermore, this definition of DD suggests a view of OT practice in this area. We would like to call this a generalist view of practice. The generalist OT in DD, from this perspective, is a therapist who has a broad knowledge and understanding of the skills a person needs to function with maximum success in the roles she or he will fill throughout his or her lifespan. The generalist's goal is to teach these skills, and he or she has the ability to do so for a variety of persons, regardless of their age or specific diagnostic category. To be most effective, however, the generalist also needs to develop special skills in such areas as, for example, the Bayley Scales of Infant Development or an intimate knowledge of the cognitive processes associated with adult decision making, problem solving and goal setting.

Another view holds that the most effective OT working in DD is a specialist. He or she develops special knowledge of the problems of patients or clients in a specific diagnostic category such as cerebral palsy, mental retardation or autism or in a special age group such as infants and develops and refines such skills within that specialty.

An apparently common belief is that the therapist who works with developmentally disabled individuals is working only with children. We know that the definition of DD states that disability is "likely to continue indefinitely" and that definition implies need for services throughout life. Most of us are also aware of individual therapists who work with adolescents or adults who are developmentally disabled. However, we would like to find out if most OTs working in DD work with children only, how many have adolescent or adult patients or clients and what programs and services we are providing for adults. We would also like to ask some questions about the reason there seems to be a preponderance of programs and services for children. Some possible explanations may lie in the organization of our health care system, which is slanted toward care for acute rather than chronic problems. A belief may exist that a developmental problem in a child is acute and therefore deserving of care, whereas the same problem, twenty years later is chronic, will change little if at all and is not worth dealing with. Some explanation may be found in today's emphasis of early intervention. Could it be because professionals find it more appealing and/or rewarding to work with children? Does the fact that the already-established structure of the education system provides a mechanism for identifying and treating developmental problems have an effect? What additional factors may be involved in this issue?

With these thoughts in mind, you the readers of this newsletter are invited to write to share your views and concerns regarding:

1. the definition of developmental disabilities; is it too vague and what problems arise as a result?

2. the scope of your own practices with respect to your roles as generalists or specialists; which do you consider yourself and how do you believe you are most effective?

3. the ages of patients or clients included in programs for people with developmental disabilities; for what age range do you provide services and what needs do you see as unmet?

4. the basic OT educational curriculum: should there be more emphasis on developmental disabilities during the entire life span?

Developmental Disabilities
Special Interest Section Newsletter; Vol. 5, No. 1, 1982

Occupational Therapy Program Development Within a Hospital Setting for Patients With Epilepsy

by Stephanie Day, MA, OTR, Los Angeles, CA

One Reed is a six-bed clinical and research unit within the UCLA Neuropsychiatric Institute (NPI) for individuals with long histories of poorly controlled seizures. Patients are referred by neurologists and admitted for extended periods of continuous seizure monitoring, the electrical (brain wave) component via telemetry EEG and the behavioral component via closed-circuit video recording. Most patients stay 2-4 weeks, but shorter or longer periods may be required to collect sufficient data. The purpose of the monitoring may be to: 1) confirm a diagnosis of epilepsy (ruling out pseudo or hysterial seizures) and to plan appropriate treatment, 2) diagnose seizure type(s) and adjust anticonvulsant medications accordingly, or 3) to evaluate the patient for surgical treatment.

Patients admitted to One Reed have ranged in age from 5 to 63 (though the majority are 16-30) and represent a wide socioeconomic and geographical distribution. Recurrent seizures are the only medical problem for some patients, whereas for others there may be a combination of difficulties, ranging from subtle deficits in learning or personality to general developmental delay, cerebral palsy or mental retardation.

Until two years ago, the staff of One Reed consisted of physicians, nurses, a neuropsychologist and neurophysiological research staff. At that time, the administration of the NPI funded a half-time occupational therapy position for One Reed, to "provide activities" for the unit because the patients complained of boredom and isolation.

In interviewing for the position, the prospective therapist spoke to some patients who were on the unit at the time. It became evident that boredom and isolation were not only hospital-induced phenomena, but were more general life problems as well. It became clear during the initial development of the OT program that, while some people with chronic seizures lead full lives with a balance of work, rest and play and are well integrated in families and communities, more patients experience a variety of problems in daily life, including social isolation and lack of "occupation." "Occupation" is used here not just in the sense of paid employment (though this is a common problem), but in the broader sense of satisfying, purposeful activity. These issues were verified in much of the rehabilitation literature on epilepsy (although there is a notable lack of participation by OT), which concludes

that seizures themselves are but a part of the problem for people with epilepsy. When combined with social stigma and other factors, they may become a major psycho-social handicap to the persons's realizing a satisfying life.

Given the wide variety of problems and age span of One Reed patients, the Occupational Behavior (OB) frame of reference was adopted to guide practice because it provided a view of the "entire developmental continuum of play and work. . ." (1). As Matsutsuyu stated, OB is "guided primarily by the sociological concept of role and socialization and by the psychological theories of achievement motivation, problem solving and personality development. Such a behavioral science base, combined with medical science and knowledge, creates a view of patients not only as diagnostic entities, but as individuals with both assets and problems in daily living" (2). This perspective provided a unified way of approaching the life problems experienced by these individuals.

A questionnaire-interview was devised by the occupational therapist to evaluate the areas of daily living in which each patient needed assistance. The problem areas identified determined the choice of activities for each patient during hospitalization.

Beginning with the child's roles as player and student, persons with recurrent seizures may experience difficulties in acquiring the skills necessary for adequate performance of their roles. Children for example, may not be allowed by their families to climb, ride a bike, skate or play games with other children for fear they may have a seizure during the activity and be injured. They may not be given chores or responsibilities in the family. If playmates observe a seizure, they may conclude that the child is "wierd" and tease or exclude the child from group activities. These children may have difficulty with attention, learning or behavior in school.

Adolescents with ongoing seizures may continue to have problems in the roles of student and player and may fall behind their peers in developing interests, values, habits and skills needed for future work (the occupational choice process), for having meaningful relationships with people of the opposite sex and in beginning to assert their independence from parents.

This developmental continuum may result in adults with not only chronic seizures, but also with deficits in daily liv-

ing skills, problems with obtaining and/or maintaining work, having satisfying leisure activities and in socialization. A theme that runs strongly throughout is that of developing independence, learning to do things on one's own, to make decisions, solve problems and to use resources. Many people with chronic seizures are overprotected by well-meaning families and are not given opportunities to participate in this developmental process. The Reed staff realized that, despite the eventual outcome of the epilepsy, these daily life problems would not disappear spontaneously and needed to be addressed.

The OT program that began on One Reed had, at all times to face the constraints of time and space, i.e., 1) the patient would be in the program (within a structured, hospital setting) only for a matter of weeks, and 2) programming must take place, on the unit, within reach of the monitoring devices (antennae for telemetry EEG and camera for video). The program was begun not only to "provide activities," but to address the major problems in the life roles mentioned above and within the historical OT philosophy, i.e., "to give opportunities. . . to work, to do, to plan and to create and to learn to use materials" (3). Its intent was to reflect the developmental stages of the patients and to develop skills that support life roles by providing natural decision-making areas for the patients, acknowledging and using existing competencies, arousing curiosity and providing opportunities for practicing skills (within the limits of the hospital) in a balanced pattern of daily living.

Activities initially introduced included: 1) occupational counseling to assist adolescents with the process of occupational choice and adults with such nitty-gritty issues as: how to choose a realistic type of work (or a meaningful alternative to paid employment), whether or how to tell a potential employer about seizures and how to deal with having a seizure at work; 2) a wide variety of crafts activites to both a) teach habits and skills necessary for adequate task performance, and b) to broaden leisure repertoires; 3) group meal planning and preparation to develop these skills of daily living and to provide opportunities for task-oriented social interaction; and 4) social games and activities to provide opportunities for social interaction, for patients to share their experiences and help one another deal with the dilemmas of daily living with seizures. Throughout

(continued)

Occupational Therapy Program Development

these activities, an attempt was made to maximize choices and decisions, to solve problems and to foster some sense of independence, autonomy and control. This may be done within as simple an issue as a child's choice of clothes for the day or as complex a project as planning a menu for a group lunch. As time went on, other OT activities were added to this initial program to meet the interests and needs of individual patients, but the overall approach has remained the same.

After some time it became clear that any small gains in skills, independence, etc. made during hospitalization would likely be eroded or forgotten upon return to home environments where opportunities to maintain them were not present. Thus began the role of the OT as family consultant and community resource person. This has meant regular consultation with patients' families to explore their aspirations

and goals for their hospitalized family member, and to assist in these plans where possible. It has meant calls and visits to numerous community agencies that might help the person attain a more satisfying life. Followup contact has been made with patients; primary physicians in the community; local epilepsy societies; regional centers; school counselors; agencies offering training in independent living, family counseling, peer support groups, opportunity for volunteer participation (a number of former patients have also come back to One Reed as volunteers), recreational activities, etc. The most recent addition to the program (with a doctoral psychology intern) has been a six-week post-hospitalization group for developing social skills in everyday interactions; e.g., how to talk to your doctor, how to talk with a potential employer, where and how to meet new people in social settings.

This has been a sometimes frustrating (e.g., waiting a year for a reasonable arrangement for storage of supplies), but, overall, a rewarding two-year period. The number of patients who can be monitored simultaneously has increased from three to four. The half-time OT now works thirty hours per week. The staff, which has been extremely supportive of the OT's efforts, now also includes a psychiatric liaison and a social worker. The program should continue to evolve, with the hope of better meeting the needs of our patients.

Bibliography

(1) Reilly, M., The educational process, *AJOT* 23:299-307, 1969.
(2) Matsutsuyu, J., Occupational behavior—A perspective on work and play, *AJOT* 25:291-294, 1971.
(3) Meyer, A., The philosophy of occupation therapy, *Archives of OT* 1:1-10, 1922.

Developmental Disabilities
Special Interest Section Newsletter; Vol. 5, No. 1, 1982

A Health Care Delivery Model for Occupational Therapy Services to Day Training Centers in New Jersey

By Christine Morse Olwell, OTR, and Sheila Smith Allen, OTR, Mountainside, NJ

Accompanying a significant decrease in residential placement for handicapped children, an evergrowing need exists for alternative community-based services for the severely and profoundly involved who are cared for at home by natural or foster parents. Such services must not only meet the complex needs of these handicapped children, they must also provide effective support systems for their families.

Within the state of New Jersey, Day Training Centers have been established in an attempt to meet the needs of severely and profoundly retarded children and their families. Initially, these facilities were viewed as day care centers. However, with changing federal and state legislation regarding education for the handicapped, school districts and parents looked toward these centers for provision of optimal daily programming, including therapy.

As a result, the Bureau of Day Training included physical and speech therapy consultation services to the classroom technicians. The technicians were responsible for incorporating therapeutic techniques into the daily classroom routine.

As parents grew increasingly aware of the utilization of ancillary services in other public schools, they began to request occupational therapy from their local educa-

tion agencies. Interested parents, in collaboration with Westfield Special Services, obtained a grant to get occupational therapy in their Day Training Center. Children's Specialized Hospital was approached to develop a working model for the delivery of occupational therapy services to severely and profoundly retarded students attending Day Training Centers in New Jersey. The pilot program was begun at Union County Day Training Center.

In looking at the complex and sometimes unique problems of the severely and profoundly retarded, the following issues became clear:

1. The families wanted to keep their children at home but were concerned with increasing difficulties in daily management.
2. These children had been medically grossly underserved.
3. The meaning of "education" for this population had to be further examined so that ancillary services could be best utilized.
4. A systematic process had to be devised that would realistically deal with the number of students in potential need of services, and would assure the quality of these services.

5. Therapeutic accountability and statistically sound verification of students' progress were needed.
6. The severely and profoundly retarded, in view of their limited rate of change, are a difficult group of students to work with.

As a basis for occupational therapy operations, a philosophical framework was formulated that took into account both the previously mentioned population-related needs and the general rationale behind the day training service, i.e., "education within the least restrictive environment." Our dual focus was designed to complement and enhance the educational process. First, a functional approach was formulated toward meeting parents' needs in relation to the home management of their children. Second, a therapeutic approach was developed to improve the students' basic sensory responsiveness and motoric abilities in order to encourage adaptive behavior.

It was our feeling that changes made in the students' adaptive behavior would not only facilitate more effective educational programming, but would make a positive impact on family life as well. Gains in basic sensory processing were thought to

(continued)

Health Care Delivery Model

lead to interactional changes that would be noted in the home as well as the classroom.

While developing this program and assuring quality services, we had to address the realities of the New Jersey personnel shortage and lack of interest in working with this population. The proposed Health Care Delivery Model therefore incorporated an OTR/COTA team with ongoing consultation provided by a more experienced OTR. This "mini-team" was established in order to facilitate intradisciplinary problem solving and to offer mutual support. In addition, it was thought that the mini-team would minimize professional isolation, a major concern expressed by program applicants.

Three delivery modes were developed for OT services so that each student, following a complete OT evaluation, could receive therapy through one.

1. *Direct* treatment in individual or group sessions.
2. *Monitoring* of positioning, adaptive equipment or classroom carryover.

3. *Consultation* regarding individual or group needs as requested by the center's staff. The responsibility for implementing occupational therapy lies with professional staff requesting consultation.

Following the development of occupational therapy delivery modes, a sound method for evaluating the validity of our philosophical premise was needed. As developmental levels *per se* were not of primary concern in programming for this population, an evaluation tool was principally needed in order to assess underlying causes of maladaptive behavior. This tool had to provide for objective gathering of data and serve as a reliable indicator of change. What evolved was a systematic assessment of the basic sensory channels. Information from this assessment was used to interpret additional data obtained from cognitive-adaptive and gross motor/reflex evaluations. Interpretive data then could be applied in the educational program.

This Health Care Delivery model, which integrated a medical model into an educa-

tional system, has now been in existence for two years and thus far our philosophical premise appears justified. The State of New Jersey, in recognizing the program's success, has created occupational therapy positions in all Day Training Centers and has made $55,000 available for specialized medical consultations. In addition, the state has encouraged its new staff to visit the Union program as well as attend our workshops so that they may develop programs based on the same philosophical premise and organizational model.

The Children's Specialized Hospital program is now in a phase-out period so that the Union Center can be self-sufficient with its own therapy staff. We are continuing, however, with the process of standardizing our sensory channels evaluation and welcome therapists interested in using our evaluation for that purpose.

In her role as chief of occupational therapy, Claire Daffner, MA, OTR, was instrumental in the initiation of this outreach program. Her support and encouragement were of great help.

Developmental Disabilities
Special Interest Section Newsletter; Vol. 4, No. 4, 1981

The Use of Games for Social Skills Training With Adolescents

**By Shawn Miyake, MA, OTR, and
Marijane Miyake, OTR, Ventura, CA**

The period of development referred to as adolescence can be characterized as a time of many changes. In the transition from childhood to adulthood, adolescents are attempting to achieve appropriate social roles, new and more mature relationships with peers, acceptance and effective use of the body, and independence along a variety of dimensions. Adolescents are also preparing for possible careers, marriage and family life, acquiring values and ethics as guides for behavior, and developing socially responsible behavior.

In this period, an adolescent struggles to define who he/she is and what is his/her place in relation to others. Developing one's own identity can be accomplished in part by the identification and acceptance of a set of values society deems important. In this way, the adolescent can begin to take into account societal values when performing certain behaviors within that social sphere. Mead offers the theoretical explanation that a person comes to understand who he or she is in relation to others through an interactive and interpretative process of comparing one's own abilities and behaviors to society's expectations for

behavior. In this fashion, one finds a place in the social structure. Developmentally disabled adolescents often have special difficulty with this developmental task because they have difficulty learning the social skills needed for appropriate social behavior. For example, a developmentally disabled individual who goes to a hamburger stand to get something to eat is sometimes observed to do the following: upon approaching the counterperson and being asked, "May I help you?", he responds, "Yes." Although this is on the surface an appropriate response, it is less than informationally complete to answer the counterperson's question. The appropriate response might have been, "Yes, I'll have a hamburger and a Coke." What the developmentally disabled individual fails to accurately recognize is the information requested by the counterperson. This in part is due to a failure of the developmentally disabled person to place himself in the role of the counterperson and understand the question in that context, one in which the counterperson is there to take food orders. Instead, the developmentally disabled person misses the point of the

social interaction and answers the question only at face value. Because the subtle nuances of social interaction are often missed, the developmentally disabled person looks less than competent, receives a negative response from other people, and may become discouraged and not attempt such interaction again.

A context within which adolescents can begin to learn social skills requisite for appropriate social behavior is the game situation. Kielhofner and Miyake have suggested that games are consistent with the "art and science" of occupational therapy and should be included as legitimate media in practice. The central concept of occupational therapy has always been that humans' use of self in everyday activities such as self-care, work and play is vital to health. As such, the use of games can be included as meaningful media for occupational therapy to use in developing skills necessary for appropriate social interaction.

Games are a form of play within which rules can be learned. Rules are internal structures which inform the individual of

(continued)

Use of Games For Social Skills

the constraints upon action learned by acting with objects and persons. The adolescent can begin to formulate constraints upon his own behavior within specific physical and social contexts by the development of such rules.

In the game situation, behaviors are mediated by the rules of the game and take into account the actions of the other players. The individual must consider the strategy of the other player and be able to take on the other player's role in order to "second guess" him. This requires the individual to consider the other person's behavior from their own standpoint or role. For instance, in a football game, the pass rusher must take into account the role of the quarterback and "think" like the quarterback does in order to guess his next action. In this way, the pass rusher is able

to tackle the quarterback before he is able to complete the play.

By using game situations such as baseball, football, and basketball, in which the understanding and performance of various roles is required, developmentally disabled adolescents can begin to develop skills in taking on others' roles in relation to their own. Again, in a football game, the pass receiver needs to consider and understand the quarterback's role in order to follow a command of "down and out." Once the command is given, the quarterback has the expectation that the pass receiver will be at the right place to receive the ball. Failure to understand the underlying message to run down the field and cut to the right may instead result in the receiver's merely crouching at the scrimmage line or running out of bounds to receive the ball. A similar

lack of understanding of the interrelationship of rules leads to the unsuccessful transaction at the hamburger stand.

Understanding of and ability to take on others' roles can be taught in games in which team members are dependent on one another. It is then hoped that learning within the game situation can lead to similar understanding in other social situations and performance of more timely and acceptable social behaviors. In summary, game situations can provide a framework within which to facilitate the development of abilities to consider others' actions, values, and role behaviors. The utilization of such media may prove to be beneficial in the teaching of social skills to developmentally disabled adolescents.

Developmental Disabilities
Special Interest Section Newsletter; Vol. 4, No. 3, 1981

The Occupational Therapist's Role in a Regional Neonatal Intensive Care Unit

By Cece Courtway—Meyers, MEd, OTR
Salt Lake City, Utah

The infant is a shaper of his or her environment. From the beginning he or she gives cues to caregivers. Premature and other high-risk infants give cues mostly through motor behavior, activity and mood. The body language of these infants is most important to observe. As occupational therapists, our training in growth and development—especially with respect to reflexes and to sensorimotor, behavioral and perceptual functions—makes it possible for us to observe and evaluate behavior and to enhance the development of premature and other high-risk infants in neonatal intensive care units.

This article describes the occupational therapy component of an ongoing longitudinal, interdisciplinary research project at the Regional Neonatal Intensive Care Unit of the University of Florida Medical Center in Gainsville. The major role of the occupational therapist in this research project is to evaluate and provide treatment to the infants enrolled in the study. (Infants are enrolled in the study by having a birth weight of less

than 1800 grams and parents who are presently residing in our funding district.)

Before initiating treatment, the occupational therapist evaluates the following aspects of each neonate's repertoire:

1. States of alertness/state changes
2. Posture, motor activity
3. Reflexes
4. Muscle tone
5. Visual, auditory and other responses, including response to handling, and consolability and defensiveness
6. Sensorimotor behavior
7. Oral functions, feeding
8. Cry

The therapist then follows routine nursery sterile procedure for handwashing, gowning, etc. The therapist checks with the infant's nurse concerning the medical condition of the infant and appropriateness of time for intervention.

Treatment is initiated for each infant in the study by providing stimulation contingent upon his behavioral

and physiological cues to the therapist. Stimulation is designed to be relevant to the individual infant's level of neurophysiologic development. The type and amount of stimulation therefore varies for each child, taking into account all aspects of his sensorimotor strengths and weaknesses. Literature on the role of stimulation in the development of prematures assisted the author in planning modes of intervention that would promote intersensory integration of the immature central nervous systems. Although the types and amounts of stimulation vary, the principles remain the same. These principles include:

1. Provide sensory input designed to stimulate *in utero* or normal postnatal development.
2. Provide experiences to facilitate normal active responses.
3. Optimize oral functioning and feeding patterns.
4. Provide graded stimulation within the infant's tolerance level.
5. Prevent secondary problems that

(continued)

Occupational Therapist's Role

would result from lack of adequate handling or active movement.

6. Provide *early* intervention to optimize function and prevent secondary disabilities.

Each infant is provided with proprioceptive/kinesthetic, tactile, visual, auditory and vestibular stimulation. Treatment emphasizes symmetry of movement and body postures, and encourages midline-oriented activities.

Proprioceptive/kinesthetic stimulation includes (mostly passive) range of motion (ROM), body-on-body movement, rolling from side to side, and joint approximation. ROM is given to all extremities, moving from proximal to distal, to help improve circulation, prevent contractures, and to provide proprioceptive feedback to infant movement and posture. Rolling from side to side provides input to the brain on change of position and awareness of movement. Joint approximation improves stability at proximal points by increasing muscle tone.

Gentle, slow rhythmical massage of the infant's skin provides tactile stimulation. The developmental cephalo-caudal and proximal-distal sequences are followed. The infant's feet are given added tactile experiences, since they are found to be hypersensitive to touch (possibly because of drawing blood from the heel). Different textures (i.e., cotton balls, terry cloth, soft flannel) are also incorporated for some infants.

The therapist provides visual stimulation by interacting with the baby face to face. Objects such as toys and mobiles (especially red ones) are also used to enhance visual fixation and tracking.

Auditory stimulation consists of talking to the infant, calling the infant by name, and using objects such as squeaky toys and rattles. Tape recordings of maternal heart sounds and classical music may also be incorporated.

Vestibular stimulation is delivered by several methods: by lifting the infant to the nursing position and rocking him or her horizontally, by rocking the infant vertically with head and trunk raised to a 45-degree angle from the bed (used mostly for those infants requiring mechanical ventilatory assistance), and by using a waterbed. The waterbed provides vestibular and proprioceptive stimulation, helps decrease skin breakdown, and helps reduce an asymmetrically shaped head caused by the infant's remaining in the same position for extended periods.

Infants enrolled in the study are provided with stimulation two to three times daily, depending upon their current medical condition and their level of tolerance to the stimulation. Stimulation is totally baby-responsive; the type and amount of intervention is completely dependent upon the cues given to the therapist by the infant. Prolonged hospitalization of some infants also requires that stimulation be graded, and that it change in response to the infant's development.

Documentation of each intervention time and of the infant's response to stimulation offers the OT a developmental hospital course of the infant. Periodic reevaluations of the infant are also done to determine changes in levels of functioning. Research to substantiate the results of intervention is ongoing in this Gainesville study.

The purpose of this article is to describe the occupational therapy component of an interdisciplinary infant/family-centered intervention project. In this study the OT provided, in addition to the evaluation and treatment described above, the following: consultation with the nursing staff and physicians to inform them of results of the infants' evaluation and of any abnormal responses to stimulation; support and instruction to parents concerning the developmental needs and appropriate stimulation for their infants; and finally, continuing educational experiences/inservices for allied health students on the growth and development of premature infants and on the role of the OT in the NICU.

Developmental Disabilities
Special Interest Section Newsletter; Vol. 4, No. 3, 1981

Occupational Therapy Involvement in a Neonatal Intensive Care Unit

By Susan R. Lutostanski, OTR
Glenview, Illinois

This article describes the occupational therapy services that are provided in the Neonatal Intensive Care Unit (NICU) at Lutheran General Hospital near Chicago. The NICU (which has recently grown to 36 beds) has provided occupational therapy services since 1977.

Before the establishment of a plan for OT involvement in the nursery at Lutheran General, the need for developmental intervention was discussed with the director of neonatology. An extensive review of the literature and contact with therapists working in similar units at other facilities followed. After the plan was approved, orientation was given to the nursing staff, and OT services were begun.

Initially, only a few infants (mostly babies who had been in the NICU for a considerable length of time) were referred for OT. Since then, the growth of the nursery has resulted in the referral of an increased number of infants in a wider variety of diagnostic categories. Infants are referred for OT services on an individual basis by doctor's order. The current criteria for referral for OT services are as follows: 1) infants hospitalized for more than 8

(continued)

Occupational Therapy Involvement

weeks or infants expected to have extended hospital stays (e.g., infants with severe respiratory problems); 2) infants who show excessive irritability or inconsolability; 3) infants having a delay in growth or weight gain; 4) infants with feeding problems that imply neurological dysfunction; and 5) infants who have abnormal muscle tone, reflexes, or poor head control.

Following referral, a clinical evaluation is done to plan treatment objectives. The evaluation also provides baseline developmental data when the infant returns for developmental screening in the NICU Follow-up Program. Five areas are evaluated: 1) reflexes: These include rooting, sucking, crossed extension, flexor withdrawal, Moro, palmer grasp, plantar grasp, primary walking, placing reaction, and Gallant response. 2) muscle tone: This is evaluated by passive and active measures for the upper and lower extremities. Passive evaluation includes use of the head-to-ear maneuver, the popliteal angle measurement, angle of dorsiflexion of the foot, scarf sign, and return to flexion posture. Active muscle tone is evaluated by righting reactions of the flexor and extensor muscles of the neck and righting reactions of the lower extremities and trunk. Allowances for prematurity are made in the evaluation of both reflexes and muscle tone. 3) visual and auditory responsiveness; These are evaluated using criteria described in the Neonatal Behavioral Assessment Scale. 4) Behavioral response to sensory stimulation and handling: These are responses to tactile, kinesthetic, proprioceptive, and movement input. This important area of evaluation indicates to the therapist the amounts and types of stimulation and individual infant is able to tolerate. Current research suggests that in NICU settings infants usually are not lacking in stimulation but are actually receiving too much, and it is difficult for their nervous systems to adequately process these stimuli. 5) spontaneous activity: This includes positions of extremities and trunk at rest (e.g., symmetrical or asymetrical): spontaneous movement of the extremities, head, and trunk; hand-to-mouth behaviors; and the infant's ability to quiet and console himself.

After the evaluation is completed, treatment is implemented. General objectives include normalizing muscle tone through inhibition and facilitation techniques, monitoring the development of appropriate primary reflexes, encouraging adaptive responses to visual and auditory stimulation, encouraging normal developmental skills, such as head, trunk, and extremity control, and improving behavioral responses and interaction with handling and other environmental stimulation. When possible, infants are seen daily during their alert periods for 15 to 45 minutes. Equipment used in treatment includes infants' toys such as rattles, music boxes, and brightly colored objects (particularly red, green and yellow ones). The therapist's face is also used as a visual stimulus. Other equipment available includes a small mat, therapy balls, rolls, and infant seats.

As part of treatment in this program, the OT collaborated with a NICU nurse clinician to design a developmental nursing care plan. This plan specifically delineates ways for nurses to encourage developmental skills. The plan is designed to take into account the type of treatment bed that the infant is in (i.e., radiant warmer, isolette, or crib). The program includes visual, auditory, kinesthetic, proprioceptive input, and positioning. Tactile intervention is evaluated on an individual basis. The nursing staff is oriented to the care plan during a two-hour inservice education program. The OT also writes and posts a bedside program for each infant.

In Lutheran General's program, working with the parents of each infant is considered of prime importance. Parents and therapist discuss the objectives of the treatment program, their infant's responses to the interaction with his environment, and future developmental expectations and the progression of skill development. Parents are encouraged to observe and become acquainted with their infant. In addition, specific developmental home programs are given to parents as a part of discharge planning. Infants are referred for follow-up therapy programs. The OT also provides developmental counseling and referral for the parents whose infant has an identifiable problem such as Down's Syndrome. Discussion of parental expectations for an infant who has had severe prenatal or postnatal difficulties that may cause later developmental problems is also available. Parents are acquainted with normal developmental milestones and progressions so that they can determine whether their child's development deviates from the norm and if so, seek appropriate intervention. The OT also consults with other medical staff on infants with range of motion problems and makes splints for orthopedic problems.

Additional participation of occupational therapy is in an NICU follow-up program with other disciplines, including speech pathology, audiology, social service, neonatology, and nursing. OT screens each child individually, using the Denver Developmental Screening Test and a test of postural reflex development. Recommendations are made and the team designs a plan for follow-up treatment. The OT also provides developmental information and guidance for parents of children in the follow-up program.

Plans for future development of OT services in the Lutheran General NICU include provision of a more systematic approach to developmental intervention for all infants in the nursery (not just those referred for services because of problems or anticipated problems). This would include encouragement of parental involvement and the education of parents on early developmental stages of sensory motor processing, reflex development, movement, and the effects of prematurity or illness on the normal developmental processes.

In conclusion, it is thought that OT services can play a key role in providing early intervention services for infants within an NICU setting. It is also thought that therapists' documentation can validate the benefits of early intervention in the Neonatal Intensive Care Infant.

Developmental Disabilities
Special Interest Section Newsletter; Vol. 4, No. 3, 1981

Practical Considerations for Developing a Therapy Program in the Nursery

By Gail Liberg, MPA, OTR,
Oak Park, Illinois

The high-risk nursery is a relatively new work setting for the occupational therapist. The following is a list of very basic, but practical points to consider when attempting to provide a new program for the nursery.

1. Before approaching the medical staff about a specific program, familiarize yourself with the level of services provided at your hospital. Services vary from the basic care of the regular nursery to the highly specialized care of the neonatal intensive care unit. The status of infants will vary accordingly, as will the need for your services. For example, the Illinois perinatal system provides four levels of care: Level IV and III centers contain the most compromised babies, as well as preemies, who will require extensive medical care including ventilator therapy and special surgeries. Level II centers may care for prematures who require oxygen but who are not excessively compromised. Level I nurseries are those whose infants need no specialized care.

2. Assess the needs of the nursery. These will vary depending upon the personnel already available and their skills. Some of the services therapists might supply include general stimulation, feeding therapy, neuro-muscular treatments for infants with abnormal muscle tone, teaching parenting skills, providing support for parents, or providing developmental follow-up testing. Nursing staff will appreciate therapists' input about special feeding techniques and positioning techniques to minimize future developmental problems.

3. Recognize the strength of the nursing staff. While the physician is ultimately responsible for the infants' health, it is the nursing staff that provides daily, 24-hour vigilance. Your concern for the infants and attempts to accommodate feeding schedules and procedures will be appreciated. Referrals may come initially from nurses who recognize the value of your service. In addition, the nurses will provide valuable information regarding the infant's medical status and family.

4. Familiarize yourself with the many medical conditions and surgical procedures special to premature and other compromised babies. Be aware of the implications for future developmental status and of contraindications for treatment. Watch monitors when treating infants with unstable cardiac or other function—and do not treat those infants you do not feel you can adequately assess.

5. Receive what training you can in assessing or treating the high risk infant. Visit centers with therapists practicing in the nursery and attend related workshops. Read available literature about infant stimulation, assessment, and treatment. Many pertinent workshops are given by perinatal centers and by nursing organizations. Experience with medical patients in the pediatric intensive care unit will provide a good basis for treatment of high risk infants. A strong background in pediatric neurological problems, neurodevelopmental treatment techniques, and maternal-infant bonding is invaluable.

6. Familiarize yourself with community agencies for referral. As you develop a program for the nursery, you will recognize the need for follow-up or treatment after discharge.

7. Realize that not everyone is suited for intensive nursery experience. The therapist working in a critical care unit may be exposed to infant deaths as well as severe illness and deformity. If you are treating these children, you will need to deal with parents' depression, fear, anger, and frustration. This is difficult if you cannot deal with your own emotions. Knowledge about grieving is important.

8. Do not jump in over your head. Providing therapy for individuals is a good way to become familiar with the nursery, be recognized by the nurses, and learn about babies and techniques. If you can arrange to test normal full-term infants and healthier preemies, this will give you a good baseline for assessment. For learning the normal variations in premature infants, stimulation treatments provide good experience.

9. If you are ready to prepare a comprehensive or aggressive program, it is helpful to work with a nurse who does discharge planning or who is interested in the babies' long-term development. This nurse may well have a better understanding of the political issues within the unit and may know how to approach issues that are less easily broached by an outsider. Any program you institute will be more effective if it is accepted by the nursing staff. For a comprehensively planned program, such as inpatient screening, you may be able to get a blanket referral from the unit director; this will ease day-to-day routines.

The above considerations are suggested as basic guidelines for the therapist who is interested in pursuing work in the neonatal intensive care nursery. Since perinatology is a relatively new and rapidly expanding field, the occupational therapist interested in this area should prepare carefully and cautiously to obtain the information necessary for adequately assessing and treating high risk infants.

Barrel Chair for Multiply Handicapped Children in a Public School Setting

By June Houston, COTA, Sequoyah School for Handicapped Children, Elizabethton, TN

Multiply handicapped children with cerebral palsy often need special seating and/or positioning chairs to enable them to maintain upright alignment during activities in school. Severely handicapped children are frequently unable to sit properly in a regular chair at a desk—it is not desirable for them to spend their entire school day in a wheelchair. This article describes one type of positioning chair that helped several handicapped children in a public school setting.

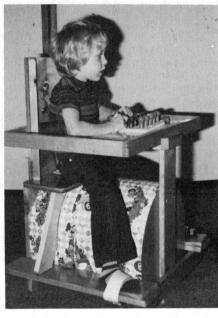

Figure I. Child positioned in hip flexion, abduction, and external rotation to break up extensor spasticity in lower extremities. Chair also aids sitting balance, freeing arms for hand activities.

The child shown in Figure I is a five-year-old boy with a diagnosis of cerebral palsy with spastic quadriplegia. Spasticity is present in the trunk and all extremities; extensor tone and scissoring of the lower extremities make seating difficult. His head control is good, but sitting balance is poor. If placed on a regular chair, he uses his upper extremities for stabilizing to achieve postural security.

To alleviate this problem, a "barrel chair" (Figure II) was constructed. A cardboard barrel fifteen inches (38.1 cm) in diameter was used as a base. The child was straddled across the barrel and measurements were taken for the following:

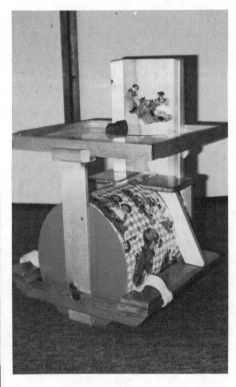

Figure II. "Barrel Chair"

1. **Back:** Straight, high back of three-quarter inch plywood, the width measured from shoulder to shoulder and the height measured up to back of child's head.

2. **Lapboard:** Length of lapboard approximately the length of the child's reach; its height allows the elbows and forearms to rest comfortably on it. Width is approximately the same as the width of chair base. Width of lapboard cutout allows for two inches (5.08 cm) between the child and edge of lapboard.

3. **Seat:** Constructed of three-quarter inch plywood. Six inches (15.2 cm) were added to each side of the barrel to stabilize child on center of barrel.

4. **Barrel:** the barrel was shortened in length, extending approximately four inches (10.1 cm) beyond child's knees.

Interior supports of wooden disks were spaced as needed inside the barrel to prevent the cardboard from collapsing with use. As finishing touches, footstraps with velcro were added to stabilize feet; the lapboard was covered with formica for cleanliness; the barrel was covered with colorful, washable contact paper; the chair was varnished and matching decals added for decoration. The lapboard easily fastens to the chair with bolts, and a lateral wing was attached on the right side of the chair over the ribcage to correct child's tendency to lean to the right side.

Finished Measurements of "Barrel Chair":

Total height of chair—33 inches (83.8 cm)
Total length of chair (front and back)—21 inches (53.3 cm)
Total width of chair at base—21 inches (53.3 cm)
Total width of chair at seat back—12 inches (30.5 cm)
Barrel circumference—15 inches (38.1 cm)
Footboard from floor—5 inches (12.7 cm)
Footboard to seat—10 1/2 inches (26.7 cm)
Width of seat insert—15 1/4 inches (38.7 cm)
Seat to top of back—17 inches (43.1 cm)
Lapboard: 23 1/2 inches wide (59.7 cm)
      19 inches deep (48.2 cm)
Lapboard cutout: 11 inches wide (27.9 cm)
      6 1/2 inches deep (16.5 cm)
Height from floor to lapboard—23 1/2 inches (59.7 cm)
Footrests: 5 1/2 inches long (14 cm)
      4 inches wide (10.1 cm)

ADVANTAGES OF THIS CHAIR

1. Provides trunk stability/sitting balance, and eliminates need for child to use upper extremities for propping, thus freeing upper extremities for hand activities.

2. Inhibits abnormal reflexes such as the Tonic Neck Reflexes and positive supporting reactions.

3. Positions hips in flexion, abduction, and external rotation, thus breaking up extensor spasticity of lower extremities and preventing further deformities (e.g., dislocated hips, scoliosis, contractures).

4. Enables child to participate in classroom activities with peers, thus increasing socialization skills and attention span for pre-academic training.

5. Chair is aesthetically pleasing in appearance and contributes to the "normalcy" of the classroom setting.

Developmental Disabilities
Special Interest Section Newsletter; Vol. 4, No. 2, 1981

The Ultimate Challenge to a Therapist's Knowledge and Creativity

By Toby J. Black, OTR, Bowling Green, KY

M.J. is a six year old girl with a diagnosis of cerebral palsy with spasticity and rigidity. Since birth, her multiple problems have confused and frustrated the professionals who have worked with her.

M.J. is the only child of a farming couple who were in their late thirties when the pregnancy was discovered. She was born at approximately 7-1/2-8 months gestation and weighed 6.5 pounds. The delivery was difficult. Her color at birth was described as pink except for her hands, feet and around her mouth. She had a delayed cry, her breathing was labored and her body was limp. A poor suck reflex was observed during breast feeding. The parents were told that the baby was probably brain-damaged.

M.J. was evaluated by an orthopedic surgeon through Crippled Children's Services when she was eight months old and was found to have poor muscle tone but no spasticity. She returned to the same clinic when she was 13 months old. At that time, she appeared to be alert and interested in her environment and her parents felt she could develop to a functional level. Her head and trunk control were poor and she was totally dependent on her parents.

By age 2-1/2, she was diagnosed as having cerebral palsy. She had fair head control but poor trunk control. The doctor suggested that the father build a standing table.

In their effort to help M.J., her parents contacted a chiropractor, who tried to help her develop better sitting posture. M.J. was also referred to a child evaluation center by CCS, in 1977. As she was totally dependent and considered to be nonverbal, the center recommended institutionalization. The parents ignored this recommendation because they felt M.J. was alert and very interested in her environment. She could communicate with her parents and showed that she enjoyed books.

In 1978, the orthopedist added spasticity and athetoid movements to her diagnosis. She could not maintain a midline position and held her head to the right. The parents enrolled M.J. in a parent-child center which offered group sessions for the parents and play therapy for their preschool, handicapped children. The center assisted the parents in buying a walker with wheels and a seat and M.J. delighted her parents by exploring the house with new interest.

I met this family at an orthopedic clinic in 1978. I had observed the mother struggling to hold M.J. on her lap. The child was trying to reach out to another child and her whole body seemed to be involved in the activity. At the medical evaluation, I observed that M.J. had a strong ATNR and she developed a rigid posture when placed on the examination table. However, she seemed to understand the doctor's commands and tried to perform the motor tasks he requested. I learned that the parents had enrolled M.J. in the parent-child center although they had not received OT or PT services. I wasn't sure what I could do for her.

In 1979, funding became available to expand a floundering infant program. I invited M.J. to attend and was surprised when the family accepted because they lived a long way from our facility.

A back X-ray showed spina bifida occulta at T_1 and mild scoliosis at the thoracolumbar junction. She was positioned in a transitchair which, with tray, would hopefully prevent further back curvature. At that time, M.J.'s means of independent mobility was rolling. She had been toilet trained by age two but she depended on her parents to take her to the toilet. M.J.'s interests were similar to those of most five year olds, she liked Mickey Mouse and McDonald's hamburgers.

M.J.'s mother investigated the local school system for school placement. They offered her a class with multiply handicapped and severely retarded children where the academic environment appeared very limited.

My therapy first attempted to improve relaxation for M.J., and I used warmth and slow rocking. Second, the focus was on preschool activities such as colors, shapes, matching and letters. For communication, she began to use her head, since it was the only part of her body over which she had some control. We got a head pointer, and although it was a poor fit, M.J. was able to use it and demonstrated that she was functioning at around a kindergarten level. A psychological evaluation showed normal intelligence—in a child who was once to be sent to an institution: I asked M.J.'s doctor to refer her to physical therapy for biofeedback training, with the hope that she could be trained to relax. She started this therapy in August 1979. In the therapy sessions, she listened to story tapes, followed by gross motor activities involving rolling and range of motion. While M.J. seemed to benefit from this approach, the results are still questionable.

In the summer of 1980, M.J. also began a special speech therapy program. She responded very well to the Bliss symbols.

There are many questions regarding the therapy approach for a child with rigid cerebral palsy as there seems to be little written on this topic. I was unable to get assistance from United Cerebral Palsy. Brain implants were investigated, but I learned that initial evaluation expense is very high and that implants may prove inappropriate for M.J. anyway. Medication was tried to improve relaxation—it made her either sleepy or hyperactive.

The parents have not been happy with their past experiences with therapy as they felt the focus was more on them than on M.J. They were her therapists for five years since qualified therapists and suitable therapy program were not available in their community. Every accomplishment M.J. made was due to their persistence.

M.J. has caused me to look closely at my role as a therapist. My focus was on medical procedures or medications which would help her relax as relaxation seemed necessary before trying to develop her ADL skills. I also see adaptive and/or electronic equipment as important in M.J.'s future. I hope that the collaboration of this little girl, her parents, doctors and therapists can help her develop into a functional, productive individual.

Developmental Disabilities
Special Interest Section Newsletter; Vol. 4, No. 2, 1981

Prone and Supine Boards for Home Use

By Nancy Thomas, OTR and Sharon Meyer, RPT, Philadelphia, PA

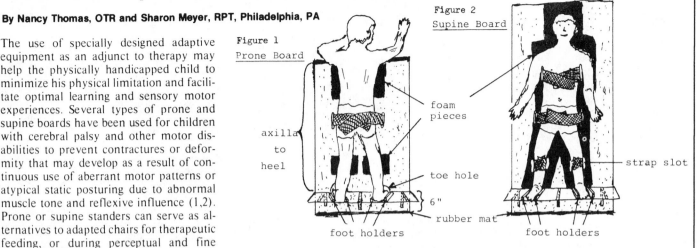

Figure 1
Prone Board

Figure 2
Supine Board

axilla
to
heel

foam
pieces

toe hole

6"

rubber mat

strap slot

foot holders

foot holders

The use of specially designed adaptive equipment as an adjunct to therapy may help the physically handicapped child to minimize his physical limitation and facilitate optimal learning and sensory motor experiences. Several types of prone and supine boards have been used for children with cerebral palsy and other motor disabilities to prevent contractures or deformity that may develop as a result of continuous use of aberrant motor patterns or atypical static posturing due to abnormal muscle tone and reflexive influence (1,2). Prone or supine standers can serve as alternatives to adapted chairs for therapeutic feeding, or during perceptual and fine motor activities, particularly in asymmetrical children. They can also assist in early, controlled weight-bearing and help provide the child with a new view of the world around him.

A simple and economical design for prone and supine boards has been developed in response to frequent parent requests. The boards were designed particularly for infants and young children to provide early and more normalized standing experiences. The simplicity and effectiveness of the design allows parents to build the boards themselves and fitting usually requires only 2 or 3 sessions with the therapist. The cost of making a board at home usually ranges from 10 to 15 dollars, making it far less expensive than commercially available standing boards. The benefits of home building include the parents' satisfaction in being in being involved in their child's treatment and the ingenuity that some parents bring to the "original designs" they help create.

The design of these boards was created with home-use in mind. Therefore, the use of a prop for free standing and attached tables for fine motor play were eliminated so they could be easily stored and used in various locations. Since each board is designed for only one child's use, it can be made with his specific needs in mind and can be custom fitted.

As seen in Figure 1, the prone board consists of a rectangular, flat piece of 1/4" plywood serving as a base. A wooden footboard is bolted to the base with 3 evenly spaced "L" brackets, screws and wing nuts. Foot holes are cut into the base where the feet hit the base. Footholders are attached to the footplate so that the feet can turn outward and so that the legs are moderately abducted, providing a wide base of support and replicating the early standing position of normal children. Foam pieces for the knees, chest and top edge of the board are cut to facilitate knee and hip extension and to prevent axillary scraping. Slots are cut into the base of the board close to the chest, hips and knees to accomodate webbing straps which can be closed with velcro. Hip abduction pads or lateral trunk supports can be added if needed. Rubber matting or a small wooden shelf appropriately angled and attached to the top prevent slipping when the board is propped against a table. (Rubber matting is usually sufficient to stop slipping for younger children).

Supine boards (Figure 2), can be constructed similarly on a plywood base with the same footplates, pads (except knees) and straps. For children whose head control is so poor that they cannot accommodate to a prone board, this small tilt table can be positioned at any angle. It must be longer than the prone board to provide head support. Supine boards have been particularly helpful in cases of severe hydrocephalus.

To measure and fit a child for the board

a. For the total length of the prone board, measure the length of the child's body from the base of the axilla to the bottom of the heel and add six inches.

b. The width should be one to two inches wider than the shoulders, on each side.

c. The footplate is placed six inches from the bottom edge of the plywood base.

d. Measure the length of the child's shoes and add one inch for the width of the footplate. Have the parents cut out the base and footplate and attach the footplate before the initial fitting. The rubber matting can also be attached before this fitting.

e. Place the child on the board and position him so that the feet are moderately spread and turned out. Draw lines on the footplate to indicate the correct position for the footholders.

f. Measure the depth of foam necessary to obtain the desired degree of knee extension and cut out the foam.

g. Draw lines on the plywood base as close to the hips as possible to indicate where the slots should be cut for the hip strap.

h. Cut foam pieces for the chest (1/4" to 1/2" as needed) and for the top of the board.

i. Show parents where to glue foam pieces, add footholders and cut slots for the hip strap. Parents should add the foam pieces and make the hip strap before returning the final fitting.

j. For the second fitting, place the child on the board and check his ability to tolerate the position and to use the hands comfortably for play. Check any lateral trunk flexion or asymetries and check for proper alignment, particularly in the lower extremities. If a child needs a chest strap, lateral trunk supports or any other modifications, add as necessary. Cover foam pieces with vinyl or cloth.

Consultation with a physician and physical therapist is advised for optimal positioning. Standing tolerance may need to be monitored and gradually increased for more severely involved children.

Acknowledgements: The original idea for prone standers was devised in Switzerland and largely promoted in this country by recommendations in Finnie's handbook and also in the Blythedale pediatric equipment book.

Bibliography

1. Connor, F.P., Williamson, G.G., and Siepp, J.M., *Program Guide for Infants and Toddlers with Neuromotor and Other Developmental Disabilities.* Teachers College Press, New York, 1978.

2. Bergen, A., *Selected Equipment for Pediatric Rehabilitation.* Blythedale Children's Hospital, Valhalla, New York, 1978.

3. Finnie, N. *Handling the Young Cerebral Palsied Child at Home.* E.P. Dutton and Co., Inc., New York, 1975.

Developmental Disabilities
Special Interest Section Newsletter; Vol. 4, No. 2, 1981

Positioning and Wheelchair Adaptation for the Cerebral Palsied

By Nancy Owens, OTR, Chalmers, IN

I. Why Adapt a Wheelchair?

1. To improve sitting posture. Because the client is in a better position to see, his outlook on life may improve (he may be stimulated to take more notice of people and things in the environment.)

2. To improve function in skills required for dressing, vocational endeavors, play, etc. Feeding ability may improve due to better overall positioning for chewing, swallowing and the digestive process.

3. Better positioning of the lungs and diaphragm allows for better breath control and speech may improve.

4. To prevent deformity (scoliosis, kyphosis, increased spasticity leading to contractures). Present deformity cannot be eliminated but additional deformity can be prevented. Good positioning *first* is of prime importance as activity done without it can lead to deformity.

5. To promote added comfort. (Clients may initially rebel against wheelchair adaptations, but those who have given them a chance for a reasonable time, have found them to add to function *and* comfort).

II. Wheelchair adaptations

1. *Hard seat:* Purpose: Prevents constant lower extremity adduction and the tendency toward scissoring which can be increased by a sagging seat. Measurement: Depth should be the length from the client's posterior buttock to the inner portion of the bent knee *less* 2-3″ (3-4 fingers' width). This provides maximal weight-bearing surface and prevents pressure behind the knee resulting in restriction of circulation in lower extremities.

Width is dependent on wheelchair with which seatboard will be used. Ideal seat width is 2″ more than the measurement of the client's widest point, either the hips or thighs. Allowance must be made for insertion and removal of seatboard if wheelchair will be folded, and for use of padding or Naugahyde.

Seat may have a U-shaped cutout at the back for those inclined toward development of pressure sores. Measurement for the cut-out should be taken in the prone position.

   a. Tip of coccyx to bed when lying prone (anterior-posterior measurement) plus 4″.

   b. Widest distance between ischii plus 2″. If a cut-out is used, a double layer of padding will be needed, or reinforcement straps can be placed over the cutout on the bottom of the seat. Webbing from lawn furniture works well for these straps.

Seatboard should be padded with a minimum of 1/2″ foam and is ideally covered with Naugahyde fastened with a staple gun.

2. *Hard back:* Purpose: Prevents slumping and possible deformity such as kyphosis. Measurement: This is dependent on the client's need. Backboard height should fall approximately 4 inches below the axilla (for measurement sit client upright on a firm surface and measure from buttocks to approximately 4 inches below the axilla; to be sure back height falls at least 1″ either up or down from the inferior border of the scapula to prevent a pressure area).

For clients with spasticity or a tendency to hyperextend at the hips and neck, a taller backboard may be needed and this measurement should be from the buttocks to the superior aspect of the skull.

3. *Footrest:* Purpose: To prevent a pattern of extension for the lower extremities and possible deformity caused by constant plantar flexion. Measurement: Feet should be at a 90° angle to the lower client's leg length should be measured from behind the bent knee (90°) to the base of the heel (with consideration for average shoe heel height) with the foot at a 90° angle to the tibia. Add 1″ to this measurement to prevent pressure due to the thigh resting on the seat upholstery. (If a seatboard is used, take this thickness into account).

4. *Lapboard:* Purpose: To prevent slumping which can lead to kyphosis, and to provide a good work or eating surface. For some people with cerebral palsy, the lapboard can also serve as a surface for placement of a communication device. There are various types of lapboards made from a variety of materials. Plexiglass is expensive, but permits added visibility. It is also more difficult than wood to cut and smooth. Lap boards are commercially available but often can be constructed at much less expense. They can be fabricated in a variety of shapes and sizes depending on the client's needs, but all should have a narrow enough cut-out to prevent the upper extremities from going under them. Lapboards should permit forearms to rest at 90° or less angle to the humerus. Half rounds may be glued on lapboard edges to prevent items placed on the boards from sliding off. Attachment of the lapboard should limit sideways and forward motion of the board. Special consideration should be made for client who propels his own wheelchair.

III. Other Wheelchair Adaptations

1. *Seatbelt:* Purpose: To encourage trunk flexion and break up overall extension patterns. A seatbelt also prevents falls from the chair. Fitting: Seatbelts can be purchased commercially, but can also be made from 2″ webbing straps or adapted from those removed from junked autos. They should pass across the acetabulum, not across the stomach or chest as this impedes digestion and breathing; it also will permit trunk flexion while other positions will not. A properly fitted belt will prevent a client from sliding down in his wheelchair. Consideration should be given to the type of fastener used to maintain the highest degree of independence possible for the client capable of this responsibility.

2. *Rolled seat:* Purpose: To provide trunk flexion if other adaptations are ineffective. Fitting: Fabrication follows the contour of the French curve. Wood slats are used for the seat and spaced equidistant to allow for ventilation. Slats are placed parallel to the seat back.

Developmental Disabilities
Special Interest Section Newsletter; Vol. 4, No. 1, 1981

Developmentally Disabled Adults' Community Participation One Year Later—Back to Square One

By Shawn Miyake, MA, OTR, and Stephanie Day, MA, OTR

Introduction

This is the first stage of a follow-up study investigating the effects of service provision and the subsequent discontinuation of such service. It describes the original intent of a community-based residential service program and the types of service which were rendered. At the program's termination, a shift was attempted from services offered by the program to available community services and supports. This report describes the shift and then looks at the clients one year later with respect to: (1) the impact the program had on their lives and (2) the impact of discontinuation of the program. Finally, certain questions are raised from the preliminary findings of the study.

Program Intent

The combined research, training and service project conducted at the UCLA Neuropsychiatric Institute lasted approximately three years. The project involved 13 mildly to severely mentally retarded adults in dependent living situations. These individuals had experienced extended institutionalization, including stays in state hospitals.

The research component of this project was designed to gain a better understanding of the social context of the mentally retarded adult and the events that occurred in their everyday lives in the natural community setting. It was hoped that this knowledge could be applied to services, in order to make them more appropriate and meaningful for the clients. The training component provided professionals with an alternate perspective on the world of the mentally retarded. It was often discovered that, although professionals had good knowledge about mental retardation, they often did not really know about the day to day living circumstances of mentally retarded persons (1). Although the approach of this project was threefold, producing research, training, and service, the service component is the focus here. This component was implemented to develop and refine a service delivery package.

Services Offered

Services were offered in the natural living, working and leisure environments of the clients and within the context of activities chosen by them. The natural living environment was comprised of renovated motels, remodeled to meet basic room and board needs of the residents. These board and care complexes were located in community settings which were predominantly business and industrial sectors. Small businesses (liquor stores, fast food restaurants, etc.) and the board and care complex made up the work environment for those residents who held some sort of job (e.g., janitor, odd job person). Finally, the leisure environment included all the community resources locally available (YWCA, parks and recreation facilities, libraries, movie theaters, etc.).

The services offered to the clients included direct training in 1) basic self-care (such as, attention to socially acceptable styles of grooming), 2) self-management in the home, neighborhood and larger community (e.g., maintaining orderly living quarters, locating and purchasing goods), 3) productive use of leisure time (e.g., involvement in purposeful activity at home and in the community), 4) social-interactional behaviors in various settings (such as attention to socially appropriate ways of interacting with persons in a variety of natural settings), 5) physical-recreational skills (enhancement of physical conditioning and recreational skills in various physical activities) and 6) discovery and use of community resources via public transportation (e.g., identifying and using a bus route to library) (2).

End of Funding

When it was clear that funding for the project would not be continued, the clients were notified of the situation and told that programming would continue for only five more months. Of the original staff of three occupational therapists, two researchers, graduate students in occupational therapy, volunteers and CETA workers, only one occupational therapist remained to "wind down" the program.

At that time, all clients were asked what activities were most important to them. Within the framework of the program already established, the primary goal of the remaining five-month period became the location of existing community resources in which the identified activities were available. The occupational therapist worked with the clients both individually and in small groups to insure that each person would be participating in at least one community-based activity at the time of program termination. Resources explored included park and recreation programs, a senior citizen's center, community colleges, adult education programs at the local high school and independent businesses. At the end of the program, more than 80 percent of the clients had been placed and were actively participating in programs in their communities.

Back to Square One . . . Almost

A follow-up visit to the community placements involved in the original project was implemented one year later to investigate the outcome of the client placements in various community activities. Upon returning to one board and care facility, it was discovered that similar services were continuing to be delivered. Further investigation revealed that a new concerned owner and newly hired professional staff, including an occupational therapist were responsible for ongoing services which were viewed by the clients as worthwhile.

A visit to another board and care facility revealed that things appeared to have returned to the circumstances observed at the beginning of the original program. Namely, the facility lacked services, staff was poorly trained or untrained for work with the developmentally disabled adult, and the clients within the facility were isolated from the surrounding community. Services which had been offered by the project staff had stopped when they left. Clients who had been placed in the various community-based programs had either dropped out or expressed dissatisfaction with the programs and they again appeared helpless and apathetic. A number of clients voiced discontent with the present state of affairs and a longing to return to the days when the project was in full swing.

Questions Raised

Although many authors/researchers are quick to publish findings on model programs or demonstration projects, little literature is available that describes how these projects/programs were "wrapped up" when the funding was discontinued. What frequently occurs is a rapid disbandment of project personnel due to the lack of funding with less than optimal follow-up or follow-through of services. The possible effects of offering services to a

(continued)

Developmentally Disabled Adults

certain group of persons and then discontinuing these services as quickly as they are started seems not to have been investigated. Certain questions can be raised around these issues.

1. How morally and ethically sound is the provision of services to mentally retarded persons living in community placements when such provision is based on funding that has no clear termination criteria and continuation of services is questionable? Preliminary findings point to the impact of such services on the lives of mentally retarded persons who typically are exposed to programs that are terminated for one reason or another. At this time it appears that when clients have experienced long-term careers of institutionalization, life-long support may be necessary to maintain gains made in the utilization of community resources.

2. Do programs exposed mentally retarded adults to another side of life, one they could not realistically achieve or participate in without continued support? It became increasingly clear that participation in many of the activities engaged in during the project could not be continued without financial support of some type or would ever be engaged in on a continuous basis without advocacy by others.

3. How is it possible to effectively end a service program which results in the least disruption in the lives of mentally retarded persons? One alternative might be the provision of at least a support person or advocate to whom the mentally retarded person can turn for the assistance required to maintain gains made in the use of community resources.

Conclusion

This preliminary study attempted to investigate an infrequently examined area of service provision, that of service termination. This is an area of increasing concern. With the proliferation of programming for developmentally disabled persons in the form of model or demonstration projects based on limited, year-to-year funding, the question is not whether to offer time limited services of questionable survival. The provision of such services to clients residing in the community is clearly a significant addition to their quality of life. The questions that remain are: 1. How can these services be offered with the least amount of disruption to the lives of persons who have already been subjected to a number of terminated programs, 2. Do chronically disabled persons, such as those developmentally disabled persons in this study, require ongoing support for the rest of their lives, and 3. Might it be more cost effective to provide such support and thus avoid rehospitalization or return to residential, institutional living?

References
1. Project Report: Upward Mobility for the Developmentally Disabled Adult, UCLA-NPI, 1977
2. Project Description: Upward Mobility for the Developmentally Disabled Adult, UCLA-NPI, 1976

Shawn Miyake is with University Affiliated Facility, Neuropsychiatric Institute, UCLA. Stephanie Day works in the Neuropsychiatric Institute, UCLA with Surgical Treatment for Epilepsy Program.

Developmental Disabilities
Special Interest Section Newsletter; Vol. 4, No. 1, 1981

Independent Living for the Physically Disabled

By Barb Tylenda OTR, Coordinator of Independent Living Program for United Cerebral Palsy of S.W. Wisconsin

Recent legislation and expanding consumer involvement are generating a new philosophy with respect to the living arrangements which should be available for people with disabilities. The traditional alternatives of remaining with family or residing in an institutional setting are no longer seen as satisfactory to the consumer.

In dealing with individuals who have developmental disabilities, it becomes evident that the existing independent/alternative living programs are primarily designed to service those adults who are mentally retarded.

United Cerebral Palsy of Southeastern Wisconsin has become increasingly aware of the adults who are severely physically involved and are dissatisfied with their present restrictive living arrangements. In 1978, United Cerebral Palsy of Southeastern Wisconsin initiated an Independent Living Program (ILP) designed to assist people with developmental disabilities who are severely physically disabled to achieve a more independent life.

The program is coordinated by a registered occupational therapist whose basic tasks are to direct client services by providing information and referral, and to assist the client in obtaining, negotiating, and coordinating those services needed to live independently, and to be an advocate for expanded living alternatives and support systems within the community. So as to avoid duplication of services, the ILP coordinator does not provide therapy and training in areas which is available elsewhere in the community.

Although the program for each person is highly individualized, the following is a "typical" sequence through the independent living program.

1. The consumer is referred to the ILP. Referrals may be made by the individual, an agency, parents or nursing home.

2. The ILP coordinator schedules an initial meeting with the consumer to evaluate and discuss the consumer's physical ability, emotional status, financial resources, motivation, and psychological readiness for independent living.

3. Those consumers not demonstrating a present potential for independent living remain in contact with the independent living and advocacy programs of United Cerebral Palsy to develop a spectrum of alternative living arrangements. Consumers demonstrating ability for independent living become clients of ILP. It is stressed that, rather than physical capabilities, the consumer's psychological readiness and ultimate ability to be responsible for coordination of the support systems necessary for independent living are the major requirements. The client need not be able to physically perform daily tasks, but must have the capability of directing others in completion of these tasks and be able to use the community resources available to enhance his or her functioning.

4. The OT assists the client in coordinating the skills and services needed for successful integration into the community. Such services and skills include but are not limited to:

   a. Obtaining accessible, affordable housing (rent assistance, HUD etc.)

   b. Obtaining attendant care (County Title XX money-Supportive Home Care).

   c. Improving Independent Living Skills

(continued)

Independent Living

A thorough assessment is performed in the areas of self-care and homemaking skills. This evaluation is performed by a therapist in an existing clinic in the community. The evaluation results are used by the ILP coordinator and the client to determine the job description for an attendant, and whether a "come-in" or "live-in" attendant is needed. The client receives training in how to advertise, interview, hire, train, and fire an attendant. Other essential skills include budgeting, banking, scheduling of daily activities, personal health care management, dealing with emergencies, and using community resources, e.g., arranging transportation. These adults have been accustomed to an environment which has sheltered, protected, and has never demanded development of skills in these areas. For this reason, a client may work with the ILP intensely for 6 months to one year before moving into the community. The ILP coordinator gradually decreases her support and releases responsibility for these areas to the consumer.

    d. Developing interpersonal skills, e.g., self-advocacy, socialization skills, etc.

    e. Coping with the emotional impact of independent living.

    f. Securing the available financial resources.

5. The client makes the transition to community living. This is accomplished by one of two methods.

    a. Direct move to client's own apartment

    b. Utilization of the apartment leased by United Cerebral Palsy to serve as a training program prior to securing client's own apartment.

Direct supervision and assistance is provided by the OTR in this setting. The average stay is 6 months.

Independent Living is an essential adjunct to existing services for people with disabilities. The OT's skills in evaluating a client using a holistic approach, coupled with knowledge of the methods and equipment which enhance functioning, places the OT in a unique position to facilitate the implementation of a successful independent living program.

Developmental Disabilities
Special Interest Section Newsletter; Vol. 3, No. 4, 1980

Adolescents and Adults With Myelomeningocele: Performance in Daily Activities and Social Relationships

By Robert J. Wolfe, Ph.D., Assistant Professor
Department of Occupational Therapy, University of Southern California

Spina bifida cystica (myelomeningocele) ranks as one of the most frequent and severe congenital defects in the United States with an incidence between 1 and 2 per 1000 (30). The disease's severity is due to its frequent simultaneous involvement of the central nervous, musculoskeletal, and genitourinary systems, often leading to severe paralysis, incontinence, physical deformity, and intellectual deficit (18, 22). Whereas before the middle 1950's most children born with myelomeningocele did not survive long, since then survival rates increased markedly due to "aggressive treatment" consisting of improved surgical techniques for early closure of the spinal defect, antibiotics, and shunting as treatment for hydrocephalus (18, 22). Currently, about half of all children born with myelodysplasia in the United States will survive into adulthood through the use of presently accepted methods of treatment (26).

Many individuals now surviving into late life stages exhibit numerous and severe physical and mental disabilities (12, 17, 18, 27). Identifying and meeting the emerging health needs of these individuals passing through adolescence and young adulthood are of current concern for multidisciplinary rehabilitation and habilitation teams. Recent research undertaken in the United Kingdom (1, 2, 5, 7, 13, 14, 31), Australia (21), and the United States (10, 15, 26, 27) has identified certain functional and behavioral problems faced by the adolescent and young adult myelomeningocele population. These studies have documented that a child's early biophysical problems increasingly manifest themselves at later life stages as deficits in activity and behavior.

This paper reviews studies relating to the "functional health" of the adolescent and young adult myelomeningocele group. "Functional health" refers to health viewed from the standpoint of the quality of a person's activities and social relationships, and not solely in terms of physical and psychological signs and symptoms, or underlying pathological processes. This is a traditional perspective within occupational therapy. Occupational therapists have been concerned with how disease, trauma, and other health related conditions may disrupt a client's performance of daily life tasks, social roles, and personal goal-directed activity. From the extant research, myelomeningocele impacts a client's performance in several life areas, which can be ordered as a rough hierarchy; performance in basic self-maintenance activities in the home, family relationships, and performance in extra-familial activities, including education, affiliations (friendships, courtship, marriage), and remunerative employment. Research findings within each general area are reviewed. In the following discussion, findings are summarized from a developmental perspective.

Self-Maintenance Activities

In Shurtleff's Seattle study of children and adolescents with myelodysplasia, significant delays were found in the group's independent performance of self-maintenance tasks compared with hypothetical normal developmental curves (28, 29). Self-maintenance tasks included urinary and stool management, dressing, grooming, feeding and meal preparation, and locomotion. On most tasks the group required significantly longer periods of time to achieve independence, commonly 17 to 18 years on tasks normally autonomously performed at 5 to 7 years of age. Developmental rates and degrees of independence were inversely associated with level of lesion. However, variability in achievement by individuals with similar paralysis indicated other unknown compounding factors were influencing why some individuals achieved independence while others with similar paralysis

(continued)

remained dependent all their lives.

A follow-up ambulation study of 56 myelomeningocele clients at Rancho Los Amigos Hospital in Los Angeles admitted prior to 1970 found that 52% were confined to wheelchairs, 9% ambulated only at home, and 36% ambulated at home and in the community (10). Very high lesions were associated with nonambulation, and very low lesions with community ambulation. Clients with midlevel lumbar lesions, by far the largest group, showed substantial variation in ambulation patterns. In the latter group important variables seemed to be mental status, spinal deformity, residual contractures, and history of bone fractures.

The self-maintenance status of myelomeningocele children may be related to disruptions in the early home environment. Parents of adolescents in a London sample reported that problems of mobility and urinary incontinence were the disabilities most disruptive of family daily routine and social life (3). Of the sample of 63 adolescents, 52% reportedly had "marked problems" with mobility, and 59% had occasional to frequent incontinence and leakage from urinary appliances. Other problems included bowel dysfunction, excessive weight gain, and decubitus ulcers. Decubiti also were frequent problems for a sample of 18 Pennsylvanians ages 17 to 31, and for Shurtleff's Seattle group (15, 28). One review indicated that 50% of pre-adolescent children with myelomeningocele were obese due to immobility, multiple operations, frequent spontaneous leg fractures, and perhaps disturbed mother-child relationships (24). Shurtleff and Sousa suggested "sick role" dependency expectations among some parents may delay the development of independence skills in their handicapped children (28). Such parents tended to overly protect the handicapped child who was perceived as being sickly and incapable of independent action. Melbourne mothers reportedly spent 2 hours a day attending to the daily needs of their children aged 5 to 10, such as dressing, feeding, and putting on appliances (21).

Family Relationships

There is some debate concerning the effects of a child born with myelodysplasia on the quality of family life and its stability. The unexpected burden of caring for a handicapped child is reported to increase a family's social isolation, to raise maternal (but not necessarily paternal) stress, and promote physical and psychological deterioration in the mother (2, 3, 21, 31, 33). In the United Kingdom, moderate financial hardships often were incurred by families, especially in the first four years (9, 25, 33). Siblings of handicapped children reportedly exhibited more behavioral problems at home and at school than siblings of non-handicapped children (31, 33). Studies have produced equivocal results concerning long-term effects of handicapped children on marital stability (20). Most research from the United Kingdom and Australia indicated no significant increase in the divorce rates over national averages among families with a myelomeningocele child (3, 21, 25), although Tew, et al. presented some contradictory evidence (32). Kolin, et al. claimed a two-fold increase of divorce among New York families with a spina bifida child (11), whereas Martin found no increases in a Missouri sample (20). The most reasonable conclusion at present seems to be this: although a severely handicapped child probably modifies normal family functioning, a poor home environment is not inevitable, and many families show great resiliance and adaptive capabilities (8, 33). In fact, Dorner found relations between adolescents with myelomeningocele and parents in the home to be close and cooperative, which he interpreted as "positive" (4, 5). However, an alternative interpretation is that such relations may not be as conducive of independence and autonomy as "adolescent rebelliousness" for certain individuals.

Performance Outside The Home

A few authors have scrutinized the performance of adolescents and young adults in activities outside the home (1, 4, 5, 7, 13, 15, 26, 28). Spina bifida patients surviving into adulthood before aggressive treatment as a group reportedly have succeeded fairly well in terms of vocational independence. Of 28 men and 23 women aged 18 to 56 years in South Wales, 36 were self-supporting in competitive employment, filling mother or housewife roles, or engaged in normal educational studies (14). Seven were partially employed in sheltered workshops or at home, whereas only 8 were totally unemployed. Over half had a secondary education; the remainder had some special schooling or home tutoring. Forty-three percent were married; most of the unmarried had never had a steady partner (13). Similarly, in a study conducted in Pennsylvania of 18 patients aged 17 to 31 years, 12 were self-supporting or attending school with prospects of being self-supporting in the future (15). Four were economically dependent upon parents or in the hospital, while two were institutionalized, receiving full-time care. In these two studies, vocational and educational success seemed related to degree of physical disability, especially deficits in mobility and cognition. Incontinence with careful management seemed no bar to establishing friendships; more important factors were early childhood and school experiences, personality, and motivation (13). However, in the South Wales sample a disproportionate number of men who had urinary diversions, penile appliances, pads, or napkins were unemployed (13).

Clients born since aggressive treatment was instituted in the late 1950's paint a bleaker portrait of extra-familial performance. Among his London sample of 46 adolescents aged 13 to 19, Dorner found severe social isolation outside of school, frequent feelings of subjective misery and depression, problems finding work or prospects of work, and preoccupying worries about the future and with prospects of unfulfilled wishes in relation to marriage and children. Only 11 were judged to have achieved satisfactory economic, social, and psychological adjustment (4, 5). Degree of handicap was not predictive of adjustment: of the 11 judged to have achieved satisfactory adjustments, 4 were minimally, 3 moderately, and 4 severely handicapped, using paralysis, incontinence, and mobility problems as handicapping criteria.

Shurtleff, Hayden, and Chapmen et al. assessed the employment and educational status of 98 Seattle clients aged 13 to 72 (26). Of 76 with intelligence quotients above 70 points, 36 were judged successful, 26 intermediate, and 12 failures. Criteria of success were self-sufficiency in daily care, and employed, a housewife, or in normal academic work; failure was defined as not self-sufficient in daily care, and unemployed with no current programs. Of 23 with IQ's lower than 70 points, all were judged "failures" by these criteria (18 were bed-care patients and 5 were in custodial care). Extended as a future assessment of the total group, 53% were predicted for "success," that is, independent in self-care and employment, and 47% were predicted for "failure," that is, dependent in self-care and employment.

These last two studies demonstrate the greater proportion of extra-familial problems encountered by the more severely affected adolescent group treated since the late 1950's. Both Dorner in London and Shurtleff in Seattle call for further information on this group of handicapped adolescents and young adults to help guide methods of intervention.

Discussion

The evidence suggests several trends in the health problems of the myelomeningocele group passing through adolescence and young adulthood. Basic problems of locomotion and urinary and stool management continue into adolescence, and development of self-maintenance skills is delayed in comparison with non-

(continued)

Adolescents and Adults With Myelomeningocele

handicapped children. However, the more pressing challenges of adolescence and young adulthood appear to lie in achieving effective and satisfying performance in the extra-familial environment. The studies of Dorner and Shurtleff suggest that particular difficulties occur in respects to affiliative relationships outside the home (friendship, courtship, and marriage), prospects for economic independence, and subjective feelings of personal satisfaction and well-being.

The problem areas are understandable in reference to a general theory of adolescent development. Normally, adolescence represents a period of preparation for independent adulthood status and role responsibilities in Western society (9). The physical changes of puberty at about 12 years of age signal the entrance of the child into a social status holding new personal and interpersonal challenges (23). From a psychological viewpoint, adolescence is said to be a period of development of a personal identity, evaluated against other "selfs" and bestowed with a degree of self-worth (6, 23). Biologically, it is a period to achieve an effective and satisfying mastery of a post-pubescent physique. Sociologically, the adolescent strives to exert increasing emotional and behavioral independence from parents and other adults, establish more maturing relationships with non-kin associates, especially other agemates, in preparation for adult roles as in marriage and family. Economically, the adolescent prepares for later productive careers through education and limited participation in the job market (9).

Adolescence may be a critical transitional period for the spina bifida child. Normally the adolescent period is one of culturally approved behavioral experimentation in new physical, social, and economic areas, during which the individual finds solutions to the challenges outlined above. The chronic disabilities stemming from spina bifida present unique problems to an adolescent during this developmental period: (1) Ambulation problems may hinder the emergence of independent performance in the extra-familial environment. (2) Urinary appliances and possible loss of sexual function infuses the patient's sexual identity with ambiguity, casts doubt on courtship capabilities, and obscures the future potential of marital and family roles. (3) The stigma of a visible handicap and restricted mobility may hinder the formation of normal adolescent peer groups and the social experimentation occuring within them. (4) Dependency-inducing relationships at home and in school may

forestall emotional and behavioral independence from parents and caretakers. (4) Low IQ's and discontinuities in childhood training due to multiple operations may compromise a person's educational and pre-vocational success, and the learning of skills facilitating independent performance. (5) The daily experiences of self-care dependency, social isolation, and sexual ambiguity collectively may create subjective feelings of low self-esteem and low self-satisfaction.

Previous research has illuminated these as areas of concern for the adolescent and young adult with myelomeningocele who is experimenting with personal and social skills for later independent living. Further descriptive research may expand this information concerning the "functional health" status of this group, helping the identification of areas of need of clients and their families during these life stages. The information can be used to guide treatment goals and methods of extant health programs. Because the effective and satisfying performance by clients in developmentally appropriate activities of daily living seems to be a central health concern, occupational therapy with its "functional health" perspective may play a significant role in meeting these emerging health needs of the adolescent and young adult with myelomeningocele.

References Cited

1. Armour, Carole (1977) A patient's view of spina bifida. Physiotherapy 63:221-222.
2. Dorner, S. (1973) Psychological and social problems of families of adolescent spina bifida patients: a preliminary report. Developmental Medicine and Child Neurology, Supplement 29:24-26.
3. Dorner, S. (1975) The relationship of physical handicap to stress in families with an adolescent with spina bifida. Developmental Medicine and Child Neurology 17:765.
4. Dorner, S. (1976) Adolescents with spina bifida. How they see their situation. Archives of Disease in Childhood 51:439-444.
5. Dorner, S. (1977) Problems of teenagers. Physiotherapy 63:190-192.
6. Erickson, Erik H. (1968) Identity: Youth and Crisis. New York: W.W. Norton.
7. Evans, F., V. Hickman, and C.O. Carter (1975) Handicap and social status of adults with spina bifida. British Journal of Preventative and Social Medicine 28:85.
8. Freeston, B.M. (1971) An inquiry into the effect of a spina bifida child upon family life. Developmental Medicine and Child Neurology 13:456-461.
9. Havinghurst, Robert J. (1972) Developmental Tasks and Education, 3rd edition. New York: David McKay Company.
10. Hoffer, M.M., E. Feiwell, R. Perry, J. Perry, and C. Bonnett (1973) Functional ambulation in patients with myelomeningocele. Journal of Bone and Joint Surgery 55:137-148.
11. Kolin, I.S., A.L. Scherzer, B. New, and M. Garfield (1971) Studies of the school-age child with meningomyelocele: social and emotional adaptation. Journal of Pediatrics 78:1013-1019.

12. Laurence, K.M. (1974) Effect of surgery for spina bifida cystica on survival and quality of life. Lancet 1:301-304.
13. Laurence, K.M. and A. Beresford (1975) Continence, friends, marriage and children in 51 adults with spina bifida. Developmental Medicine and Child Neurology, Supplement 35:123-128.
14. Laurence, K.M. and A. Beresford (1976) Degree of physical handicap, education, and occupation of 51 adults with spina bifida. British Journal of Preventative and Social Medicine 30:197-202.
15. Levin, G.D. (1974) Functional evaluation of eighteen adult myelomeningocele patients. Clinical Orthopedics 100:101-107.
16. Lipsitz, Joan (1977) Growing up Forgotten: A Review of Research and Programs Concerning Early Adolescence. Lexington: Lexington Books.
17. Lorber, J. (1968) The child with spina bifida: medical, educational, and social aspects. Physiotherapy 54:390-397.
18. Lorber, J. (1972) Spina bifida cystica. Results of treatment of 270 consecutive patients with criteria for selection for the future. Archives of Disabilities in Childhood 47:854-873.
19. Mahoney, Florence J. and D. Barthel (1965) Functional evaluation: the Barthel Index. Maryland State and Medical Journal 14:61-65.
20. Martin, P. (1975) Marital breakdown in families of patients with spina bifida cystica. Developmental Medicine and Child Neurology 17:757-764.
21. McAndrew, Irene (1976) Children with a handicap and their families. Child: Care, Health, and Development 2:213-218.
22. Morrissy, Raymond (1978) Spina bifida: a new rehabilitation approach. Orthopedic Clinics of North America 9:279-389.
23. Muuss, Rolf E. (1975) Theories of Adolescence. 3rd edition. New York: Random House.
24. Rickard, R.D., M.S. Brady, E.L. Gresham (1977) Nutritional management of the chronically ill child. Congenital heart disease and myelomeningocele. Pediatric Clinics of North America 24:157-174.
25. Richards, I.D.G. and H.T. McIntosh (1973) Spina bifida survivors and their parents, a study of problems and services. Developmental Medicine and Child Neurology 15:293-304.
26. Shurtleff, D.B., P.W. Hayden, W.H. Chapman, A.B. Broy, and M.L. Hill (1975) Myelodysplasia—problems of long-term survival and social function. Western Journal of Medicine 122:199-205.
27. Shurtleff, D.B., P.W. Hayden, J.D. Loeser, R.A. Kronmal (1974) Myelodysplasia: decision for death or disability. New England Journal of Medicine 291:1005-1011.
28. Shurtleff, D.B. and J.C. Sousa (1977) The adolescent with myelodysplasia. Development, achievement, sex, and deterioration. Delaware Medical Journal 49:631-638.
29. Sousa, J.C., L.H. Gordon, D.B. Shurtleff (1976) Assessing developmental daily living skills in patients with spina bifida. Developmental Medicine and Child Neurology, Supplement 18:134-142.
30. Stark, G.D. (1977) Spina Bifida. Problems and Management. Oxford: Blackwell.
31. Tew, B. and K.M. Laurence (1973) Mothers, brothers, and sisters of patients with spina bifida. Developmental Medicine and Child Neurology, Supplement 29:69-76.
32. Tew, B.J., K.M. Laurence, H. Payne, K. Rawnsley (1977) Marital stability following the birth of a child with spina bifida. British Journal of Psychiatry 131:79-83.
33. Walker, J.H., M. Thomas, and I. T. Russell (1971) Spina bifida and the parents. Developmental Medicine and Child Neurology 13:462-476.

Functional Vision

By Pat Glass, OTR

This past year I attended a workshop conducted by the staff of the Model Vision Project, Peabody College of Vanderbilt University. Participants consisted of special education teachers, teacher aides, vision teachers, occupational, physical, and speech therapists. The course was the outreach phase (third year) of a research project being conducted at the Kennedy Center. The project staff has compiled information on how to evaluate multihandicapped children with visual problems that are functioning developmentally under five years. More emphasis is placed on the sensorimotor period (0-2). Assessments and information included the areas of functional vision, cognitive development, gross and fine motor, speech and language, and mobility. They also address the areas of working with parents, positioning and handling, dealing with behavior, team work, writing individualized educational programs (IEP) and rights of the handicapped. Much of the information has been published in seven books available from Stoelting Publishing Co., 1350 South Costner Ave., Chicago, IL 60623.

The publication that I found most helpful is *Functional Vision Inventory for the Multiply And Severly Handicapped* by Beth Langley. The book gives detailed instruction on how to assess a child's vision in the areas of awareness of visual stimuli, fixation, convergence, shift of gaze, tracking, near and far vision and peripheral field.

There are two assessments in the book. One is a short screening and the other a more detailed inventory. The test items are various toys and common objects that can be collected from what is on hand or purchased at local stores. I spent $15 to collect additional items needed for my kit. I put mine in a small suitcase so it could be easily transported when I consult in schools and homes.

Once the visual screening is completed, it may have several uses. If the child fails the test (4 items or more), visual training may be indicated. The form with the findings can be sent with the child if you feel a referral to an opthalmologist is indicated. It is also a reference for progress and gives subjective and objective information. This inventory should be combined with at least a cognitive assessment prior to setting up goals.

The booklet also includes information on eye abnormalities, positioning, effects of reflexes on vision, glossary and many suggested activities for remediation that incorporate cognitive development, fine coordination, form and color perception and visual perceptual organization. These areas all in turn help develop functional vision.

Therapeutic Feeding Programs

By Peggy Stratton, OTR, and Kathy Graci, OTR

The following articles related to feeding programs for the profoundly retarded are currently implemented at J.N. Adam Developmental Center or West Seneca Developmental Center.

A Therapeutic Feeding Program was initiated in 1974 at West Seneca Developmental Center with 55 residents (ages 6-16 years). All of the residents were diagnosed as profoundly retarded with multiple physical handicaps and all displayed major difficulties in eating (i.e., tongue thrust, excessive food loss, choking). The focus of the program was to increase the ability to effectively take in food/liquid and improve nutritional status of these residents.

Initially, a feeding evaluation was completed for each resident by an OTR through observation of oral functions during the noontime meal. Included in the evaluation in addition to observable feeding problems was positioning, muscle tone, reflex patterns, head control and a feeding history. In collaboration with physical therapy, any adjustments in positioning were addressed to assure optimal relaxation and alignment.

Goals were established based on the oral evaluation; with implementation emphasis on positioning, jaw control, thickened food and liquid and adapted utensils.

In order to successfully implement the program, in-service training was given to all living unit staff on day and afternoon shifts. A card for each resident indicating the feeding goal and related feeding techniques was posted on the living unit above the food chart. Occupational therapy and physical therapy staff were used to feed those residents requiring the most therapy and amount of time to feed. This not only relieved living unit staff—allowing extra time to feed other residents and provided individual therapy to the most difficult feeders—but helped to set a consistent example of therapeutic techniques to other staff.

At the present time, the program continues with each resident being reassessed on an annual basis. Results indicate continuing progress in all areas of oral function with active lip control progressing most rapidly and areas of tongue control and chewing showing more limited changes.

Liquid Intake Program

In the development of a therapeutic feeding program in the pediatric unit of the West Seneca Developmental Center, it was noted that certain areas of oral function showed less progress. These same areas also showed the greatest problems in the implementation of therapeutic feeding techniques. The sipping and swallowing of liquids was one of these areas. Although the use of correct positioning, jaw control, thickened liquids and cut-out glasses was conveyed to living unit staff, only sporadic progress occurred primarily due to lack of consistency.

A liquid intake program was initiated with a group of 15 residents on a one-to-one basis with the occupational therapist four days per week. The use of thickened liquids, desensitization techniques and jaw control was used to improve problems included jaw thrusting, lip retraction, poor lip closure and tongue thrusting.

The program has shown slow but significant success with the most improvement noted in a decrease of jaw thrusting and improvement of lip closure. Consistent use of all components of the program: thickened liquids, desensitization techniques, jaw control and adaptive equipment appears to be the key to the program.

Further information may be obtained by writing the authors at J.N. Adam Developmental Center, Perrysburg, NY 14129.

Developmental Disabilities
Special Interest Section Newsletter; Vol. 3, No. 3, 1980

Treatment Programs for Children on Gavage Feedings

By Paula Manthei, OTR

The following is a brief discussion of information the author found useful in establishing treatment programs for children on gavage feedings.

The assessment process entailed more than a checklist of feeding skills. To plan intervention, information was needed on the child's nutrition, health and physical status, past feeding history, present oral motor skills, gross motor skills and positioning needs, hand skills, general cognitive and social developmental levels. It was also critically important to assess the child's primary feeder, her perspectives, needs and interaction patterns with the child.

The child's age, length of time on gavage feedings, present levels of functioning, and highest level of feeding attained before initiation of gavage feeding were factors affecting the transition to oral feeding. Older children (3 to 5 years) who had eaten normally previously generally regained skills rapidly once they regained consciousness and some motor control. Babies who had not achieved developmental milestones in feeding and had been on tube feedings for several months presented more of a challenge. They required much more patience and time.

In deciding to initiate oral feeding, medical clearance was obtained and the child's other skills were evaluated. The program usually began after the child could handle his secretions, cough spontaneously, and showed some signs of reaction to his environment. Soft, pureed foods were tried initially. With children 2 years or older, flavorful table foods worked better than bland baby foods. Some infants spent several weeks at this stage, getting accustomed to the solid foods. More difficult children were sometimes fed 3 times daily with initial oral intakes of only several tablespoons. Children were rarely fed for longer than a 45-minute period.

As a child showed more ability to swallow pureed foods, crisp, starchy foods were introduced; then foods that required more chewing; and liquids. With infants older than 8 months, the process of moving from spooning liquids to introducing cup drinking proved to be easier than re-introducing the bottle.

The author found the most effective oral motor therapy techniques were using her hands for jaw control and lip closure, and using teething biscuits, spoons and soft foods for desensitization. It was felt that the use of food was more effective and normalizing than some textbook techniques (brushing, vibrating). With neurologically involved children, positioning significantly influenced oral motor performance.

When possible, parents and therapist worked closely together. Some mothers were very active in their child's program. They found their child's return to oral feeding to be exciting. Mothers were counseled extensively while working with the therapist on feeding.

As the child progressed with oral eating, feeding schedules were established with the team. Records of food and fluid intake were kept. The team decided whether to reduce the tube feedings gradually or to withhold tube feedings entirely, considering the child's physical status, nutritional needs, and fluid intake.

The program became an ongoing assessment of the child's potential to eat orally. Due to some children's problems or limitations, or family factors, tube feedings sometimes remained the most viable alternative. That decision was generally made, however, after a trial period of several weeks, giving the child every possible chance.

Developmental Disabilities
Special Interest Section Newsletter; Vol. 3, No. 2, 1980

Treatment Procedure for Dysphagia

By Margaret E. Bartley, OTR and Sherry H. Pries, MSW

The following case study was completed to demonstrate the effectiveness of a combined sensory integrative and behavior modification approach to dysphagia.

The case history of L, a four year old female student of Special School District of St. Louis County, Missouri, consisted of tracheoesophageal fistula, poor swallowing coordination, esophageal stricture, abnormal motility pattern of the esophagus, mechognathia, coloboma of the retinal discs, and a marked hearing loss. She had been fed via a gastrostomy tube since birth with intermittent and unsuccessful attempts at oral feedings. Behaviorally, L presented herself as manipulative, capable of producing autonomic responses such as drooling, sweating, and respiratory changes when placed in situations which she found aversive. Total body tactile defensiveness, especially strong at the face, and vestibular defensiveness were present. L's history and behavior, and the professional literature suggested that the child may have been suppressing autonomic digestive responses due to behavioral and sensory integrative dysfunctions. It was hypothesized that through conditioning and sensory integration, the child could be transferred from tube to oral feeding.

DiScipio (1978) briefly outlined a three-phased behavioral treatment of "conditioned" or learned dysphagia including 1. shaping by positive reinforcement of psychomotor components of oral feeding behavior, 2. a contingency plan making tube feedings contingent upon oral feedings, and 3. massed learning trials. The present case study seemed to fit into his classification of dysphagia and Illingworth's (1969) categories of structural and neuromuscular dysphagias. Her tactile and vestibular defensive behavior could be generally associated with Ayres' description of sensory integrative dysfunction, although standardized sensory integrative scoring was not possible. Autoshaping research (Hearst and Jenkins, 1974, and Siegel, 1977) suggested that a response to stimuli presented to a subject causes the subject to perform the operant response without specific instructions or conventional training, seemingly an automatic response. In his work on reciprocal inhibition and systematic desensitization, Wolpe (1958) reported that autonomic

(continued)

29

Treatment for Dysphagia

functions can be manipulated by external environmental stimuli.

Considering Illingworth's (1969) identification of three steps in the mechanics of swallowing, L's feeding program was developed from research in sensory integration and behavior modification. Sensory integrative treatment included general tactile and vestibular stimulation throughout L's day and oral desensitization at feeding times. Autoshaping procedures were used to elicit food reaching, grasping, and consuming behavior. Positive stimuli, such as vibration,

play, light on/off, food in her tube, talking and rocking were used to reinforce those identified behaviors appropriate to the end feeding goal. Twice daily feedings allowed many learning opportunities. Tube feedings were used contingent upon oral behaviors until it became apparent that L did not associate relief of hunger with the oral intake of food.

Conditioning and shaping procedures and sensory integrative therapy resulted in increased oral intake of food and decreased autonomic responses inhibiting oral feeding.

L presently cooperates with oral feeding at school lunches, and actively assists in bringing the spoon to her mouth. At home, tube feedings continue, as she manipulates the home environment through her autonomic responses to feeding stimuli. Currently, home visits are a part of the therapeutic intervention.

Further information may be obtained by writing the authors at Deaf-Blind Program, Litzsinger School, 10094 Litzsinger Rd., St. Louis, MO, 63124.

Developmental Disabilities
Special Interest Section Newsletter; Vol. 3, No. 2, 1980

A Feeding Assessment

By Florence Yossem, MA, OTR

The process of feeding is truly a fascinating one. Manipulation of the oral musculature is complex and interesting, as we must learn a coordinated pattern of breathing, sucking and swallowing. Long before the production of speech sounds the development of these primitive reflexes are necessary. In feeding the action is suck and swallow with the inhibition of respiration. The inhibition guards against excessive coughing and choking. We use our lips to purse, to suck, to close on the spoon and to drink from a cup. We use our tongue to move food particles about in the mouth and to clean our lips. We move our jaw in a rotary fashion in order to chew our food before we swallow. At this point an intriguing division begins as air is swallowed down into the pharynx, the larynx, the trachea and into the lungs. Food enters the pharynx and splits off into the esophagus and down into the stomach. If all goes well we swallow without choking.

With neurological dysfunction, there is often a lack of maturation within the central nervous system, the tactile and kinesthetic being the most prominent sensations found lacking. Damage to the motor cortex, as well as feedback sensation from areas of movement, leaves an individual with tremendous interference and isolation. Abnormal reflexes are frequently prominent and add to the difficulties already present. Facilitating normal responses and breaking up the abnormal reflexes is a prime concern for the therapist.

One of the ways we can evaluate for oral deficiency is through observation. We need to observe body posture and the oral and body reflexes, as well as the feeding processes of suck, swallow and breathing. We need to look at the mouth—is it open or closed? Is there drooling and is there a coor-

dinated swallow? What food does the patient eat and is it mashed or cut up fine? Is there coughing or gagging? Where is the tongue during the eating process and do the lips close on the cup or is there much spilling? What is the patient's behavior pattern during a meal—is he rigid and rejecting? How long does he take to eat? If dealing with a child, it's important to know how many bottles per 24 hours are consumed and if a pacifier or spout cup is used. Also, in what position is the patient when eating—where is his head, trunk, hips and feet, etc.?

The following oral-motor, pre-speech feeding evaluation completes the picture. It considers the total person, primitive or pathological; child or adult.

1. **Facial Expression**: The first item considered. Does out patient have fine motor control with localized movement? Is the face expressionless, flaccid, perhaps almost primitive? What is the muscle tone? Is there asymmetry with a drooping eye or lip?

2. **Reflexes**: Are considered next. Does our patient have an ATNR and, if so, is it bilateral or to the right or to the left? Is there a Moro reflex? What about extensor tone? Also, of primary concern are the oral reflexes—the rooting reflex (which should disappear at approximately 3 months), the suck-swallow reflex (disappears approximately 3-5 months) and the gag reflex (diminishing approximately 7 months when chewing begins).

3. **The Jaw**: At rest the jaw should be lightly closed. When in motion, it should demonstrate horizontal and rotary movements. It is not at all uncommon to see malocclusions:

4. **The Lips**: At rest the lips will seem lightly closed. When in motion they possess a full range of fine movements. Many of our

patients have hypertonic (retracted) or hypotonic (floppy) lips. Isolated movements for pursing or kissing will, therefore, be lacking.

5. **The Tongue**: Normally rests on the bottom of the mouth and is extremely flexible with fine coordinated movements. With the handicapped, we frequently see a thrusting and/or protruding tongue, or one which rests between the open teeth or presses against the alveolar ridge. Movements will then be gross with little or no laterality.

6. **Oral Digital Stimulation**: Next we need to look at our patient's response to oral digital stimulation. What is the reaction to stimuli on the face, on the outside gums and within the oral cavity? Is our patient hypetonic or hypotonic?

7. **Dental Development**: An important consideration. What do the teeth and gums look like? White puffy gums may indicate an excess of medication requiring attention. The hard palate is generally seen as high and narrow in the mouth of a cerebral palsied individual.

8. **Breathing Pattern**: This needs to be coordinated and effortless. Feeding and respiration go hand in hand as patients need to learn to suck, swallow and breathe in a rhythmical pattern. We need to observe whether breathing is shallow or blocked by spasms. It is perhaps reversed with the patient talking on inhalation instead of exhalation?

9. **The Voice**: Requires listening to in order to determine intonation and loudness. What sounds do we hear, what words? After all we learn to coo at approximately 2 months.

10. **Positioning**: Next we need to look at what kind of a chair is used for feeding—

(continued)

A Feeding Assessment

where is the patient's head, shoulders, hips, knees and feet? Are the hips back in the chair with the knees flexed at 90 degrees? Are the feet stabilized? What sitting balance is possible and is there any self-feeding? Are the elbows stabilized on a lap tray or table? Is the patient free of the burden of his body enough to be able to used his hands independently?

11. **Feeding Behavior and Positioning:** May be observed while the patient is eating a snack or a meal. Can he bite, chew, purse on a cup, or eat independently? Do abnormal reflexes interfere? What about behavior, rigidities and temperament? What feeding utensils are used and are they adapted?

12. **Foods:** What foods are eaten? Are they regular table foods or are they mashed, chopped or pureed? Are they nutritious and is the meal well chosen?

Together with the above evaluations (visual and oral-motor) are numerous other evaluations and assessments that need to be utilized. I shall not go into them here. However, it is important to note that we are not only dealing with feeding problems, we are dealing in truth with a whole being. Our evaluation must also consider an assessment of the environment—the schools, therapist, caretakers and teachers—the hospital, nurses and therapist aides—the home, housekeeper, siblings and relatives. One section of my evaluation includes recommended therapeutic management *and* behavior management. In order to fulfill all of the therapy requirements, every person associated in the daily life of our patient needs to be considered. How much motivation is present? What is the time element for the feeder? How skilled is the caretaker and how much patience does he/she possess?

There are numerous other questions and hopefully some of them will emanate from the individual testing and working with the patient. The end result needs to be a composite of all that is required to fully evaluate the total individual.

Developmental Disabilities
Special Interest Section Newsletter; Vol. 3, No. 2, 1980

Evaluation of Oral-Motor Functioning

By Linda King-Thomas, MHS, OTR,
Division of Occupational Therapy
School of Medicine, Wing B-207H
University of North Carolina
Chapel Hill, NC 27514

The evaluation process is crucial to the implementation of any therapeutic program. Baseline information must be recorded in order to be able to adequately measure progress. The University of North Carolina (UNC) Feeding Assessment has been developed utilizing "The Pre-Speech Assessment" by Suzanne Morris,[2] "Ten Steps to Oral Assessment" by C.A.D.R.E. Center,[1] and personal experience with handicapped children with feeding problems. The following is a summary of the assessment form.

Feeding History: It is extremely important to gather information regarding the type of diet, position the child is fed, equipment, and the primary concerns of the parent/teacher. The time required to finish a meal and/or current weight may become measurement indicators of progress and need to be recorded before intervention. By identifying the environmental situation surrounding the mealtime both at school and at home, it will be possible to assess the most appropriate time to introduce therapeutic intervention. For example, if a parent or teacher has other responsibilities during mealtime, such as supervising siblings or feeding five severely handicapped children in 45 minutes, perhaps a snack time would be the most appropriate time to introduce therapeutic techniques. After the history is recorded, attention can focus on the child.

General Observations: While the child is resting or playing, take notice of motor patterns and spontaneous behavior. Does the child have facial asymmetry or an open mouth pattern? What is the respiration pattern? Explore the oral area in order to observe the condition of the teeth and gums. If a high arched palate is present, it becomes important for the child's safety and oral hygiene that no food remain on the roof of the mouth after meals. If the child drools, try to determine the basis for the excessive drooling. Remember drooling is normal when a child is cutting teeth and learning to walk.

Postural Mechanisms: The oral area tends to reflect the muscle tone and motor patterns of the body. General observation of spontaneous behavior and handling can provide valuable information about muscle tone, reflex activity and motor control. This information is then used to determine the best position for feeding. The position of the hips is often a key area in controlling the motor patterns of the jaw, tongue and lips. By reducing extension tone through hip flexion, abnormal patterns such as jaw thrusting, tongue and lip retraction can be inhibited.

Affect and Attitude: Behavior problems are frequently observed during mealtimes, e.g., stealing food, leaving the table, throwing a utensil, etc. Determining the basis for behavior problems, if possible, can be useful in deciding which treatment approach to use. Behavior management programs are more successful when the behavior is under voluntary control. Neurologically based behaviors such as hyperactivity and tactile defensiveness would tend to respond more to a sensory integrative approach utilized prior to mealtime. Often the child with strong motivation and perseverance can compensate for poor skills.

Oral Sensitivity: Hypersensitivity as well as hyposensitivity can interfere with the feeding process. Hypersensitivity in the facial area may result in a hyperactive gag reflex, and/or increase in abnormal muscle tone.

Voluntary Control of Oral Mechanisms: Imitation of tongue and lip movements provides information on motor control and motor planning abilities.

Oral Reflexes: Oral reflexes provide a foundation for oral-motor functioning and also contribute to the development of the parent-infant bonding. In normal development, reflexes are seldom obligatory. The infant can move in and out of reflex patterns and does not become locked into a reflex. It is important to determine if oral reflexes and oral-motor patterns are delayed or abnormal. For example, a phasic bite reflex which persists beyond five months is a delayed reflex, however, a tonic bite reflex (strong closure of the jaw with difficulty in releasing the bite) is never normal.

Feeding Patterns: The quality of movement and coordination of the lips, tongue, and jaw are extremely important in developing sucking, swallowing, and chewing skills. A thorough understanding of normal oral development is necessary to be able to identify poor coordination, poor quality of motor patterns, and to determine if movement patterns are delayed or abnormal. Patterns which are not observed in the normally developing infant and therefore considered abnormal are: jaw thrust, jaw retraction (excessive), tongue thrust, tongue retraction, poor tongue action controlled by intrinsic muscles, lip retraction, weak or inefficient sucking, very slow or inactive swallowing.[3]

(continued)

Oral-Motor Functioning

Self-Feeding: Identification of the components of self-feeding skills through activity analysis helps to identify each step needed for successful completion of the task. Visual-spatial skills, and eye-hand coordination are important foundations for functional activity and should be considered when analyzing the quality of the movement pattern.

At the completion of the feeding assessment, it would be useful to summarize the child's strengths and weaknesses in order to utilize the strengths in an intervention program. By organizing primary deficits and establishing treatment priorities, a therapeutic program can be developed and implemented.

Therapists are encouraged to use the UNC Feeding Assessment in their clinical practice and urged to send feedback to the author to help with further revisions. Copies of the evaluation form can be obtained by sending a self-addressed envelope and $.35 to the author.

Bibliography

[1] C.A.D.R.E. Center. Ten Steps to Oral Assessment. 1977. Available from C.A.D.R.E. Center. I.S.D. No. 911, 430 N.W. 8th St., Cambridge, MN 55008.

[2] Morris, Suzanne, Pre-Speech Assessment. NDT Course, May-June, 1979.

[3] Wilson, Jan (ed.). Oral-Motor Function and Dysfunction in Children. Conference proceeding, University of North Carolina at Chapel Hill, 1978. Available from Division of Physical Therapy, School of Medicine, Wing C, 221-H, University of North Carolina, Chapel Hill, NC 27514. $10.00.

Developmental Disabilities
Special Interest Section Newsletter; Vol. 3, No. 2, 1980

An Interdisciplinary Approach to Eating Problems

By Anne Barry Jolles, OTR

Ms Jolles is an assistant supervisor in the Childrens Hospital Medical Center Department of Occupational Therapy located at Wrentham State School.

The eating problems of the developmentally disabled, institutionalized population are complex. They may include aspiration, oral motor deficits, body position, malnutrition, behavior, limited hand usage, obesity, assorted medical problems, equipment, etc. Most clients are referred for a combination of the above problems. We have found that the clients rarely warrant the services of less than three disciplines. Given the intensity of the eating problems at this facility, and the number of clients needing services, the need for an *interdisciplinary approach and a corresponding management system* was recognized and has developed into our present system. There are now approximately 60 professionals comprising 6 Feeding Teams at Wrentham State School. There is one Main Feeding Team and 5 Mini-Feeding Teams.

The role of the Main Feeding Team is primarily administrative. This includes developing policy/procedures, facilitating departmental and groundswide communication, support and education of Mini-Feeding Team members, and training of new employees. The teams consist of members from the following disciplines: occupational therapy, physical therapy, nursing, psychology, speech and hearing, nutrition, and mental retardation assistants. Representatives from medicine, dental and pharmacy are available on a consultative basis.

The role of the Mini-Feeding Team is to provide comprehensive feeding evaluation, interpretation and monitoring of results to direct care staff, direct care staff support, and training. Input from the teams has also been given in regard to dining room environmental factors, i.e., seating plan, noise levels, table setting, etc.

Three of the Mini-Feeding Teams are located in the units where the most severely involved multiply handicapped people live. The additional two teams service the population which is less severely physically involved. The responsibilities surrounding meals does not rest solely with feeding teams. There are currently many programs operating which meet the general needs of the population. This then frees team members to concentrate efforts where their expertise is most needed. We have learned that stationing the teams in the units where clients live has enabled the followup of recommendations, facilitation of staff support and continued education to direct care staff to be done more efficiently and consistently. We have also provided for groundswide coverage through a "Float Mini-Feeding Team."

The occupational therapist, physical therapist and speech therapist on the Feeding Teams evaluate oral motor abilities and oral structure. The occupational therapist and physical therapist assess body position and upper extremity function. Utensil use, adapted feeding equipment and social skills are also evaluated during this time. The evaluation form was compiled by the Occupational Therapy Department and the Physical Therapy Department.

Much Team effort goes into reiteration of recommendations, support and education of direct care staff as to specific client needs. Others training efforts include:

1. A slide-tape presentation to new employees comprising feeding team structure/function and proper feeding techniques.

2. Laminated individual client photographs and program description for severely involved clients which can easily be referred to by direct care staff.

3. Availability of feeding team members at the three meals.

Also, the feeding team in collaboration with the Respiratory Therapy Department and Staff Development have provided an inservice series for long-term employees who may have missed out on the new slide-tape presentation at employee orientation. The content of this inservice includes: the effects of abnormal muscle tone in the eating process, body position during the meal, the physiological effects and complications of aspiration and training in the obstructed airway maneuver. In order to maintain quality services, the Main Feeding Team continues to coordinate educational experiences not only for mental retardation assistants, but also for the professionals on the Mini-Feeding Teams. There is an ongoing lecture series covering a wide variety of topics of interest to members.

All staff in the Department of Occupational Therapy currently participate in some aspect of the feeding process. Besides valuable contributions during interdisciplinary evaluations, Certified Occupational Therapy Assistants and Occupational Therapy Aides, under the supervision of a Registered Occupational Therapist are directly involved in the therapeutic feeding programs with the more severely involved clients. COTAs and OTAs have also made a large impact on social refinement and dining room environmental improvements.

Now having this system in place, we are able to see vast improvements in the quality and consistency of care. In regard to client care, we generally note a decrease in the number of aspiration incidences and im-

(continued)

Eating Problems

provement in nutritional status. Benefits to clients are found in the increased carry over of feeding team recommendations by direct care staff. Examples of this include improved positioning, equipment use and staff/client interaction during meals.

We have discovered that in developing this interdisciplinary approach, much of the success can be attributed to factors inherent in this process. Examples of these include routine involvement of direct care staff, well defined tasks and clear cut goals. Also, direct care staff are rewarded by measurable client gains upon following of recommendations. The Mini-Feeding Teams fit into the system well to provide input into an existing activity.

Professionals on the teams report that the support, identity and education have been very beneficial to their service delivery. Although some of the disciplines historically were not involved in feeding they have broadened skills, gained new skills and applied their expertise to meet the multiple needs of the developmentally delayed person at mealtime.

Bibliography For Treatment Of Dysphagia
By: Margaret E. Bartley, OTR, Sherry H. Pries, MSW

Albe-Fessard, D. and **Fessard, A.,** Thalamic integration and their consequences at the telencephalic level. In G. Moruzzi, A. Fessard and H. Jasper (Eds.), Progress in Brain Research, Volume 1, Brain Mechanisms. New York: Elsevier Publishing Company, 1963.

Ayres, A. J., Sensory Integration and Learning Disorders. Los Angeles: Western Psychological Services, 1972.

DiScipio, William J., Kaslon, K., Ruben, R. J. Traumatically acquired conditioned dysphagia in children. Annals of Otology, Rhinology and Laryngology, 1978, 87, 509-514.

Hearst, E. and **Jenkins H. M.** Sign-tracking: The stimulus-reinforcer relation and directed action. Austin, The Psychonomic Society, Inc., 1974.

Illingworth, R. S. Sucking and swallowing difficulties in infancy: diagnostic problem of dysphagia. Arch Dis. Child, 1969, 44, 655-664.

King, R. B., Meagher, J. N., and **Barnett, J. C.** Studies of trigeminal nerve potentials. Journal of Neurosurgery, 1956, 13, 176-183.

Melzack, R. and **Wall, D.** Pain mechanisms: a new theory. Science, 1965, 150, 971-979.

Morris, S. E., Program Guidelines for Children with Feeding Problems. Edison, N. J., Childcraft Education Corp., 1977.

Mountcastle, V. B. and **Powell, T. P. S.,** Central Nervous mechanisms subserving position sense and kinesthesis. Bulletin of the Johns Hopkins Hospital, 1959, 105, 173-200.

Mueller, H. A., Facilitating feeding and prespeech. In P. H. Pearson and C. Ethun Williams (Eds.), Physical Therapy Services in the Developmental Disabilities. Springfield: Charles C. Thomas Publisher, 1972.

Siegel, R. K. Stimulus selection and tracking during urination: autoshaping directed behavior with toilet targets. Journal of Applied Behavior Analysis, 1977, 10, 255-265.

Wolpe, J. Psychotherapy by Reciprocal Inhibition. Stanford, University Press, 1958.

Developmental Disabilities
Special Interest Section Newsletter; Vol. 3, No. 1, 1980

Programming for the Head-Injured Client

By Connie Hoeke, OTR

Connie is a graduate of Temple University and is currently working at the Regional Comprehensive Rehabilitation Center for Children and Youth in Pittsburgh, PA.

This article provides a brief overview of the rehabilitation program offered to head trauma clients at the Regional Comprehensive Rehabilitation Center for Children and Youth with a focus on occupational therapy services. The majority of these clients begin in a residential program and then may be transferred to a day and/or outpatient program.

Services offered to individual head-injured patients vary to some degree depending on their specific needs. The schedule which follows, however, provides an overview of the typical services offered.

7 AM *Morning Activities of Daily Living.* This is primarily done by child care workers trained to work with head-injured clients. Consultation and evaluation services are available from occupational therapy as needed.

8 AM *Breakfast*

8:30 AM Reality Orientation Session carried out by speech language therapist. This session is for those clients who are able to process information but who remain in a state of confusion. Orientation to person, place, time (including their schedule) and their condition are emphasized. Clients functioning at this level carry a log book with them in which all daily events are recorded. This book is reviewed with the client throughout the day to stimulate recent memory and improve orientation.

9-11:30 AM; 12:30-3 PM *School and Individual Therapy Sessions.* A school program is available with teachers skilled in working with learning problems common to the head injured. Individual therapy sessions (OT/PT/ST) also occur during this time as well as a social service group (or individual contact) which provides clients with a specific time to talk about what has happened to them.

11:30-12:30 AM *Lunch.* Depending on the client's specific needs, this may be a therapeutic feeding program carried out by OT/PT/ST feeding team, a supervised or independent eating situation or the client may be involved in the OT Meal Preparation Group. This group emphasizes both organization and skill.

3 PM *Auditory Processing—Thought Organization Group.* This group is for patients with moderate to severe deficits in information processing, memory, thought organization, attention, and judgment. Group activities are done under guidance of a speech/language therapist that addresses these problems areas.

3:30 PM *Structured Activities and Community Reorientation Group.* Short projects are performed in the group, i.e., cooking, games, simple functional craft tasks, that emphasize organization, sequencing, memory, safety and judgment. Clients are also taken on community excursions. Crossing the street, purchasing items, asking for information, use of public services are some of the areas stressed. This group is run by the occupational therapy department.

4 PM *Free time*

5 PM *Dinner*

6 PM *Unit Programs.* These may include swimming, games, sport activities, community outings. They are carried out by child care workers.

In addition to the noon time and afternoon occupational therapy groups, most clients are also seen daily on an individual basis. These individual occupational therapy sessions incorporate reality orientation and organization but also focus more specifically on motor and visual perceptual needs of the client. Improving upper extremity function, bilateral skills, motor planning, or specific visual perceptual/memory difficulties are common goals. Joint treatment sessions may be done with speech and/or physical therapy.

For the head-injured client who is just coming out of a coma, occupational therapy is involved in carrying out a stimulation program geared at eliciting and heightening motor responses. Specific, appropriate responses are the objectives and a well-structured session is imperative.

The Head-Injured Client

By Mark Ylvisaker, Speech Language Pathologist, CCC

If all summaries of patients with severe head trauma were gathered together in one assembly, it would not be easy to see what these people had in common. There would be quadriplegics, right and left hemiplegics, and those with no physical involvement at all; some would have a hearing impairment; others a visual field deficit; others no sensory loss; some would be talking nonstop in grammatically well-formed and perfectly intelligible sentences, while others would be completely nonverbal. Why, then, do we consider this a useful diagnostic label around which to structure a coherent integrated rehabilitation program? The thread which knits this diverse group together can be stated singly: generally depressed cognitive functioning. More challenging, however, is a perspicuous explication of this unifying theme. For the purposes of this article, cognitive functioning incudes the following areas: orientation, memory, perceptual processing, thought organization, and judgment. Throughout this discussion it must, of course, be remembered that the head injured is of equal importance to the head injury in predicting outcome.

Orientation: In the early stages of recovery most patients evidence some degree of disorientation to person (Who am I? Who are the people around me?), place (Where am I? Where do I belong?), time (What day is it? What time of year is it? How long since my accident), and condition (What is wrong with me? Why can't I ride my bike and play football?). In severe cases, orientation returns slowly and only with patient guidance by family and staff. Orientation to condition may never be more than superficial.

Memory: Remote memory (memory for pretraumatic events and people) usually begins to return with recognition of family members and often returns relatively quickly. Immediate recall (e.g., digit span) may or may not be significantly depressed, but is particularly important only for children in the early grades. Of primary concern is the frequently long-lasting deficit in short-term memory. This poses a major obstacle to school learning as well as to the efficient conduct of one's affairs at any stage of life.

Perceptual Processing: It is extremely common for head injury patients in the middle and late stages of recovery to process simple auditory information (e.g., words or short sentences) and simple visual information in an age-appropriate manner. However, with increases in length and/or complexity of the stimuli, processing may deteriorate precipitously. The difficulty is related in part to inadequate figure/ground mechanisms and in part to an extremely slow rate of processing that makes complex material particularly difficult to handle.

Thought Organization: The more abstract levels of thought—categorizing, sequencing, drawing inferences, distinguishing details from main idea—are typically impaired in head-injured individuals. This affects the patient's ability to actively structure himself around a task (e.g., cooking, crafts) as well as his ability to passively organize material in his mind for purposes of effective learning and organized expression of ideas.

Judgment: A common residual deficit observed in otherwise well-recovered head-injured patients is inadequate safety judgment (e.g., crossing streets, participating in dangerous sports) and social judgment. Due to a depressed awareness of the nuances of social reality, head injury patients may fail to effectively merge into their previous social world.

Implications: The survivor of severe closed head injury, particularly those with no observable physical deficits, pose a challenge to professionals and family alike. They may look, talk and walk exactly as they did before their accident. Their problems are not easy to see, for them or for others. Insufficiently aware of the residual impairment to memory, information processing and thought organization, they and their superiors wonder why they are failing at school or on the job. This failure easily leads to a punitive response from superiors and a behavioral maladjustment in the individual. This history has repeated itself countless times in the past and can be altered only by informed and dedicated professionals. . . .

Article Review: Psychological Testing of Severely Head-Injured Patients

Two articles on "Cognitive Recovery After Severe Head Injury" appeared in the *Journal of Neurology, Neurosurgery, and Psychiatry*, 1975, 38. The following are brief summaries of both articles.

1. "Serial Testing on the Wechsler Adult Intelligence Scale," by Ian A. Mandleberg and D.N. Brooks, pp 1121-1126.

Beginning in 1968, forty head-injured patients were studied at Glasgow University to look at the course of recovery of cognitive functions. The Wechsler Adult Intelligence Scale (WAIS) was used. All subjects were more than 15 years of age and had post-traumatic amnesia (PTA) (time of injury to recovery of orientation to time, place and person) more than four days. Only two subjects were women. A comparison group of 40 noninjured men was established.

The first administration of the WAIS was given when the patient emerged from PTA. Patients were tested in time blocks relative to their injury and dependent on whether they were out of PTA. Intervals were 0-3 months, 4-6 months, 7-12 months, more than 13 months. Therefore, it was possible a subject was only tested once, but could have been tested up to four times, depending on when he came out of PTA. It was concluded in the study that practice did not affect the WAIS scores of the head-injured sample used.

Testing revealed a trend toward more deficit in Performance than in Verbal subtests in initial testing. Verbal scores more quickly returned to the level of the comparison group also (within about one year). Recovery in Performance IQ continued over about three years.

". . . the cognitive abilities of the head-injured patients as a group eventually
(continued)

Psychological Testing

returned to normal levels, despite the severity of their injuries as assessed by duration of PTA." (1125) These findings suggest that "duration of PTA does not predict cognitive outcome." (1126)

2. "Wechsler Adult Intelligence Scale During Post Traumatic Amnesia," by Ian

Mandleberg, pp 1127-1132.

Thirty-two adult severely head-injured patients were given the WAIS at Glasgow University. They were divided into two matched groups; Group I was first tested while in PTA, Group II was first tested when out of PTA. On initial WAIS testing, scores

from Group I were significantly lower than those of Group II. More deficit was found in the Performance than in the Verbal subtests. At follow-up testing Group I had substantially caught up with Group II on the WAIS.

Developmental Disabilities
Special Interest Section Newsletter; Vol. 2, No. 4, 1979

Pre-Vocational Training for Mentally Retarded Adults

By Bettina Beckman, MEd, OTR

The following article outlines a variety of pre-vocational training programs for mentally retarded adults at the Fernald State School in Waltham, MA. These programs have been developed and implemented by members of the occupational therapy department in conjunction with psychologists, educators and rehabilitation counselors. They constitute one part of a continuum of services to our clients that ranges from basic skills training to placement in competitive employment.

The focus of our pre-vocational programs is on the total client, his interactions with the environment, his peers, staff, and the task at hand. This differs from vocational training, where the emphasis is on work-related issues. Because of this "total person" approach, occupational therapists have been a key in the development and implementation of pre-vocational programs.

Pre-vocational training at Fernald is divided into three major areas. These are evaluation, pre-vocational programming and on-the-job training. Each area has been designed to meet the specific needs of the client and to facilitate his movement into a vocational training program. Each area will be described separately.

Evaluation. When a client has had no previous training experiences, or when he is in need of a major program change, he is referred to a formal evaluation. This evaluation consists of a four-week placement in

one of 11 sheltered workshops or four on-the-job training sites located at Fernald. During this time, an occupational therapist assigned to the evaluation observes the client's daily performance in the following areas: quality and quantity of work, fine and gross motor activities, functional academic skills, social skills, and work habits and attitudes. Using standard tests, department-developed batteries and live work, the OTR assesses the client's skills, learning style and motivational reinforcers. At the completion of the evaluation, she refers the client to the appropriate day program, based on his performance, interests and programmatic needs. She then assists the new program staff to develop specific training objectives and implement the treatment plan.

Pre-vocational programming. Five pre-vocational programs at Fernald serve approximately 80 clients. These programs are staffed by occupational therapy assistants and vocational instructors; the staff-to-client ratio averages 1:4. OTRs function as consultants to each pre-vocational program. In this role, we perform evaluations, assist in setting client objectives and program goals, implement a variety of therapeutic activities, and supervise staff. Each pre-vocational program runs four hours a day, and is broken down into components 20 to 45 minutes in length. The components include table-top or simulated work activities, gross motor training, pre-academic and functional academics

training, and socialization. The socialization component ranges from cooking to current events discussions to community experiences. The goal of the pre-vocational programs is to assist each client to reach his potential for successful independence in his community.

On-the-job training (OJT). A number of on-the-job training sites at Fernald and in the Waltham community provide pre-vocational training for 40 clients. OJT work areas such as the greenhouse, cafeteria/restaurant, housekeeping crew, and clerical pool have proved to be excellent program areas for clients who have not yet been exposed to the "working world" or who have not succeeded in the more traditional sheltered workshop setting. Staffed similarly to the pre-vocational programs, OJT programs can be structured, or unstructured, to meet the needs of each client. Flexibility in both activities and expectations is key to the client's success, and his relationships with staff, peers and the work itself are used to teach appropriate work habits and attitudes and specific vocational skills.

We are very excited about the role of occupational therapy in pre-vocational training. Through pre-vocational training, much progress has been made in assisting the mentally retarded adult reach his maximum level of independence in society.

Developmental Disabilities

Special Interest Section Newsletter; Vol. 2, No. 4, 1979

Assessment of the Pre-Vocational/Vocational Client

By Pat Marvin, OTR, Johnstown Rehabilitation Center

The pre-vocational and vocational evaluation roles for the OT can be one of the most challenging in the field of occupational therapy. These roles offer routes and challenges for creativity well beyond what is considered a normal day's work. The therapist must integrate her role with that of the vocational counselor and the vocational evaluator to move the client into functional productivity. . . work!

The first stage in the evaluation centers on the physical capacities of the client—an area unique to the evaluation process for the OT. An excellent assessment has been developed by Susan Smith of the Woodrow Wilson Rehabilitation Center. A copy of this can be found in the new *Willard and Spackman's Occupational Therapy*, 5th ed., pp. 213-218. This is a very detailed analysis and corresponds with the *Dictionary of Occupational Titles*.

Along with the physical capacities evaluation, the activities of daily living status is judged as well as sensory deficiencies, visual-perceptual limitations, and communication techniques. Also, an emotional picture is formulated and integrated with the motivational factors, e.g. self-image, financial status, pain tolerance, etc.

Lastly, within this stage the work history is noted. This gives the evaluator an insight into the interests and skills of the client as well as the stability of the work background.

The second stage calls for the occupational therapist to have an awareness of the standardized tests that are commercially available. These tests will allow a greater accumulation of knowledge to assist the client in a vocational choice. Many of these tests can be administered by the OTR once an adequate knowledge of procedures has been learned. Others are given by the psychologist or the trained vocational evaluator. It is imperative, if the OTR is the principal evaluator, to know what to look for in standardized testing and what tests to use to find out the information that is required. The following is an edited list of available tests:

A. *Achievement and Intelligence Tests*
1. Army General Classification Test
2. Basic Skills in Arithmetic Test
3. Differential Aptitude Test
4. Full Range Picture Vocabulary Test
5. Gates MacGinitie Reading Survey
6. General Aptitude Test Battery
7. Metropolitan Achievement Tests
8. Minnesota Paper Form Board Test
9. Otis Quick-Scoring Mental Ability Test
10. Peabody Picture Vocabulary Test
11. Revised Beta
12. Haptic Intelligence Scale for Adult Blind
13. School and College Ability Tests (SCAT)
14. S.R.A. Reading Record
15. Terman-McNemar Test of Mental Ability
16. Tests of General Ability (TOGA)
17. Tiedeman Arithmetical Knowledge and Information Tests
18. Turse-Durost Shorthand Achievement Test
19. Wide Range Achievement Test
20. Peabody Individual Achievement Test
21. Wechsler Adult Intelligence Scale
22. Audey Test of Cognition Limited
23. Culture Fair Intelligence Test

B. *Dexterity Tests*
1. Bennett Hand Tool Dexterity Test
2. Crawford Small Parts Dexterity Test
3. Minnesota Rate of Manipulation Test
4. Pennsylvania Bi-Manual Work Test
5. Purdue Peg Board

C. *Interest Tests*
1. California Picture Interest Inventory
2. Geist Picture Interest
3. Kuder Performance Record

D. *Special Abilities Tests*
1. Bennett Mechanical Comprehension Test
2. Bennett Stenographic Test
3. IBM Aptitude Test for Programmer Personnel
4. MacQuarrie Test for Mechanical Ability
5. Maitland-Graves Design Judgment Test
6. Meier Art Judgment Test
7. Minnesota Clerical Test
8. O'Rourke Mechanical Aptitude Test
9. S.R.A. Clerical Aptitude Test and Mechanical Ability Test
10. Turse Clerical Abilities Test
11. Bausch and Lomb Occupational Vision Test

E. *Personality Tests*
1. Bernreuter Personality Inventory
2. California Test of Personality
3. Minnesota Multiphasic Personality Inventory
4. Vineland Social Maturity Scale
5. Mooney Problem Check List
6. Rotter Incomplete Sentence Blank

The third stage is the work sample try-out where once again the occupational therapists' creativity is displayed. The work samples consist of small units of actual job tasks or simulated units of equal value. Inclusive in this stage is the use of one or more of the many commercial evaluation systems. The McCarron-Dial Work Evaluation System, the Singer Vocational Evaluation System, the Valpar Component Work Sample Series, The Tower System and the Talent Assessment Programs are but a few of the many commercial systems available for use.

During the third stage, the OTR is often called upon not only to develop the simulated tasks but also to do a basic activity analysis of the work job. Here the OTR completes a comparison analysis of the job requirements and the physical capacities of the client.

In the fourth or last stage of pre-vocational/vocational training the job try-out becomes an actuality. Now the OTR is called upon to use her expertise in adaptive equipment as well as other areas to help this experience become a valid, positive and productive achievement. At this point mobility systems may have to be finessed, architectural barriers modified, tools adapted to special situations, self-care systems adjusted for work schedules, specialized strengthening programs instituted, and social support systems established.

Finally, the status of WORK—the foundation of occupational therapy—is achieved.

Developmental Disabilities
Special Interest Section Newsletter; Vol. 2, No. 3, 1979

Assessing an Assessment Tool

by Wendy Coster, MS, OTR

Proper use of an evaluation instrument depends on the clinician's having a thorough understanding of the instrument—of its construction, applicability, administration, and interpretation. The fact that a particular test is widely used or covers areas of interest to us does *not* necessarily ensure that it is an appropriate method to use with a particular client or that the questions we are asking can be answered with its scores. Even in situations where a particular test is the definite choice, either because of its stated function or because no other instrument is available, knowledge of the test's strengths and weaknesses is of great importance when drawing diagnostic conclusions from its results. This article is a review of important areas to consider to assist therapists in assessing evaluation instruments. As it is brief, references are given at the end which can provide greater detail on any area of particular concern.

Among the important areas to be reviewed are:

A. *Purpose of Test:* What is the stated purpose of the test—what population (age, functional state, etc.) was it designed for and what areas does it intend to examine? What conclusions, according to the authors, can be drawn from its results?

As one reviews standardization, reliability, and validity, consider whether there is solid data backing the stated purpose and function or whether, in fact, the instrument does something quite different from what was intended or does what was intended too poorly to be useful.

B. *Standardization:* Has the test been standardized? If so, was the sample adequate? Was it representative of the population at large? Were sufficient numbers of subjects included at each age?

If the test is not standardized, on what basis are scores given?

C. *Reliability:* How consistent is the test over time (test—retest) and how consistent are items with one another (internal consistency)? Test—retest provides a measure of whether, if the test were repeated, the scores originally obtained would remain approximately the same. Reliability may be reported for individual subtests as well as for the instrument as a whole. Test—retest reliability may vary considerably for different age groups, making this factor important to consider when interpreting results for a particular client or selecting the instrument for use with a particular age group.

Standard Error of Measurement (SEM) may also be reported for subtests. This statistic indicates the range within which an individual's "true" score would fall if the test was repeated a large number of times. The SEM is very important to consider when drawing diagnostic conclusions from a test or subtest that uses a "cut-off-point" in determining normality or abnormality.

Internal consistency provides a measure of how well all items in the instrument or subtest measure the same thing. Internal consistency is important in assessing how interpretable a particular score will be.

D. *Validity:* Does the test actually measure what it says it does? A variety of validity measures may be considered. "Face validity" may be examined directly by each clinician by looking at the items considering whether they look like they are measuring what they should. "Content validity" examines the author's theoretical or empirical rationale for choosing their items. "Construct validity" examines the extent to which a test measures a particular theoretical construct or trait i.e., intelligence or strength. "Criterion validity" gives information on the extent to which scores on the test are in agreement with (concurrent validity) or can predict (predictive validity) some particular measure or "criterion."

These are the major objective pieces of information which can be reviewed. They will, of course, be supplemented by more subjective (but also useful) information such as experiences of other clinicians using the test, appeal of the test to different age groups, etc. The composite of all such information should enable one to make truly informed choices when selecting a test instrument and sound interpretations of the results obtained.

References

Anastasi, A. *Psychological Testing* (4th ed) NY: MacMillan Co. 1977.

Buros', Oscar K. (ed) *The 7th Mental Measurements Yearbook,* Highland Park, NJ: Gryphon Press 1972.

Cronbach, L., *Essentials of Psychological Testing* (3rd ed), NY: Harper and Row 1970.

French, J. and Michael N., *Standards of Educational and Psychological Tests and Manuals,* Washington, D.C. American Psychological Assn. 1966.

Mehrens, W. and Lehmann, I., *Measurement and Evaluation in Education Psychology,* NY: Holt Rinehart and Winston, 1973.

Developmental Disabilities
Special Interest Section Newsletter; Vol. 2, No. 2, 1979

Spotlight on COTAs in the Baltimore County Public School System

The COTAs in Baltimore County Public School System were hired in August 1977, originally under a federal grant made available after the passing of Public Law 94-142. At present, three COTAs hold positions in three special education schools in this county. The grant expired after one year and the COTA salaries were accepted into the county budget.

Guidelines for all COTAs were developed last year by the therapists. COTAs must:

1) have completed satisfactorily an occupational therapy assistants curriculum approved by the American Occupational Therapy Association;

2) be certified and hold current certification with said professional organization; and

3) be licensed to assist in the practice of OT under the supervision of/or with the consultation of an OTR whose license is in good standing.

Maryland's licensure law was passed in July 1978. The law will go into effect in July 1979.

Providing direct services is a major responsibility of the COTA. This is done in

(continued)

COTAs in Baltimore County Public Schools

collaboration with or under the supervision of an OTR, although the OTR need not be on the premises for treatment to be carried out. Consultations between OTR and COTA are held at least weekly.

COTAs are involved in the overall screening of new pupils; attending pediatric, orthopedic, and team conferences when applicable; serving as resource people to teachers and parents; scheduling parent conferences and home visits when needed; and providing input with teachers and other therapists concerning the student's program. These services are rendered under the supervision of an OTR. COTAs as well as most other school personnel must be available to assist with and attend school activities as required by the principal.

Each child seen in therapy has an individual therapy plan (ITP) to be included in the individual educational plan (IEP) for the year. This is compiled by the case manager who is usually the teacher. The ITP is discussed with both parents and teachers, and is updated throughout the year.

OT assistants prepare report cards for pupils at mid-term and at the end of the school year. It is imperative that the COTA maintain current records as defined by the school district.

The OT assistants help supervise and train aides, volunteers, and other health workers, and also contribute to the learning of OT students involved in clinical experiences.

Itinerant services are provided to regular schools which, through the placement of students in the least restrictive environment, have students they feel will benefit from therapy. After approval from the supervisor of Special Education, an assessment/ evaluation is performed by the itinerant OTR. The student may be scheduled for OT services once or twice weekly. The itinerant COTA carries out some of the therapy sessions after consultation with the OTR.

One major problem that exists within the school system is that there often is no employment category solely for the COTA. Salary is based on that of an instructional aide, although COTAs do not function in an aide capacity. Assistants are given an identity within their own schools and OT departments, but confusion often arises concerning meeting attendance, form completion, and employment benefits.

The COTA is a viable part of the team approach and provides valuable input to the child's OT program. Under the supervision of an OTR, COTAs help with the recognition and remediation of children with spatial needs. They provide therapy techniques that encourage the child to perform, and enhance the child's opportunity to develop and use the abilities needed while minimizing the disabling effects of handicapping conditions.

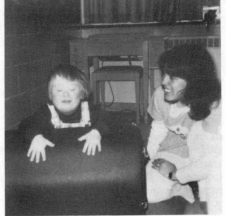

Nancy Rehmeyer *is employed by the Baltimore County Board of Education, Special Education, State of Maryland. Ms Rehmeyer's primary assignments are at Rolling Road School, which services children with mental and/or physical handicaps or developmental delays; and Campfield Elementary School, which has both regular and special education classes. A primary responsibility at Rolling Road School is with the newly established parent-infant program serving infants 0-2 years old. Ms Rehmeyer is presently serving as COTA representative on the Executive Board of Maryland Occupational Therapy Association.*

Developmental Disabilities
Special Interest Section Newsletter; Vol. 2, No. 2, 1979

The Roles of Occupational Therapy in the Baltimore Public School System

By Meridith Garitee Muehleib, OTR
(Meridith is an Occupational Therapist with the Baltimore County Public School System)

The "Education for All Handicapped Children Act of 1975" (PL94-142) has been a major steppingstone for occupational therapists practicing in the public school systems. Because of this legislation, programs that did not previously receive the services of an occupational therapist are now receiving those services, and many programs that had minimal or adequate services have been able to expand to include new populations of students. PL94-142 includes the "related service" of Occupational Therapy "as may be required to assist a handicapped child to benefit from special education." ?4:17. The major goal of any occupational therapist in a school system is to prepare students for learning and to help the student perform optimally in the learning environment.

The role of occupational therapist in the schools can be paralleled to the levels of service that are optimally provided within the special education system. The level of service to be provided to a student is based on the individual needs of the student, and the amount of intervention that is necessary to provide the student with those skills that will allow him or her to function within the learning environment. Occupational therapists should be involved in all levels of service that are provided by the local education agency.

The first level, *Level 1*, is that of consultation within a regular education program. This level involves working with teachers, and administrators without direct service to a student. At this level, the occupational therapist can work to orient teachers to various handicapping conditions, to demonstrate adaptive equipment, and to direct teachers to texts and other relevant information.

Level 2 is the "resource level." Students within a regular education program are not given direct service, but the progress of an individual student is monitored. An occupational therapist may work in this capacity, particularly in the case of a student placed in a regular classroom program who needs special equipment in order to perform optimally.

Level 3 is the level at which itinerant serv-

(continued)

Roles of Occupational Therapy

ice is provided within the regular education program. The occupational therapist provides direct service to an individual student, and also maintains contact with the teacher and administrator.

Level 4 is also an itinerant service level, but the direct service is provided to the student in a special education program within a regular school. At this level, the occupational therapist can provide direct therapy while the student benefits from a less restrictive environment than a special school.

Level 5 is the traditional role that occupational therapists have played in the school

system at the level of special education facility. The advantage of this type of service model for the occupational therapist is that it allows for constant contact with the student, other therapists, other team members, administrators, and families. The disadvantage of this service model is that it is a very restricted environment.

Level 6 is the residential care facility which is another direct service model that occupational therapists have traditionally worked in.

By using the levels of service models to identify the roles of occupational therapy in the school system, more non-traditional

roles can be examined. The parallel between less restrictive environment and increased independence demonstrates the importance in following an individual student through to his or her level of optimal functioning, and greatest independence. Occupational therapists need to re-examine their public school systems and move into the roles of providing itinerant, resource, and consultative assistance in regular education, so that more students will be able to leave the special school service models, and move into the regular education system.

Developmental Disabilities
Special Interest Section Newsletter; Vol. 2, No. 1, 1979

Occupational Therapists in Action: Lynne Pape

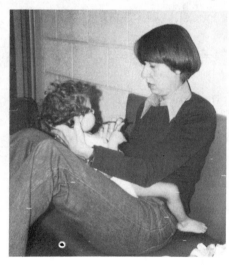

Lynne Pape is the occupational therapist at St. George Developmental Center which is a part of the Cuyahoga County Board of Mental Retardation in Cleveland, Ohio. St. George's is funded through Title I monies and provides service through day programs to those individuals who have been diagnosed as mentally retarded or developmentally delayed.

The concept of early intervention in mental retardation is basic to the philosophy of the St. George Developmental Center; 80 percent of its population is under six years of age. These children are physically and/or multiply-handicapped, and display neuro-motor dysfunction. In addition to direct

therapy, consultation is provided to the infant stimulation classrooms.

Assessment focuses on the quality of motor skills (gross, fine, and oral motor). A problem solving analysis of the whole child is primarily aimed at defining what is interfering with normal development. Establishing a developmental level in terms of motor milestones is not emphasized.

Individual programs are developed, based on each child's specific needs. All treatment goals are written in *observable* and *measurable* objectives. Although it is difficult to state all therapeutic objectives in measurable terms (i.e. development of head and trunk control, normalization of tone, etc.) this method of treatment planning assures that goals are set at an appropriate level, and facilitates tracking progress results. Goals emphasize working towards improved *overall* function; the development of individual isolated skills is not stressed.

The overall philosophy of treatment is based on the concepts of Neurodevelopmental Treatment (NDT). Specific treatment goals include normalization of tone, development of normal postural reactions, (righting, equilibrium, and protective), improved oral motor and feeding abilities, maintenance of quality gross and fine motor control, promoting proper positioning through adaptations and use of specific adapted equipment, and the development of age-appropriate skills. Comprehensive therapy is provided throughout the child's day

and incorporates handling techniques which emphasize total body responses. A specific exercise program, designed to improve isolated body parts, is not integral to this treatment approach.

Whenever possible therapy is integrated into the child's classroom. This approach has proved invaluable in providing consistency of treatment, and maintaining good communication between teachers and therapists. Teacher and therapist together plan how to incorporate therapeutic goals into the educational setting. The therapist is readily available to answer questions, provide input, implement and re-evaluate each child's objectives.

Parents and caretakers are an integral part of our program and are utilized when possible within the classroom setting. We are delighted that parents have recently begun taking a more active role in planning programs for their child (possibly as a result of PL 94-142). Therapists work with parents in discussing and demonstrating appropriate handling techniques which can be incorporated into the child's daily home routine. These discussions are supplemented by home visits when it is indicated by the needs of the child.

To insure comprehensive programming, an interdisciplinary approach is utilized within the program. Staffings done twice a week are attended by the teachers, occupational therapist, physical therapist, speech therapist, social workers, and outreach worker.

Developmental Disabilities
Special Interest Section Newsletter; Vol. 2, No. 1, 1979

Clinically Speaking

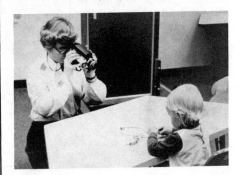

Rita R. Hohlstein, *MS, OTR is Section Head of Occupational Therapy at the Diagnostic and Treatment Unit of the Waisman Center on Mental Retardation and Human Development, a UAF. Her duties include classroom and clinical teaching, research, administration and service.*

The need for good evaluation tools or methods is well known and understood by occupational therapists. Two common ways to respond to this need exist. One is to go to published and/or standardized tools and accept that they are "good" because they are widely used and accepted by others. The second is to take items considered important from these same tools and add additional items believed to be necessary for the evaluation of populations served by the individual therapist. Both of these methods

credit the theoretical basis on which the items were founded as being accurate and worthy of promulgation.

I believe that occupational therapists should contribute to information about human function and not just continually use information contributed by other professions. In an attempt to do this I designed and am implementing a longitudinal study of the development of prehension in normal and handicapped infants and children. The need for this study became evident after my clinical experience caused me to question the validity of existing prehension evaluations used by occupational therapists. My library search revealed that most tests of prehension for infants and children were based on the work of Henry Halverson. In a cross-sectional study Halverson (1931) presented infants with one inch red cubes and filmed their responses. From these data he labeled the different grasps he observed and formulated a developmental sequence of prehension which was utilized by Gesell (1941) in his Developmental Schedules. I wanted to determine if infants and children in the 1970s followed the previously described developmental sequence for prehension as well as investigate if the size and shape of objects presented to infants influenced the type of grasp used. To answer these questions 10 normal children were filmed in

their own homes monthly during their first year of life and then biannually until they were six years old. A parallel study has been initiated with developmentally disabled infants and children to compare their development of prehension with that of normal children.

The data from the first year of the normal infants challenge Halverson's basic concepts. He suggested that a small number of prehensile responses can be observed, labeled, and linked to a specific age. He advocated the use of non-descriptive terms such as hand, inferior forefinger, and superior forefinger grasp. An analysis of my data revealed that the infants were consistent in the specific grasp used with a given object only 25% of the time. Yet the infants clearly demonstrated a developmental sequence in the evolution of prehension within the time frame 4-12 months. The sequence identified in this cinematographic research was:

1. uses the whole hand in an unspecialized manner;
2. uses parts of the hand—beginning to develop specialization;
3. uses pads of the distal phalanges (tips of the fingers) in a specialized manner.

These data were presented at the AOTA Conference in Milwaukee and are on videotape available for loan.

Developmental Disabilities
Special Interest Section Newsletter; Vol. 1, No. 2, 1978

Occupational Therapists in Action: Peggy Smith

Peggy (Margaret M. Smith) is the pediatric occupational therapist at The New York Hospital in New York, NY. She is also an assistant instructor and member of the Board of Directors of the Neurodevelopmental Treatment Association. The pediatric program at NY Hospital services both in-patients, including the neonatal intensive care unit, and out-patients, the majority of which are infants with neuro-motor and/or sensory-integrative deficits.

In the developmental process, we are what we do, before we are what we say, before we are what we write. Before the age of eighteen months and the development of complex verbal language, the child's ability to react and to exert influence of the environment is measured primarily through his level of mobility and manipulation. Dur-

ing this time, analysis of motor behavior is the best method of evaluating the developmental process: assessing both how the infant responds to and operates on the environment.

When doing an assessment, many factors have to be taken into consideration. Gestational age and medical history can cause considerable variability in early development. An infant's behavior at any one time can be markedly altered by physical needs and environment, e.g. the assessment of oral-motor reflexes and responses can be completely different in the same pre- and post-feeding infant.

Their motor behavior is the end product of many different systems of integration, e.g. some babies with suspected primary neuromotor deficit in the clinic evaluation at NY Hospital were ultimately labeled sensory

integrative deficit following diagnostic therapy, when it became evident that the movement responses were secondary to problems organizing tactual and vestibular information.

At last, schedules of development are beginning to be replaced by process and quality oriented assessments, although sensitive and standardized tools remain to be developed. As the evaluation and treatment focus moves away from milestone achievement and toward quality of performance, the therapist is forced to better understand the normal developmental process. For this author, the research done by Lois Bly, RPT, which analyzes the components of normal movement and the process of motor development, has been invaluable to her understanding of neuromotor development,

(continued)

Occupational Therapists: Peggy Smith

both normal and abnormal. This information is currently incorporated into the teaching of normal development within the Neurodevelopmental Treatment (NDT) courses, and Lois is planning to publish this material in the near future.

The infants who require the specialized medical treatment of the neonatal intensive care unit at NY Hospital make up a population at high risk for developmental disability. Early detection of disability within the nursery and perinatal followup clinic can facilitate early intervention, particularly with infants with neuromotor deficit.

From the total population of this author's ICU, there were originally four groups of babies requested for referral. The requisite conditions were the following: 1. abnormal tone or posture, i.e. inappropriately hypo- or hypertonic infants. 2. sensory deficits, e.g. infants with visual and hearing impairments, peripheral nerve injuries, brachial plexus injuries, etc. 3. feeding problems, i.e. babies who have difficulty nippling when age and/or medically appropriate. 4. congenital abnormalities, e.g. cleft lips and palates, meningomyeloceles, congenital amputees, etc. Interestingly, the medical and nursing staff have initiated referrals on two other

groups—the "behavior" problems, i.e. too lethargic or hyper-irritable babies and the "chronic" babies, i.e. meaning all babies with a hospital stay exceeding four weeks.

Babies on the unit are seen on an almost daily basis with nursing and parental carryover as appropriate. The therapeutic milieu frequently serves to ventilate the parents' concerns about their child's developmental prognosis which are usually surpressed by the focus on day to day medical and surgical conditions.

After discharge, the infants are followed at the perinatal clinic at one month and then subsequent (usually three months) intervals as necessary. At these visits each infant receives an evaluation of neuromotor development, basic sensory-motor responses, feeding behavior and home adjustment.

Of the babies requiring intervention, the largest group are those with neuromotor deficit. The average age for initiation of therapy is between three to six months when abnormal tone and movement patterns become evident to the trained observer, although most children are not labeled with diagnoses until the end of the first year.

Treatment focuses on the following:
—normalization of muscle tone and de-

velopment of mobility.
—facilitation of the automatic movement responses of righting responses, protective extension and equilibrium reactions.
—development of graded control with the automatic movements through appropriate activities.
—development of voluntary movement and of the age-appropriate skills of feeding, manipulation, etc.
—parent/caretaker support and training, through demonstration and practice, of appropriate handling.

The program, as it now exists, is serviced by approximately three positions: one and one-half physical therapists and one and one-half occupational therapists. Each is highly skilled in the assessment and treatment of the infant; there is significant role-blurring between the two professions. Although there is generally only one therapist involved with each parent and child, there are frequent case reviews to redefine the child's needs and problem-solving sessions to integrate each profession's expertise in formulating the treatment plans. Videotaping has been particularly helpful in accomplishing these reviews and as a visual record in documenting change.

Developmental Disabilities
Special Interest Section Newsletter; Vol. 1, No. 2, 1978

A Developmental Approach to Home Activities for Infants

By Ellen Tessler, M.S. Ed., OTR

Along with the early identification of at risk infants, there is also increasing awareness of the effectiveness of timely intervention. With knowledge of normal development and sensitivity to the mother-infant relationship, the occupational therapist can play a significant role in early intervention.

While more and more very young infants are being referred to center-based stimulation programs, the primary responsibility for care remains in the home.

The infant is born with capabilities in both sensory and motor modalities. By helping the primary caregiver recognize the kinds of stimulation that an infant seeks and the kinds of responses elicited, therapy can have maximum impact on the developing infant.

An example of a developmental approach for the first twelve months follows. By roughly identifying stages on the basis of motor development parents can be given concrete suggestions to stimulate their child at its level of development.

Stage I.

Main features: Gaining oculomotor con-

trol. Vision and hearing become functionally related. Gets hand or object to mouth. Grasps with hand and object in view. Hand watching.

Materials to use: Visually interesting objects. Mobiles. Patterns with contrast between light and dark. Objects to follow with eyes (yarn, flashlight, rattles, etc.).

Stage II.

Main features: Gaining more head and upper trunk control and increasing arm and hand use. Mouthing objects. Swiping with fisted hands. Grasps with just toy in view. Visually directed reaching. Clutching.

Materials to use: Objects that can be acted upon. Mobiles to hit. Hanging toys. Chime balls. Squeaky toys. Rattles. Textured toys. Mirrors. Sponges for water play.

Stage III.

Main features: Increasing trunk and finger control. Can sit and creep. Transfers objects. Drops object to reach for another. Good aim when reaching. Thumb opposition. Finger feeds. Releases object on surface. Pat-a-cake. Hits objects together.

Materials to use: Items for reaching, banging, exploring. Cause and effect games and toys (switches, jack-in-box, pull strings that make something happen, music box). Textures to explore. Box full of small, safe objects (clothespins, plastic lids, spools, silverware). Measuring cups. Blocks.

Stage IV.

Main features: Greater mobility; ready for standing and walking with support. Does things with intention. Throws toys. Deliberate release. Searches for hidden objects. Putting things together.

Materials to use: Objects and games to encourage movement and planning. Balls. Blocks. Pop-beads. Water and sand toys. Old magazines to tear. Containers to fill and empty. Stacking and nesting toys. Things to take apart.

Often, just some general guidelines like these are enough to add interest and spontaniety for the parent while she follows through with positioning and handling instructions given by the therapist.

Developmental Disabilities
Special Interest Section Newsletter; Vol. 1, No. 1, 1978

Occupational Therapists in Action: Joyce Flora

It has become increasingly obvious that an absence or interruption in the visual system has an overwhelming effect on development. Attempts to substitute or augment that system with other types of sensory stimulation prove extremely difficult and, in this writer's opinion, fall short of the input provided by vision. There is an obvious difference between those students with congenital visual losses as opposed to losses occuring after the developmental process was well on its way to maturation. Mannerisms seem to be much more frequent in the congenitally blind child and include a variety of rocking, finger flicking and eye poking behaviors. There is a strong suspicion (by this therapist and Antje Price, consultant to the program) that many of these mannerisms are "sensory behaviors", directly related to vestibular and tactile processing problems. (Several students have demonstrated decreased frequency and intensity of rocking after SI treatment).

Evaluations of the developmental level of students is an ongoing process. The SI clinical observations are used, where applicable the PRN test is administered, and some adopted versions of the SSCIT have been presented to the "testable" students. A. Price designed a form board for the MFP Test which has been interesting to use; and the Kinesthesia Test is sometimes adopted with tactile locations at the reference point. Frequent observations of the children in various settings (class, dorms, play, art, gym) and the test data, including developmental sequencing, forms the base from which therapy is planned and implemented.

It's difficult to identify any "most significant" problem seen in therapy. However, these clinical situations have interested this therapist during the past two academic years:

—High incidence of tactile deficits; a permanent problem for the hypo and hyper-responsive children, whose entire world is based on tactile input. Braille requires fine discrimination, and bilateral coordination, working in a totally cooperative effort. Many of the children have difficulty with crossing midline and dealing with their hands functioning in different ways at the same time, perhaps because so many of their pre-academic and academic activities are done bilaterally.

—Very abbreviated, or absent, periods of crawling and quadrupedal play. This is particularly interesting in relationship to the high numbers of hypotonic youngsters. Like other handicapped children, the blind seem to be "put into" situations rather than using their motor resources to get from place to place, activity to activity.

—Without the visual motivator, stimulation for play is limited, object relationships suffer, concepts and perceptual development appear diminished. If there is damage severe enough to cause visual loss, often other sensory systems are also affected and thus inadequate, inconsistent sensory feedback is provided.

—Postural insecurity seems to be a permanent problem for many of the students; it is manifested at both ends of the spectrum: the "no stops" kind of child, the child fearful of any movement in space. To work through the postural insecurity, it has become apparent that there is a great need for a consistent trusting relationship between student and therapist. Their need for a supportive atmosphere is extremely high. It is with great hesitation that many of these children surrender their secure upright orientation to space.

—Many of the children at the school are masters in the art of verbal avoidance. They seem to use their best skill (talking) to avoid activity and/or explorative play. Especially with the young child, this lack of appropriate play seems to be related to ADL skills that are below age expectancy. Of course none of these relationships can be even remotely considered exclusively. The numerous and sometimes prolonged hospitalization these, and most multiply handicapped kids experience, strongly influence the sensory-motor/psychosocial development. Common to all of these children, regardless of the primary diagnosis, is the absence of that visual component which makes working through the problems much more difficult. They do not have the visual reference . . . a "check-up" system that gives perspective and security to "who I am" and how my world is put together.

For the past two years OT intervention has primarily been 1:1 treatment. Group has been attempted, but really requires a lot of additional hands to keep the activities moving smoothly. There is a need for more intervention in the classroom, with the child care workers who are responsible for a lot of the "free time" activities. There is also a need for additional input with regard to feeding programs — oral and hand/mouth skills — many oral apraxias and defensive behaviors have been observed. For the "upper school" students there is an activity of daily living class — which emphasizes acquisition of self care skills. The relationship between the ADL instructors and OT has been beneficial, the role of OT being via "underlying preventative" treatment: awareness of body parts, relationships and bilateral integration (as opposed to teaching actual ADL skills).

Thus far involvement with parents has

been minimal due to scheduling the volume of students seen. There is a definite need for early intervention and rapport with the parents of these extremely complex children. As ICP's continue to stimulate more parental involvement it is hoped that there will be the opportunity to further define the OT services provided to students and these families.

On the whole there has been only one group of students that have proved to be *totally* frustrating to this therapist: several adolescent deaf-blind boys. Their responses to an SI approach have indicated more disorganization than organization; for the most part they are receiving a lot of pre-voc activities and are functioning in very structured, closely supervised situations. Their movement quality is not refined; some display primitive reflex activity, many are rigid, and some are toe-walkers. Teachers see OT as *surely* being able to intervine . . . the OT is questioning the value of trying to interrupt a repertiore of activity that enables them to function. A very supportive atmosphere has made implementing OT at WPSBC a very positive experience. The students are amazingly complex and treatment, as in any OT department, is based on the individual assets and liabilities of the student. The approaches vary — SI seeming to emerge as a principle method, with very encouraging responses.

The formation of a Motor Development Team which meets twice monthly, enables the staff to communicate about many of the sensory motor and education components of the children's individual programs. The emphasis is toward a more concentrated "team approach" to the management of these children. The school is looking forward to continued growth and specialized programming as more multiply handicapped, visually impaired children are identified as needing early intervention and treatment.

Joyce is the occupational therapist at the Western Pennsylvania School for Blind Children in Pittsburgh, PA. This school provides comprehensive education programs for legally blind children on both a residential and day student basis. The children often have more than a visual handicap; they may also be mentally retarded, physically handicapped, brain damaged, learning disabled, emotionally disturbed, and/or speech and language impaired.

Joyce has offered to be a central resource person for DDSS on the blind child. Please send her both questions and information that you are willing to share. Send them to: Joyce Flora, Western Pennsylvania School for Blind Children, 201 North Bellfield, Pittsburgh, PA.

Developmental Disabilities
Special Interest Section Newsletter; Vol. 1, No. 1, 1978

Development of the Congenitally Blind Child

There has been increasing awareness of the role sight plays in stimulating normal motor and emotional development. The external stimulation provided by vision is thought to be the motivational factor causing the developing infant to reach out and to move from one position to another. Because of this, it is not uncommon for the blind child to skip, or be delayed in, some of the normal developmental milestones. Therefore, some of the basic building blocks for later cognitive-sensory-motor functioning are often missing.

In addition to mobility, the unsighted child is delayed in exploratory activity. Sound may be used as an initiating stimulus for exploration, but not until approximately 10 months of age (the sighted child usually begins swiping at objects at 3 months of age). The significance of this is obvious when it is noted that without intervention, until the blind child learns to reach on sound cue, s/he does little reaching out and self initiated exploratory movement.

The blind child usually develops postural stability (i.e. head and trunk control) within normal ranges of development, but is delayed in the mobility aspects. This results in the blind child going through development in a series of plateaus. During these plateaus, in which "nothing seems to be happening", and the child does not seem to be making any gains, the child is at *serious* developmental risk, both physically and emotionally. Some of the typical periods of plateau are:

● When placed prone, the child is unlikely to bring arms forward or raise head until after 5 months of age.

● Once child progresses to sitting unsupported s/he often remains in that position, not moving in and out of positions to prone, supine and stand, and back to sitting.

● Creeping is tremendously delayed and often skipped altogether.

● Once child learns to take steps with hands held, the next step, taking steps independently, is quite delayed.

When examining the developmental progression of the blind child, one must also consider that the blind child must give up a major portion of his/her physical contact with the tangible world every time s/he takes a developmental step. This makes moving from lying, to sitting, to stance, a much more threatening experience for the blind child because s/he receives much information about the surroundings from physical contact.

These early developmental deviations affect all aspects of the child's cognitive-sensory-motor and emotional development. The development of body image and self concept, which is greatly enhanced by vision in the sighted child, is also significantly delayed. It is obvious that intervention with the blind child is needed as soon as blindness is suspected or diagnosed. These children need an environment rich in auditory, tactile and movement experiences to minimize their developmental deficits.

Developmental Tendencies With The Congenitally Blind Child

I. *Gross Motor Development*

A. Milestones usually occurring at 'normal' age in blind child:
   sits alone momentarily,
   rolls from supine to prone,
   sits alone steadily,
   takes stepping movements when hands are held,
   stands alone.

B. Milestones usually delayed in the blind child:
   elevating self by arms in prone,
   raising self to sitting,
   pulling to stand (on furniture),
   walking alone across room.

II. *Social-Emotional or Behavioral Differences Between Blind and Sighted Child*

A. Spontaneous movement (child often very passive):
   0-4 mo. — if turns head side to side, usually keep centered,
   4-8 mo. — does not explore or reach out for toy nearby.

B. Self-concept:
   object permanence difficult to establish, differentiating self from environment harder.

C. Peer relationships:
   parallel play difficult without vision, difficulty initiating contact and in knowing when is accepted.

D. Social Behavior:
   difficult learning appropriate and acceptable behavior.

Developmental Disabilities
Special Interest Section Newsletter; Vol. 3, No. 3, 1980

Test/Book Review: A Prescriptive Behavioral Checklist for the Severely and Profoundly Retarded

This book was written by Dorothy Popovitch, MA, an instructor in the Department of Educational Psychology at West Virginia University. It was published in 1979 by the University Park Press of Baltimore, MD. The volume (431 pages) presents a series of checklists that are meant to be diagnostic tools as well as prescriptive curriculum guides for planning an operant conditioning educational/therapy program.

The checklist include the following:

Motor Development
   Head and Trunk Control — 5 items
   Sitting — 4 items
   Hand-Knee Position — 4 items
   Standing — 6 items
Eye-Hand Coordination — 51 items
Language Development
   Attending — 6 items
   Physical Imitation — 6 items
   Auditory Training — 11 items
   Object Discrimination — 16 items

Concept Development — 12 items
Sound Imitation — 9 items
Physical Eating Problems — 7 items

The items on the checklists are not given an age level but are organized in a developmental sequence.

Each item in the checklist is worded as a behavioral objective with a specifically defined criteria. The instrument lends itself well to use in a setting where the therapist is responsible, with the educational or residen-

(continued)

Test/Book Review: Behavioral Checklist

tial staff, for writing instructional objectives for the developmentally disabled client's IEP or rehabilitation plan. The objectives are in turn broken down by task analysis into small "teaching steps" with implementation explanations. A conditioning approach is taken for instructing and charting these steps. The author has taken an approach of avoiding the use of technical language and jargon, thus attempting to make the task analysis steps easily used by parents and aides. This would seem to make the behavioral checklist particularly useful to occupational therapists in situations where, due to job description or large numbers of clients, they are acting primarily as consultants rather than as direct service providers.

The concepts of behavioral objectives ("object is behavioral only if it describes an observable act") and task analysis ("sequenced so that easy steps occur before more difficult ones") are explained briefly but in an easily understood manner in Chapter 7 of the text. All of the narrative chapters of the book are presented in a self-instruction format with questions to be answered and case studies to be solved at the end of each chapter. The answers are provided at the back of the book. This would seem to make it useful to the OT who, because of locality or other obligation, is unable to attend continuing education on the subject matter. The self-instruction format also lends itself well to instruction of aides and/or parents.

Unfortunately, the author did not specifically mention occupational therapy or occupational therapists in the book. A physical therapist was mentioned as assisting in the development of the motor coordination checklist. Also, a cautionary note is included prior to the motor development checklist and the physical eating problems checklist to "seek out the approval of your physical therapist before beginning these activities." Although I would have much preferred the wording "your physical therapist and/or occupational therapist," the caution to seek out therapy input is well taken as the material is aimed at the severely and profoundly mentally retarded and no mention is made of any additionally handicapping conditions.

It is my feeling that individuals with additional difficulties such as cerebral palsy could possibly benefit from parts of the checklist, but the program would of necessity have to be modified and individualized with the assistance of a therapist. There are particular parts of the physical eating problems task analysis steps and implementation methods involving icing, brushing, and physical intrusion into the oral area that in my opinion should be carefully monitored by an OT or perhaps a speech therapist skilled in this area.

The author tested the checklist in a day care center in Mt. Clemens, MI, and in a community program in West Virginia, and stated "31 samples of inter-rater reliability on the checklist"—on the eye hand coordination checklist attaining a rate of 99%, and on the various sub-areas of the language development checklist attaining rates of from 90%-98%, depending on the specific sub-area involved. Reliability checks were not taken on the motor development and physical eating problems checklists since they were trained through the physical therapy department.

The text chapters cover many areas. Among them:

1. The definition of operant psychology
2. The instructional cycle of behavioral objective to: stimulus, to: response, to: reinforcer
3. Methods of assessment and rating including timing and materials
4. Training methods
   a. Determining the operant level or the last step in the task analysis that the student can initially perform
   b. Establishing reinforcement preference
   c. Bridging or going from response to reinforcement
   d. Schedules of reinforcement
   e. Use of three types of prompts (physical, gestural, and verbal) and fading of prompts
   f. Advice on aide and parent training methods including role playing
5. Data collection—specific data collection sheets provided with detailed instruction for filling out at each training session including type of prompt, reinforcer, and number of correct responses.

On the whole, this text material is written in a very readable fashion and could be very useful to the OT not well acquainted with operant techniques. With the present demand for specific objectives evidenced today in many therapy settings and the need for measurable results of intervention the use of the checklists and data collection sheets may be a valuable aid to the occupational therapist.—*Betty Scanlan, MA, OTR*

Developmental Disabilities
Special Interest Section Newsletter; Vol. 2, No. 4, 1979

Test Review: 50-Hole Beaded Pegboard Test

By Edith DeEtte Huffman. M.Ed, OTR

I. Reference Data
   Title: 50-Hole Beaded Pegboard Test
   Age Range: Adults
   Equipment: 1 ID 3681 wood pegboard 6"x6"
   1 ID 3690 box (1000) plastic beaded pegs
   Stopwatch
   Source: Pegboard and pegs from:
   The Formative Years Inc.
   Box 130-1 R.R.3
   Westbrook, CT 06498
   (203) 399-7928
   Stopwatch: Meyland Stopwatch Co.
   264 West 40th St.
   New York, NY 10018

II. Description
   This test measures hand dexterity in terms of the time it takes a subject to put fifty pegs in a board. Fifty 7/8 inch pegs are inserted into each side, 3x6 inches, of pegboard. It measures other factors such as concentration, endurance, ability to follow directions, vision and concept of speed. A 100-hole pegboard is divided vertically through the center by a black magic marker or tape to separate it into halves. The pegs are placed in the box which is positioned on the same side as the hand being tested. The subject fills in the right half of the board with the right hand, and the left side with the left hand. Each side is timed separately. This test includes placement of pegs only, not removal.

III. Standardization
   A. Standardization Sample: $n = 100$
      Subjects were mild to severely mentally retarded residents of several Intermediate Care Facilities in the age range of 18-69 years with 41.6 median age.
   B. Reliability: $n = 10$
      Test-Retest Spearman's rank-difference Rho correlation reliability coefficient:
      Right = .82   Left = .71
      (continued)

Test Review: Pegboard Test

C. Validity:

The 40% of the subjects who scored above the mean for the right and 45% of subjects who scored above the mean for the left hand were considered by the staff of these facilities as having greater potential for intensive programming and the eventual goal of placement in a sheltered workshop. It was found that scores on this test were good predictors of potential for simple vocational tasks and participation in craft programs.

D. Statistical Data
1. Right Hand

Number	100
Median	305 seconds
Mean	344.36 seconds
Standard Deviation	166.17 seconds
Range	130-997 seconds

2. Left Hand

Number	100
Median	353 seconds
Mean	375.72 seconds
Standard Deviation	189.25 seconds
Range	131-1415 seconds

Score = Number of Seconds

IV. Discussion

This test is a quick way to discover many important aspects of a mentally retarded adult's functional ability. The test must be administered in a quiet room where there are no distractions and it must be carefully demonstrated to the subject prior to administration of actual test. The individual should be retested at regular intervals as a measure of improvement of hand coordination, speed and attention span.

Norms are available by sending 30¢ and a self-addressed stamped envelope to: Edith DeEtte Huffman, M.Ed, OTR, 339 North Rutan St., Wichita, KS 67208

Developmental Disabilities
Special Interest Section Newsletter; Vol. 2, No. 1, 1979

Test Review: Denver Developmental Screening Test

I. Reference Data:

Title: Denver Developmental Screening Test

Authors: Wm. Traukenburg, M.D. & J. Dodds, PhD.

Publisher: University of Colorado Medical School

Age Range: 2 weeks — 6 years

Purpose: early detection of delayed development

II. Description:

105 items were selected from 12 existing developmental and preschool tests which could generally be categorized into 4 areas of functioning: gross-motor; fine-motor adaptive; language; personal-social.

The test form indicates in graph form at which ages items were passed by 25%, 50%, 75% and 90% of the standardization sample. Over-all results are then categorized as Normal, Questionable, or Abnormal according to established criteria. The test is not designed to give separate scores in each category.

III. Standardization:

a. Standardization sample: n=1036 children between ages of 2 wks and 6.4 years; children with high risk of developmental abnormality were excluded.

b. Reliability: n=186. Test-retest agreement +97%. Sample reflected racial, ethnic, and occupational groups of Denver, CO.

c. *Validity: (Criterion-related) Correlation with other tests.

Bayley
  n=96 (mean age 19 mos.)   r=.81
Stanford-Binnet
  n=156 (mean age 54 mos.)   r=.74

* This represents data from revised edition to the best of our ability to glean from the literature. Reports are confusing and information difficult to obtain.

Discussion

This discussion will focus primarily on some of the cautions and limitations of DDST usage. The authors caution against using the DDST as a *diagnostic* devise: it is intended only to alert the examiner to a developmental problem which needs further examination.

One important factor which can influence a child's performance on the test is inherent in the test's standardization which was based on the population of Denver, and the sample reflects a significantly higher proportion of children from professional families. The examiner must therefore, use caution in interpreting scores—particularly language scores—of children from other economic and social backgrounds.

Another limitation is the test's reliance on the mother's report for scoring many of the items. This can potentially increase or decrease reliability of results; i.e. they may be more accurate because mother's report is based on observation of the child over time or less accurate if she is not a good observer or doesn't report areas of difficulty.

Performance on the DDST can be significantly affected by factors such as the child's motivation, fatigue, anxiety due to strange surroundings and unfamiliar examiner, dependency/hostility in mother-child relationship, etc. Because of this variability and because the DDST, over-all tends to over-select children as *questionable* or *abnormal* (as much as 42%) we recommend screening be repeated before referring children for further evaluation. The potentially high over-selection rate is further strong support for not using the DDST to diagnose abnormality.

Developmental Disabilities
Special Interest Section Newsletter; Vol. 1, No. 2, 1978

Test Review: Developmental Programming for Infants and Young Children

This three-volume set includes Volume 1, *Assessment and Application,* a manual which describes *Profile* administration and program development; Volume 2, *Early Intervention Developmental Profile,* an assessment instrument for children from birth to 36 months; and Volume 3, *Stimulation Activities,* a collection of sequenced activities geared to *Profile* items.

The set was compiled by staff members of the Early Intervention Project for Handicapped Infants and Young Children which operated from 1973 to 1976 at the Institute for the Study of Mental Retardation and Related Disabilities, University of Michigan, Ann Arbor, MI, and served as a basis for the project's curriculum. The materials were published by the University of Michigan Press after completion of the project and are now available from this publisher.

The *Profile* contains six developmental sequences which normally emerge between birth and 36 months of age. Major milestones in the areas of language, gross motor, fine motor, social/emotional, self-care, and cognitive development are presented in three-month intervals which reflect normal developmental patterns attained in the first three years of life. The gross motor scale and the feeding section of the self-care scale reflect a body of knowledge which constitutes the basis for the current treatment of cerebral palsy in infants and young children emphasizing neurodevelopmental theories and reflexive development. The cognition scale provides landmarks in the development of sensorimotor intelligence described by Piaget and focuses specifically on the acquisition of the concepts of object permanence, causal relationships, spatial relationships, and imitation during the first two years of life. The social/emotional scale reflects current theory on the emotional attachment between the mother and child and child's gradual acquisition of ego functions during the first 36 months of life.

The *Profile* is not a standardized instrument; it has not been validated on normal children. Therefore, it is intended to be used to supplement to, not replace, formalized evaluations. The age range and selection of items used in the *Profile* are based on the developmental norms standardized or described by various researchers in the field of child development as referenced in the bibliography. The *Profile* can be administered in forty-five minutes or less by an interdisciplinary team with combined expertise in the areas of physical and/or occupational therapy, speech and language pathology, and psychology and/or special education. Each section of the *Profile* requires disciplinary knowledge and skills on the part of the evaluators, skills that one member of the team can ultimately teach to other members of the team. Thus, each member can learn to administer the entire *Profile* by using other team members and the manual as resources.

The *Profile* provides a structured approach to therapeutic programming for children whose developmental levels are between 0 and 36 months. It can help the evaluator to determine the child's present skill levels, as well as his relative strengths and weaknesses in each of the six areas, and to project which skills will emerge next. This information is then used to develop objectives to focus on the skills which are projected to appear next in the child's repertoire. Play activities are selected for each objective as the mode for stimulating and supporting emerging skills. Thus, the *Profile* helps professionals choose objectives and activities which are developmentally appropriate for each child's functional level and developmental patterns and rate. Each *Profile* can be used four times to allow the evaluators and parents to see the child's progress from one evaluation to the next. The final page of the *Profile* provides a chart on which to graph the child's developmental skills in the six areas evaluated.

Stimulation Activities contains instructions for developing objectives for individual children and activities for meeting the objectives.

Volume 1, *Assessment and Application,* describes validation studies of the *Profile* with handicapped children during operation of the project. Possibilities for standardizing the *Profile* on a population of normal children are now being explored. — *Martha S. Moersch, M.Ed., OTR, FAOTA.*

*This three-volume set is available from The University of Michigan Press, Ann Arbor, MI (1977), $15.00.

Developmental Disabilities
Special Interest Section Newsletter; Vol. 1, No. 1, 1978

Test Review: Motor-Free Visual Perception Test

I. Reference Data
    Title: Motor-Free Visual Perception Test
    Authors: Ronald P. Codarusso, EdD., Donald D. Hammill, EdD.
    Publisher: Academic Therapy Publications, 1539 Foruth St., San Rafael, CA 94901
    Date: 1976, 1974, 1972
    Cost: manual $4.50 Kit:
    Test administration time:
    Age designed for: 4-0 to 8-11

II. Description:
    Based on research, five categories of visual perception were selected which the authors feel are the most prominent theoretical constructs of visual perception.

    They are: spatial relationships, figure — ground, visual discrimination, visual — closure, visual — memory.

    There are a total of 36 non-motor visual perceptual tasks required of the child.

    The standardization population was 881 *unselected* normal children aged 4-8 in 22 states.

(continued)

Test Review: Perception Test

III. Reliability

Type	No. tested each age group	Total tested	Reliability Coefficients	Overall reliability coefficient
Test-Retest	20-45	162	.77-.83	.81
Split Half	53-332	881	.81	
Kuder-Richardson	53-332	881	.71-.82	.86

—Statistically significant at .01 level —

IV. Validity

Content: Description in manual brief but consistent with what they claim to measure

Construct:

A. Age differentiation N40 — significant at .01 level

B. Correlation with other tests:

visual	Frostig .38—.60 overall	.73
	Metropolitan Readiness	.31—.40
	Durrell Analysis	.46
non-visual	Metropolitan Readiness	.05—.50
	Stanford Achievement	.03—.42
	Durrell Analysis	.33—.46
	Slossen Intelligence	.31

This seems to back up authors claims that it measures primarily non-motor visual tasks; therapists will note the highest correlations are with Frostig form constancy, spatial relationships, and eye-motor coordination. No comparisons with Ayres tests are available. Validity appears to have been done, as convenience permitted, i.e. scores already available, rather than designed to find out specifics about this test.

Discussion:

The MVPT merits some consideration by those therapists in need of a motor-free visual perceptual test. Though the standardization sample was unselected, the N was adequate. Reliability correlations are good, higher than any other motor free visual perceptual test, and comparing favorably with the Berry VM1, Frostig and WISC. (Approx. same reliability as Ayres DC, somewhat better than SV and PS).

Validity information is less impressive. Description of content validity is scanty. Age differentiation is fair, only based on N of 40. MUPT correlates more highly with visual-motor tests than school readiness or intelligence tests, a good sign it is measuring what it proports to measure. **Only** one article comparing use of MVPT with a visual motor test with (the Gestalt test) motor impaired children is available (Newcomer, P., and Hammill D. "Visual Perception of Motor Imparied Children: Implications for Assessment" Exceptional Children 39 (1973) 335-336) *No predictive validity is noted.* Interpretations are thus limited to observable, scorable behavior.

It is too new (1972) to have been reviewed by Buros. Some clinicians report it to be a useful tool with developmentally delayed adults, and in determining existance and severity in stroke patients (no age norms though).

The other excellent features are the large number of visual-perceptual areas tested, though the number of items in each category is small, and the fact that the test is designed to be given in isolation. Therapist does not have to worry about pulling out only a couple of subtests from a whole battery and thus possibly distorting standardization.

2

Gerontology
Special Interest Section

Gerontology
Special Interest Section Newsletter; Vol. 6, No. 2, 1983

Assessing Self-Care Status

By Teepa Snow, MS, OTR

As therapists we are all aware that it is important for all care-givers to be knowledgeable concerning the older person's self-care status. The ability to perform tasks independently means a great deal in terms of level of care determinations, use of restraints, staff time, amount of supervision, the family's ability to provide home care, and the person's ability to participate in leisure and social activities.

There are at least three subskills associated with self-care abilities. These are cognitive skills, physical abilities, and temporal awareness. To perform self-care tasks independently, the cognitive skills of clients must be such that they can initiate, participate in, and conclude the task in a properly sequenced fashion. The physical demands vary greatly for each activity, but all tasks comprise fine motor, gross-motor, balance, perceptual and sensory skills that must be mastered to successfully complete the task. The older person must also be able to use "time" information appropriately. The clients' perception of time must be consistent with those of others in the environment so that they can accurately follow the established routine.

Unfortunately, these three subskills are difficult to assess independently, since the "whole seems to be greater than the sum of the parts," or at least different! We have all seen people who are able to get up, get dressed, and fix breakfast in their own home, but are unable to even find their underwear in the nursing home. By far, the most "realistic" assessment would be to arrive at clients' residences as they wake and observe their behavior throughout the day. At the same time one must realize that this only allows the therapist to identify what clients DO, not necessarily what they CAN do. This scenario is also "unrealistic" in terms of therapist time and resources. The next best thing would seem to be to combine client and care-giver reports and sampled activities. The activities selected should reflect areas of difficulty as well as areas of skill. One method for evaluating self-care status is simulation. In this fashion one can choose tasks and have necessary props on hand prior to the assessment.

There are a multitude of "ADL Scales" described in the literature. Testing and scoring performances vary among the tests, but tend to fall into four major groupings. These are:

1. Timed performances — tasks are scored on the basis of time taken to complete the activity.

2. Level of independence — tasks are scored on the basis of independence in completion. A diversity of categories can be used to rate independence (dependent, semi-dependent, independent versus full assist, partial assist, physical prompts, verbal prompts, independent).

3. Subskills independence — tasks are broken down into parts of performance and then based on levels of independence as stated above (for example: putting an arm through a sleeve hole).

4. Time performances and level of independence — tasks are scored both by ability to perform independently and by the length of time taken (staff and client) to complete the task.

The fourth group of ADL Scales offers promise for therapists who want to use the screening evaluation as a baseline measure and as a yardstick for changes over time during intervention. The ability of the assessment data to reflect both losses or gains in independence and changes in requirements of staff/care-giver time is useful for many reasons. One can use the results to justify additional treatment time or to document further needs for services, as well as to indicate to all the abilities of the client. Administrators, nurses, physicians, caregivers, third party reimbursers, and the client can all benefit from this information in different ways.

The tasks chosen should be somewhat client-population specific. Clients in nursing homes may require different testing items than community-based elderly. There are many tools which have already been selected out as tasks for different settings. In all cases, the tools need to be tested in different settings to determine whether the tasks are representative of the client's abilities or whether the tasks need to be modified to better identify strengths and inabilities. Items commonly used are: transferring, toileting, eating, walking/wheelchair mobility, dressing, communication, bathing, and telephoning.

One strategy for assessment is to select subtasks from these headings. Activities such as drinking from a cup and cutting meat might be used for eating tasks. Another strategy is to observe the activity as it is usually performed and rate it in context. In either case it is important to remember that in screening the goal is not to test everything, but to choose some tasks that may reflect performance skills. The performance test should be standardized and made as realistic as possible to ensure that progress during treatment is being measured and so that any new learning that occurs can be applied to the real-life situation. The screening should not be used in isolation when developing an intervention strategy. It can however, serve as a starting point.

The screening process can also be used to identify the at risk elderly. The early identification of this population would enable the care-givers to help develop a "safety net" to have services ready to come into play or to start a therapeutic program to prevent injuries, accidents, or episodes of acute illness resulting from neglect or inactivity. Additional support systems can then be activated before the situation becomes irreversible or critical.

In conclusion, because self-care status is so important to everyone working with an older person, there is a need for all involved to speak the same language and to have the same goals and plans for the client. A critical part of beginning to interact with other caregivers is to develop a common data base and to have common definitions for all items being used. A self-care screening assessment that is somewhat flexible, but identifies the client's abilities and the amount of help and time needed to perform selected tasks is a good starting point. These measures can be used to reflect changes in performance over time. Changes may

(continued)

Self-Care Status

be identified as resulting from activity programs, therapeutic interventions, care-giver training, increased socialization, or improved routinization of tasks. Much research is beginning to come to light regarding the effects of all of the above on older persons' abilities to care for themselves. YOUR use of an ADL Scale as a data collection tool can be the start of your research efforts as well as a simple way of charting a client's progress.

REFERENCES

Bruett, TL & Ouer, RP. "A Critical Review of 12 ADL Scales". *Physical Therapy* 49:8 857-61.

Potwin, AR et al. "Simulated Activities of Daily Living Examination". *Archives of Physical Medicine and Rehabilitation*. Oct. 1972, 476-498.

Gerontology
Special Interest Section Newsletter; Vol. 6, No. 1, 1983

Assessing Mental Status

By Teepa Snow, MS, OTR

Why Assess Mental Status?
Mental incompetence and changes in mental status are frequently the major deciding factors in the institutionalization of the elderly. Problems are identified in the areas of safety and independence when one's cognitive processes are impaired. Family members, and older persons themselves, commonly have difficulty in identifying changes without prompting. The picture presented is often confusing regarding the kinds of changes that have occurred and the time frame for their occurrence. I have found that the simple evaluation that looks at orientation to person, place and time does not adequately identify degrees of memory loss, types of cognitive deficits, and perceptual or sensory changes that effect the population I work with.

As therapists, there is a need to assess the mental status of the elderly in a gross, quick, yet accurate fashion to ensure an effective and appropriate treatment program. The older person's ability to follow verbal and manual instructions, the ability to make safe and independent judgments and decisions, concentration abilities and attention span, emotional stability and variability, ability to recall information from the immediate environment, the recent past, and the distant past, as well as the ability to serve as a reliable informant are important variables in determining a treatment plan and setting goals with the client.

Factors that effect the performance and quality of mental activities include:
- *brain dysfunction*—due to traumatic injury or a chronic, progressive disease process, such as head injury, cerebral vascular accident, Alzheimer's disease, or Parkinson's disease;
- *psychiatric illnesses*—such as depression, schizophrenia or paranoia;

Teepa Snow, MS, OTR, works for the Program on Aging, School of Medicine, University of North Carolina at Chapel Hill.

- *sensory dysfunctions*—such as presbyopia, cataracts, macular degeneration, presbycusis or impaired depth perception;
- *environmentally induced problems*—such as dehydration, malnutrition, drug overdoses or interactions, social isolation or sensory deprivations;
- *social expectations* by caregivers and family members regarding "old age stereotypes," senility, roles, alteration or continuation of life-long behavior patterns in different environments, or willingness to tolerate new learning with its positive and negative outcomes and side effects.

Baseline and subsequent measures of mental status are important for the identification of acute versus chronic conditions, reversible versus irreversible brain damage, and sudden versus gradual changes in function. Therapists should not underestimate their ability to have an impact on the older person's quality of life by helping to accurately recognize mental status changes (positive or negative) as they occur and report them to appropriate caregivers for the reassessment of the appropriate treatment measures.

How to Assess?
There are a variety of tools available to assess the mental status of older persons. Some of the more popular tests are: the "Mini-Mental State," by Pfeiffer, the "Screen for Organic Mental Syndromes," by Jacobs, an objective measure of mental status by Kahn and others, the "Set Test" developed by Issacs and Kinnie, and the FROMAJE by Libow. In my practice, I have found the FROMAJE, combined with the Set Test, to be of assistance in assessing the mental status of my older clients. I would like to take this opportunity to share these tools with you.

The FROMAJE comprises seven parts: function, reasoning, orientation, memory, arithmetic, judgment and emotional state. It follows a structured interview format and has proved to have an 80 to 90 percent

concordance with psychiatric diagnoses. The results of the evaluation are to serve as a guide and not as a diagnostic label concerning the mental functioning of the patient. The FROMAJE takes about 10 to 20 minutes to administer and, if necessary, can be completed in several sessions. Rapport with the client should be established before administering the assessment and a statement similar to the following should be made: "I am going to be asking you some questions now. Some will seem very simple and easy, while others may seem quite difficult. Answer them as best you can and we can talk about the ones you have difficulty with after we are finished."

Function
The first parameter to be tested is function. This refers to individuals' mental ability to maintain themselves in the community and in the home or to return to that setting. This score should include consideration of the person's ability to get meals, eat meals, behave in a socially acceptable fashion, dress appropriately and meet financial obligations. Information from family members, the client, caregivers and therapist observations should be used to rate this area.
Rating (points):
1=Mental function is adequate, no at-home support needed.
2=Due to mental impairment, some at-home support is needed at least part of the day or week.
3=Due to mental impairment, 24-hour at-home support is needed.

Reasoning
Ask the client to explain the meaning of a proverb or saying. If the client's education or cultural background does not reflect this skill, try to use other sayings that are appropriate. Samples are: "The early bird catches the worm," or "A stitch in time saves nine."

(continued)

Mental Status

Rating:

1=Good explanation of proverb; gave general connotations of proverb.

2=Some semblance of meaning given, but with some incompleteness, or was unable to generalize.

3=Completely unable to assign any meaning or a totally incorrect explanation.

Orientation

1. Time:

   a. "What day of the week is it?" (If necessary give choices.)

   b. "What month is it?" ("Is it June? July?") "What is the date?"

   c. "What year is it?"

2. Place: "Where are you now?" ("Is this your home? Your daughter's home? The doctor's office? A hospital, a nursing home?")

3. Self: "What is your name?"

Rating:

1=Generally accurate, minor mistakes in time, place or self.

2=Significant error in one area: time, place or self.

3=Significant errors in two or three areas: time, place or self.

Memory

1. Distant (change questions to match cultural or educational differences):

   a. "Who was the U.S. President during WW II who was in a wheelchair?"

   b. "What U.S. President was assassinated during the early 1960s?"

   c. "What year were you born? Where were you born?"

2. Recent (ask questions about function and happenings in the last 48 hours and questions for which you can obtain the correct answers):

   a. "What did you eat for breakfast?"

   b. "Where were you yesterday?"

3. Immediate:

   a. "What questions did I ask you about the U.S. Presidents?" (Change if above questions were different.)

   b. "Remember the numbers 4, 12 and 18. I will be asking you to repeat them in the next few minutes." (Minutes later.) "What numbers did I ask you to remember?"

Rating:

1=Generally accurate and made only minor errors in distant, recent or immediate memory.

2=Significant error in one area: distant, recent or immediate memory.

3=Significant error in two or three areas: distant, recent or immediate memory.

Arithmetic

1. "Count back from 100 to 90."

2. "Subtract 7s from 100."

3. "Count from 1 to 20."

(Note any cultural or educational differences that would influence this area. Allow clients to use paper and pencil if that is helpful to them.)

Rating:

1=Generally accurate and made only minor errors.

2=One significant error, not related to educational or cultural differences.

3=Two or more significant errors, not related to educational deficits.

Judgment

1. "At night, if you need some help, how can you obtain it?"

2. "If you are having trouble with your neighbor, what can you do to improve the situation?"

3. "If you see smoke in a wastepaper basket, what should you do?"

Rating:

1=Generally sensible responses.

2=Demonstration of some poor judgment.

3=Shows extremely poor judgment.

Emotional State

Observe the client's manner during the interview. Ask the client about crying, sadness, optimism, suspiciousness, delusions, mood swings, hallucinations and future plans.

Rating:

1=Emotional state seems reasonable and appropriate for the client's situation.

2=Client gives evidence of extensive or inappropriate depression, or grandiosity.

3=Client has extremely unreal or inappropriate ideas (delusional, hallucinatory behavior, extreme depression or suicidal ideas).

Total FROMAJE Score and Interpretation

All points are added together to form the total score:

7 or 8=Client does not display significant abnormal behavior or mentation.

9 or 10=Client displays symptoms of mild dementia or depression.

11 or 12=Client displays symptoms of moderate dementia or depression.

13 or more=Client has symptoms of severe dementia or depression.

An emotional rating of 3 when other factors are ranging in the 1 to 2 rating serves to highlight depressive symptoms and indicates a need for further evaluation in this area.

The second instrument I would like to share is the Set Test. This assessment evaluates the client's fund of knowledge regarding common, ordinary categories. The test is performed by asking the older persons to name as many items (or 10) as they can recall in each of four successive categories or sets—colors, animals, vegetables, towns. One point is awarded for each correct item offered for a maximum score for all categories of 40.

In healthy older people a score of 25-40 is considered in the normal range, a score of 24-15 is indicative of some mental impairment (depression, dementia, confusion, paranoia or other affective or mental dysfunction), a score of 0-14 is indicative of moderate to severe dementia or depression.

The results of this evaluation can provide the therapist with some data concerning the individual's ability to recall information and ability to categorize information. With the more severely involved older client it may serve as a measurement tool for the effectiveness of reality orientation groups. The categories can be chosen to reflect areas of interest or new learning. Physical prompts or verbal assists might also be used to ascertain the limits of the individual's abilities in using environmental information to help in mental manipulations.

So What?

The accurate appraisal of a client's mental status can reduce the risk of inappropriate treatment planning and can identify changes that may have come about subsequent to a treatment intervention. Accurate and periodic re-evaluation can speed the identification of older persons who have experienced acute, reversible dementias or brain dysfunctions. These assessments can be used to document the progress of clients in the community or nursing home setting and to assist in the determination of level of care needed by the individual for safe functioning. This information is also helpful to the family, who is often undecided about whether or not "mother can be left alone" or whether "daddy just isn't safe doing his own cooking anymore." Family members frequently wonder whether their relative is "just being stubborn" or whether the older person is really helpless.

Although these screening tools are only a starting point, they can serve as an aid in the identification of problems and allow the therapist an opportunity to intervene to cope with the deficit.

REFERENCES

Libow L: A rapidly administered, easily remembered mental status evaluation: FROMAJE. In Libow & Sherman (eds) *The Core of Geriatric Medicine*, St. Louis: CV Mosby Co., 85-91, 1981

Issacs B & Kinnie A: The set test as an aid to the detection of dementia in old people. *Brit J. Psychiat* 123: 467, 1973

Kahn R et al: Brief objective measures for the determination of mental status in the aged. *Am J Psychiatry* 117: 326, 1960

Pfeiffer E: A short portable mental status questionnaire for the assessment of organic brain deficit in elderly patients. *J Am Geriatric Soc* 23: 433, 1975

Jacobs J: Screening for organic mental syndromes in the medically ill. *Ann Intern Med* 80: 40, 1971

Gerontology
Special Interest Section Newsletter; Vol. 5, No. 4, 1982

Occupational Therapy and Pharmacy: Adapting Drug Regimens for Older People

By Betty R. Hasselkus, MS, OTR and Steven F. Bauwens, PharmD

The elderly in this country are major consumers of prescription and nonprescription drugs. A disproportionate 20-25% of all prescription drugs are currently consumed by this age group, which comprises only 11-12% of the general population. It has been estimated that prescription drug usage by the elderly will increase to 40-50% as the elderly population grows to represent 17-20% of the overall population by the year 2010. Approximately 25% of patients over age 65 consume six or more prescription drugs daily! An estimated 40% of these drug users are dependent on their medication to be able to pursue desired and necessary activities of daily living.

Compliance and noncompliance are terms used to describe a patient's medication-taking behaviors. Compliance, strictly defined, is taking the right drug according to prescribed instructions in the right dose at the right time. This has long been identified by pharmacists as a major problem in geriatric health care. Noncompliant behaviors may include: discontinuing a drug before the desired therapeutic effect is seen, taking a medication prescribed for another individual, administering an inappropriate dose due to difficult or confusing directions, misunderstanding directions or inability to properly measure the correct dose, i.e., liquid preparations. Other important factors include: storing drugs in containers labelled for another drug, concurrent unsupervised use of over-the-counter (OTC) drugs or alcohol, all of which may cause potentially significant drug interactions.

Many factors contribute to noncompliant behaviors. The patient who has multiple prescribing physicians and who uses multiple pharmacies is at risk for drug misuse through conflicting instructions about drugs and uncoordinated medication planning. The hearing and visual impairments of many older people may compromise the understanding of instructions and labels. Economic factors, educational level, motivation and culturally imbued life-long attitudes may have an impact on drug-taking behaviors.

It is a mistake to regard compliance as a problem of the *elderly* and to focus only on *their* medication activities. In reality, drug compliance is also closely related to the health providers' behavior as they provide communication and instruction regarding the prescription and monitoring of the drugs. Since most older people live in the community and have primary responsibility for their own daily care, medication taking becomes an activity of daily living (ADL) task that requires assessment and intervention, similar to other ADL skills such as bathing and dressing. Further, as the elderly continue to increase in numbers and the cost of traditional institutional care continues to escalate, it seems desirable and necessary to ensure that the elderly individual remains independent. The occupational therapist can work effectively with a clinical pharmacist in adapting medication routines that promote safe, accurate and independent drug use by the elderly. This seems particularly important since repeated inconsistencies in drug taking can lead to decompensation of a chronic disease state requiring repeated hospitalizations, which ultimately may result in institutionalization of the elderly person or death.

These authors worked together as members of an Interdisciplinary Geriatric Training Program located at the VA Hospital in Madison, Wisconsin. The interdisciplinary health team served a population of 100 outpatient veterans in the Madison area, offering a home care service and an outpatient geriatric clinic. Students from medicine, social work, nursing, nutrition, OT, PT, and pharmacy all trained with the program. Medication management was a high treatment priority for every patient. This included a detailed drug history, careful assessment of the need for and dosage of all existing medications, OTC drug usage patterns and idiosyncratic habits, screening for visual, hearing and cognitive abilities, and ongoing monitoring of compliance and levels of knowledge about the drugs.

Modification of drug taking systems for patients to promote independence and compliance tended to require highly individualized approaches. For some patients, the commercially available plastic drug dispenser with a pill compartment for each day of the week provided a simple and effective memory help and medication organizer. More often, however, such a pill dispenser had to be further adapted: more readable labels on the compartments, taping together 2 or 3 dispensers for the person who takes medication more than once a day, or allowing for more than one dispenser in the home, e.g., one on the kitchen table for mealtime medication and one at bed side for night medications. Variations of this dispenser system were also created using labeled envelopes for each day, muffin tins, hospital medication cups or egg cartons.

Medication dosages and time schedules were simplified and consolidated as much as possible so that the patient was not required to remember several different sets of instructions. A medication *might* be as efficacious taken once a day in a larger

(continued)

MEDICATIONS	SUN	M	TU	W	TH	F	SAT
ASPIRIN 1 TABLET taken in morning							
PROBANTHINE 1 TABLET 3 TIMES A DAY breakfast lunch dinner							
WEEK							

Flow sheet design by Mary Lenling

Adapting Drug Regimens

dose or as taken three times a day in smaller doses. Each patient's already established life style and daily routine was considered in order to use, whenever possible, existing patterns of activity and habits that might enhance compliance. With cognitively impaired patients, it was especially important not to impose marked changes on their drug systems unless absolutely necessary. One gentleman kept all medications on his kitchen table with a large manila envelope to serve as a divider between his pills and his wife's. His wife had been dead for three years! It became apparent, however, that his "system" would totally collapse if his wife's medicines were discarded. Somehow they provided significant cues and memory aids, enabling this man to administer his own medications. The only change we instituted was to remove, with his permission, his *own* out-dated or no longer prescribed drugs.

Large-lettered labels and bright-colored adhesive stickers were used to assist the compliance of visually impaired patients. Sometimes the colored stickers were affixed both to the pill containers and to a medication flow sheet the patient used as a daily checklist. This system proved to be particularly helpful to one patient who was anomic following a CVA. At times the bright-colored stickers were only placed on a *new* medication to serve as a reminder of the change.

Students seemed to be particularly inventive about creating adaptive medication aids. An occupational therapy student made a large-lettered one-week flow sheet with simple clear instructions for a cognitively impaired patient (see illustration) using commercially available rubdown letters. A nursing student, struggling to help a patient understand a fairly complicated prednisone tapering schedule, finally devised a calendar chart on which she drew each day's dosage in pill-colored dots—pink dots for the pink 1 mg. pills and white dots for the white 5 mg. pills. The patient had both the colored dots (e.g., 2 pink and 2 white) and the written dosage (12 mg.) as reminders each day.

Perhaps the piece de resistance was offered by a pharmacy student who was working with a patient who had a history of alcohol abuse. Both vitamins and a diet supplement had been prescribed to improve this patient's marginal nutritional status. The diet supplement came in pop-top cans and the patient seemed to be able to readily incorporate opening a can into his daily routine! But the vitamin pills went unnoticed day after day. Finally, this ingenious student simply *taped* 2 vitamin pills to each can of diet supplement and from then on the patient remembered his vitamins!

Working with the elderly patient to bring about understanding, compliance and independence in drug regimens is obviously an important part of geriatric health care. The adaptation of drug taking methods and behaviors to promote independence—in spite of physical and psychosocial changes associated with aging and disease—is a natural extension of the occupational therapist's concern for activities of daily living. Collaboration with a clinical pharmacist greatly enhances the OT's potential contribution in this arena and therapists should be encouraged to develop such cooperative ventures to maximize the overall health care of the elderly.

Suggested Readings:

Lundin, D. Medication taking behavior of the elderly. A pilot study. *Drug Intell Clin Pharm*, 1978, 12:518-522.

Pratt, C. C., Simonson, W., and Lloyd, S. Pharmacists' perceptions of major difficulties in geriatric pharmacy practice. *The Gerontologist*, 1982, 22:288-292.

Raffoul, P. R., Cooper, J. K., and Love, D. W. Drug misuse in older people. *The Gerontologist*, 1981, 21:146-150.

Atkinson, L., Gibson, I., and Andrews, J. The difficulties of old people taking drugs. *Age Aging*, 1977, 6:144-149.

Lamy, P. P. Misuse and abuse of drugs by the elderly. *Am Pharm*, 1980, 20:14-17.

Gerontology
Special Interest Section Newsletter; Vol. 5, No. 3, 1982

The Occupational Therapist and In-Service Education in Nursing Homes—A Focus on Canada

As an OT consultant, employed by Community Therapy Services in the Westman region of Manitoba, I have the opportunity to provide service to 6 nursing homes located in this area. The homes vary in size from 30 beds to 260 beds; only 2 of the 6 homes have inservice coordinators; the other 4 homes rely on the director of nursing for planning staff education. These facilities are primarily located in rural areas and many of the staff are recruited locally. Their educational backgrounds are extremely varied ranging from professional training to those with little opportunity for training other than that given on the job. Some staff complete a 6-week program designed for a health care aide by the community college in the area.

One of the common concerns expressed by health professionals today working with the elderly in these settings is the need to change care from "good, custodial, antiseptic medical treatment" to care that emphasizes the "quality of life" with respect for human dignity, independence and individuality. Inservice education is one of the avenues that can be used to promote this change. All staff need to be involved in this process, that requires change in traditional roles and attitudes toward the care of the elderly. As an OT consultant I participate in team meetings and inservice programs working with staff to facilitate staff growth and promote change in staff approaches to care of the elderly.

I am a firm believer in the principles of adult education and try to apply these in inservice programs. Effective learning takes place when: adults are actively involved in the learning process; the material is relevant to their daily work; the adult's own background is integrated into the learning experience; the learning is a pleasant experience with rewards given for success to encourage further learning.

Let me describe some of the approaches I have used for inservice. Frequently the learning goal concerns attitude change and I have found role playing or sociodrama an effective tool. This method by definition is a "technique in which people spontaneously act out problems of human relations and analyze the enactment

(continued)

In-Service Education—Focus on Canada

with the help of other role players and observers." This method brings attitudes and feelings before the total group and can later be used as a focal point for group discussion. It is very important to identify a problem of common concern to the group in their daily roles.

To give you an example of how this method can be used: One day the director of nursing in one of my homes greeted me with, "Win, I've tried everything to get my staff to encourage residents to do things for themselves. They still insist on making residents dependent — in self-care, etc. Help me"!

This problem resulted in an inservice session where role playing was used to illustrate a common situation in nursing homes. A brief history of a new resident was given before the role playing. The scene takes place at 7:00 a.m. when the resident is wakened by a staff member and then washed and dressed, i.e., made dependent on staff. The dialogue uses phrases frequently heard in nursing homes — "I can do that faster"; "Let me do it"; "That dress will do," etc. The scene culminates with the resident bundled into a wheelchair and whisked off to the dining room while protesting that she is quite able to walk short distances with her cane.

Immediate feedback should be given by the "actors." The audience was then divided into buzz groups, and, after appointing their own recorders, specific questions were handed out to be discussed. These included analyzing the role playing and correcting errors and suggesting more appropriate approaches; identifying the needs of the elderly, etc. When the total group reassembled, reports were given by each recorder. This stimulated lively discussion concerning attitudes and helped staff gain a different perspective on their approaches to the residents.

In another setting this method was used to promote change in staff attitudes concerning the "over use of safety devices" (restraints). It is gratifying to note a significant decline in using safety devices in this particular setting with a changed attitude in allowing residents increased freedom.

I have not yet attempted using this technique with residents themselves but think it could be useful in changing the attitude of some residents who inform staff frequently "You're paid to look after me."

A second approach I have used involves patient simulation. This method can be used when teaching staff skills related to self-care, i.e., feeding and dressing. Staff are assigned specific disabilities common to the elderly, e.g., impaired vision (eye patch); stiff joints (newspaper splints); use of one hand only, etc. This not only provides training in self-care but also heightens staff awareness of some of the difficulties residents have in executing these tasks. Time is always allotted at the end of the practical session for group discussion, which frequently involves problem solving for specific residents.

Demonstration is a method used frequently for inservice education where the learning goal is related to attaining a specific motor skill, e.g., correct lifting procedure, passive exercises, etc. We are fortunate in having many excellent slides that can be used to enhance the learning process. Demonstration is always followed by practice to give the participants feedback on their performance. If time permits staff may then apply the technique on the ward with a resident. The session usually ends with a discussion of problems related to performance, clarification of any misunderstandings, and problem solving with residents, etc.

I like to include audiovisuals in the presentations because I can see exciting potential for their use in presenting inservice programs. We are fortunate to have access to a wealth of slides, transparencies, posters, etc., which are certainly very helpful. In this age of technology one of the exciting prospects, which we are just exploring, lies in the production of one's own videotapes using a TV camera (portapak), e.g., if you were doing an inservice on correct lifting and transfer techniques, one could tape staff performing on the job and later play back their performance and give staff the opportunity to analyze their own technique.

Another way this could be used

would be to tape "live" sessions of specific techniques, e.g., reality orientation, and then share these tapes with other facilities for staff education.

The possibilities of using videotapes are only limited by one's ingenuity. They are valuable for giving a person feedback on their own behavior as mentioned in relation to lifting and for giving a group a common experience. They may also be used as a focal point for group discussion and to inform families (Family Night) of some programs and techniques used in nursing homes.

I recently read Alvin Toffler's book *The Third Wave* and, if his predictions for the future are correct, we will need to capitalize on the available technology to make our inservice programs effective learning experiences. I am sure some of you are much further along in this area and can share your experiences with us later.

I would like to pass on to you the following information, based on research on the learning process. People remember:

10% of what they read
20% of what they hear
30% of what they see
50% of what they see and hear
80% of what they say
90% of what they say and do

This is a helpful guide when one is selecting a method for presenting an inservice.

These few examples of methods used for inservice were selected to illustrate the contribution of an OT to staff education. There are many other techniques and one needs to develop a repertoire by experimenting and evaluating their effectiveness as a learning experience. Participation in staff training programs by the OT consultant should include inservice, team meetings, etc., and also, working directly with the staff on the wards to gain their cooperation in the process of change to become teachers, encouragers, friends rather than caretakers and "doers for." This combination gives the elderly new hope and meaning in their lives.

— *Win Grayston, OTM*
620 Frederick St.
Brandon, Manitoba

Gerontology
Special Interest Section Newsletter; Vol. 5, No. 3, 1982

Retired People Are Not Senile Simpletons—A Focus on Denmark

The heading is from an 80-year old old-age-pensioner's diary. He is not young any longer. His legs are not what they used to be. Holidays or study tours to foreign countries are something to read about in books. All the same he was among the first to enroll when we planned a strenuous tour to Strasbourgh. He made the trip "colours flying" like 29 other retired people from Viborg, Denmark.

"Challenge and engagement keep us young and active." This is also true for retired people. In spite of old age we can achieve things. We are not senile simpletons. We need each other and meet new challenges together.

This is the motto of the study circle in which retired people in Viborg have taken part for a number of years with great interest and enthusiasm. The formalities are taken care of by LOF, an organization concerned with adult education, and the writer, a former occupational therapist, is employed as leader of the study circle. What we have done and why it has turned out to be a success we would like to relate to you in the following paragraphs.

Study circle and tours

One means loneliness — two means togetherness — three means the solidarity of a group.

Twenty people form a group/study circle, and at present four such groups exist. We meet once a week in the study of the local library and talk and talk and talk: someone has read the local newspaper and found something of interest, someone else does not understand the young generation, and another member is inviting fellow members to join him for a lecture or for a trip to the pictures. Topics are in abundance, and my job is to sort out the topics for discussion, the inspiration is mutual.

Our meetings usually start with these improvised discussions and talks while we drink coffee from thermos flasks brought along by the members. However, usually we take up one special topic for closer discussion at the meeting.

Schools, terror, legal systems, etc.

Do you remember your school days? Were children and youngsters nicer then? We spent several mornings discussing this topic. The members took turns telling about their childhood and school days — the nice things and the not so nice things.

They brought to light old school books and long forgotten photos. We compared the teaching methods of yesterday and today, and we actually went out to take a look at schools today. This caused new discussions and comparisons with the "good old days." But one excursion was not enough. We visited a folk high school, a school for handicraft, a school for kindergarten teachers, the local center for educational material, etc. The Tvind school in West-Jutland was such an interesting experience that we had to go there twice for a whole day.

Another topic for discussion was violence and fear and our legal system. We read almost every day about bag-snatchers and old people being knocked down in the streets. Is there more violence today than when the old were young? Many members of the group are afraid to go out at night. We tried to get to the bottom of this problem, went to the local police station where we were welcomed with coffee and cake, and were told that life was considerably more dangerous in the "good old days" with highway men and gypsies. Our minds were set at rest. However, we wanted to see a criminal in real life. So, we went to the local court room to hear a case against a young man who had crashed a bottle on the head of a friend in a pub. We were even more reassured. The "criminal" was an ordinary person — a young boy who had had a little too much to drink.

We have discussed a number of other topics: local planning, nuclear energy, pollution, nursing homes, agriculture, advertising, literature, castles and manors, etc. After the group discussed the topics thoroughly for several mornings, we make an excursion to the actual place, well prepared. The members themselves arrange the excursion by bus.

The experiences of several of the excursions have been put into writing. We have written newspaper articles about our activities and journalists from newspapers and the broadcasting corporation have come to see us.

Major study tours

Our discussions and short excursions inspired us to go even further. We live in the country far from Copenhagen — especially for a retired person. We therefore decided to visit our capital together.

A normal pension is insufficient for this kind of luxury so that we wrote applications for money to the county authorities, to the banks, to various charitable trusts, etc. Many refused to help, but we kept on and at last we succeeded in raising the funds for a 4-day trip to Copenhagen for 24 retired people. Among other things, we visited the Parliament, the television studios, the Royal Theatre, the Memorial Park for the victims of the German occupation, and had a meeting with retired people from Copenhagen. Two nurses took part in the trip and we all reached home safe and sound.

This trip opened new vistas: we spent a week at the Folk High School at Haderslev, and a week in Gotherburgh, Sweden, where we made a radio broadcast.

And finally, we made the big jump: we went to Strasbourgh in France to visit the European Parliament.

The idea had come to us through a radio broadcast about farmers in the Common Market countries. We had already seen slides, heard lectures, and been discussing pro and con. The information bureau of the Parliament in Copenhagen gave us assistance concerning travel costs. We went by train, stayed at third class hotels, carried our own luggage and endured a lot of hardships, which, however, made the trip even more unforgettable.

Lectures in the morning, briefings in the afternoon, unfamiliar food, discussions in the evenings. The old people coped with it all. Our preparations at home were of immense help. The politicians complimented the group on this insight. We were not senile simpletons.

After the trip a film was made that we now show to other interested groups. Reports and photos took up

(continued)

Retired People—Focus on Denmark

more than 100 pages. "An open door-day" after the return with photos, plates, radio transmission and French pies gathered several hundred visitors. We have proved to ourselves that we could cope with the biggest challenges.

Why do we tell you this? Because we want to tell you that old age does not necessarily mean years of senility, but, on the contrary, is an invitation to take up new tasks, new challenges. Bad health or minor complaints are forgotten or nonexistent when an informal and inspiring 'being together' with others leads to an engagement in the surrounding world.

Being retired is the third stage of a person's life. It must be lived fully like the two preceding ones and this way its brings good health and happiness to all retired people.

— Ulla Brita Gregersen

Gerontology
Special Interest Section Newsletter; Vol. 5, No. 2, 1982

Functional Ability of Elderly People—A Focus on Sweden

By Birgitta Lundgren-Lindquist

As the number of elderly people in the community increases it is important to gain detailed knowledge about functional ability in higher ages and to try to influence these abilities through training or to make the environment meet the needs of the elderly. Both from the individual's point of view and from that of the society it is important for elderly people to be able to stay in their home milieu with or without help. Relevant knowledge about functional problems among the elderly can only be obtained through systematic studies of individuals. Current studies on elderly people conducted by the Department of Geriatric and Long-Term Care Medicine, University of Goteborg, Sweden, are obtaining this information. The first phase of the population study "70 Year Old People in Gothenburg" was carried out in 1971 and 1972. It was a comprehensive longitudinal study with a far-reaching survey of the social and medical constitution in this age group.

A representative, systematic sample of 70-year-old people in Gothenburg was obtained for examination during the period they reached their 70th birthday. In 1976 and 1977 when the subjects were 75 years old a further examination was done as well as more recently in 1980 and 1981 when the subjects were 80 years old.

I have been given the opportunity to participate in the current study in which 550 subjects will take part. I am performing a study of Activities of Daily Living among the elderly. A functionally oriented interview is included in the study, where I, among other things, obtain information about the ability and actual performance of different activities of daily living, especially pertaining to the home milieu, personal hygiene, physical activities and previous occupation. Functional skills are tested to attain baseline information in the following manner:

1. Manual ability is tested in various tasks of importance for an independent ADL function.
   A) Pulling out and inserting a key into a lock.
   B) Pulling out and inserting an electric plug into a socket.
   C) Screwing in an electric light bulb.
   D) Inserting a coin in a slot.
   E) Dialing numbers 0-9 on a telephone.
2. Pronation and supination of the forearm is studied with a water pouring test.
3. The reach of the upper extremities is studied when the subject tries to lift a glass and to place a one kilogram weight on shelves of varying heights.
4. Maximal static strength (MVC) is measured in key grip, transversal volar grip, elbow extension and elbow flexion. The submaximal endurance time at 50% MVC is also measured.
5. The ability to rise from a sitting position is studied when the subject rises and sits down on chairs of various heights.
6. Ability to open different types of screwtops on jars and bottles is measured with equipment which has been used by the Swedish Packaging Research Institute. The jars correspond in size and weight to the ones which are frequently found in daily housekeeping.
7. Muscular coordination in hand and arm is measured with Molbech's clothespin test. This test consists of 50 clothespins with metal tips which the subject grasps, opens, and fits into 50 pairs of holes at maximal speed.
8. The examination of functional ability in hygiene activities takes place in a standardized bathroom. This type of bathroom and layout frequently occurs in the apartments of elderly people in Gothenburg. In the bathroom different functions are studied. Standing by the sink washing hands and face, the ability to sit down and stand up from the toilet, the ability to get into the bath and sit down at the bottom of the bath, and the ability to stand up and climb out of the bath. Evaluation includes time taken, movement patterns, stress, strain, and heart rate to identify difficulties experienced. The subjective amount of strain is estimated by means of Borg's scale and the heart rate is registered by telemetry of ECG.
9. Heart rate, time required, effort expended, and stress are also

(continued)

Functional Ability—Focus on Sweden

registered during spontaneously demonstrated, as well as maximal speed exercises of walking 30 meters in a corridor and stepping up and down stairs of various heights.

An extremely important question is what relation aging in itself has to a decreased functional capacity because of changed habits and reduced activity in elderly people. Another important question concerns the potential influence of training for functional ability as compared to improvement of performance with changes in the milieu.

For practical reasons and for technical development it is important to be able to identify the important determinants of function in an aim to achieve improvement of the functional ability. It is hoped that these studies will supply support in order to achieve more flexible solutions so that elderly people can remain in their home milieu for longer periods of time. Maybe, for example, there is an advantage in having a shower stall rather than a bathtub?

My hope and expectation is that these studies will contribute knowledge and form a basis to achieve changes in attitudes of the persons working in home health services, bringing them a more realistic view about the real functional ability of the older individuals.

Birgitta Lundgren-Lindquist
Dept. of Rehab. Medicine
Sahlgrenska sjukhuset
413 45 Goteborg
Sweden

Gerontology
Special Interest Section Newsletter; Vol. 5, No. 2, 1982

Occupational Therapy in Psycho-Geriatrics—A Focus on Holland

By Joos van den Hoek

The author of the following article works as an OT at the Psychiatric Centre St. Bravo, in Noordwijkerhout, in Holland. One of the four departments of this center is that for geriatric care, consisting of an intake unit and four units for further treatment. After a year and a half experience in the intake unit, she describes the possibilities for OT in this field.

OT is one of the disciplines in the treatment team working in the intake unit; in addition, there are a geriatrician, nursing staff, a psychologist, a social worker, a priest, a physical therapist, and an activities worker. The unit can take 27 patients: they are all elderly people (65+) who can no longer manage life in their home situations because of disturbed behavior.

In general we are involved with two different groups of patients: people who develop behavior disorders as a result of incipient or advancing dementia, and people who are decompensating for psycho-social problems.

In the first group we are concerned with a demonstrable deterioration of the brain functions (e.g. visible on an EEG). The second group concerns social problems such as depression, mourning, or loneliness, all of which are closely connected with the consequences of aging in our society.

Patients usually stay in this unit for two to three months. The questions we are confronted with during this period are: what has caused the disturbed behavior (observation); can we influence the causes and how (treatment); what living situation will be most appropriate for the patient (advice for the future).

In the course of the patient's stay each discipline has its task, and uses its own means and views to formulate its assessment of the three aspects mentioned. I shall give a general description of the procedures followed in the intake period, with emphasis on OT.

On admission, the necessary medical and nursing arrangements are first made (medication, assistance with personal care); then general observation of the patient takes place for two to four weeks. This consists of: a physical and psychiatric check-up (geriatrician); psychological test (psychologist); gathering information on the home situation and the people who are close to the patient (social worker); a check-up of the functions of the patient in daily life activities and general activities (OT); if necessary, examination of the functions of the neuromuscular system (physical therapist); observation of the behavior and general functioning in the residential unit (nursing staff). The priest and the activities worker have important tasks for the welfare of the patient during his/her stay: spiritual support and recreational activities.

In principle the OT observes each patient; if therapy is refused or if the need for nursing care dominates, OT information is lacking in the total observation picture. Therefore, a check is made with each new patient concerning which functions, necessary for personal care, are intact, and what the highest attainable level of independence for that patient is in personal care.

In general this is washing, dressing, eating and drinking, and toileting; sometimes independence in housekeeping and cooking are important too.

This information is obtained by accompanying the patient on two or three mornings while the individual is washing, dressing and breakfasting. I then write up where the problems lie, what help is necessary, and what approach I advise to the nursing staff for further attendance of the patient. The areas identified as important to understanding the problems are:

motor functions: mobility of the joints, general mobility, eyesight, hearing.

(continued)

Psycho-Geriatrics—Focus on Holland

mental ability: consciousness of actions, spatial orientation, general orientation, idea of the right order of actions, understanding of instructions, efficient use of objects.

attitude: interest, independency, wish for independence.

Disturbed mental abilities are the greatest problem for these patients; besides this, their own attitude is very important. Someone who really wants to take care of himself will make good use of instructions and will manage, in spite of decreased general awareness and orientation. Someone who is too depressed to find satisfaction in any exertion, will not have enough energy to do things independently, in spite of advice and instructions.

After their treatment most patients will stay in surroundings where there is some degree of nursing and care. The level of independence in regard to personal care will determine to what kind of institution a person will go. For instance, in a home for the elderly, one must be independent in regard to personal care, whereas hot meals and household help are provided. In nursing homes there are often different levels of care, where patients are placed in accordance with need for assistance.

Besides the observation of ADL functions, I have the task of finding out how people react to the activities available to them. This indicates the extent to which they can cope with their lives with their intact and disturbed functional abilities. Obviously, several aspects are important: the objectively demonstrable disordered cerebral activities, the personality of the patient, his background and former way of life—thus, both physical and psycho-social factors.

An opinion is formulated on these aspects while working with clients in the observation group in the OT room. The first contact with the patient is when I invite him for an individual talk. I then tell him about the therapy program and obtain his case history. In this way we each get a general idea about each other and we make appointments for therapy. Most patients feel OT to be threatening; often they realize that demands are going to be made and that they may be confronted with their problems and incapacities. For that reason I consider this first contact of essential importance as a basis for

further observation and treatment.

I see shock when someone sees all the craft materials and products, and hastily tells me he never was handy and has had bad sight for years. Another patient walks around with interest, finds a few balls of wool and says: "My dear you've no idea how many cardigans, scarfs and socks I have knitted in my life!" In both cases I get useful hints about the best activities to offer these patients.

The activities I use are determined by age, physical condition and interest, and are also aimed at allowing me to obtain relevant information. The way a patient approaches an activity gives me information on that person's: method of working, personal preferences, willingness to accept a task, level, degree of independency, insight, general awareness, use of materials and utensils, understanding of instructions, speed, concentration, care for the finishing touch, self-criticism, application and enthusiasm. In addition, specific aspects of the physical condition like the eyesight, coordination and mobility affect the way a person does things. There are also indications of the mental condition of the patient: orientation in time, person and space, the imprint and memory, the approachability and the verbal power of expression, insight to the situation and state of health.

Finally, the psycho-social functions: interest in one's surroundings and one's response to them, how contact is made with others, one's own will, the proprieties, moods, the concept of the future. I evaluate all the above points by providing the people in the observation group with a program of individual and group activities on three mornings. The activities are simple woodwork, wickerwork, weaving, handwork, (knitting, crochet, needlework, embroidery), leadwork, leatherwork, parlor games, typing, and household activities.

At the end of this observation period I write an observation report and an ADL report, with my conclusions, recommendations for further treatment and my opinion on the patient's potential. Both reports are intended to inform the other staff members on my views and help to determine the plans we then make together for the treatment to be given.

During treatment we distinguish two

general groups. The people we expect to be able to live more or less independently in their own home, in a home for the elderly, or in a sheltered psychiatric residential unit, and the people who will have to be taken care of in a nursing home. We aim at resocialization for the first group. In the second group activation, social adaptation, and limitation of institutionalization symptoms are the most important aims. The OT does not work directly with the latter patients; the activities worker and the nursing staff organize these patients' activities.

My task with the patients of the resocialization group is to provide each patient with an individual activity aimed at leisure pursuits. They come to OT in groups of five to eight people on three afternoons a week. I work towards the return home of these patients after their treatment by making demands of their independency and by introducing, as a subject of conversation, the possibilities and difficulties of making worthwhile use of their free time. The techniques I use are the same I mentioned for the observation group, with the accent on the personal interest of the patient and practical feasibility when returned home.

In addition I set up an individual program with activities for some of the patients, which is intended as a rehearsal for functioning in their own homes after discharge. Being at home in this context means being away from the protective, caring atmosphere of the hospital unit, without people around all the time. No nurses or therapists who keep an eye on everything and are there to take immediate action if anything goes wrong. In such an activity program I may tell the patient to go shopping for a hot meal and to cook it. If necessary I provide some help initially at the completion of treatment. In the end the patient does it all alone. I discuss the problems the patient expects beforehand, how he wants to handle the task and how it worked out in the end. Housekeeping and leisure pursuits are subjects that also come up in these talks; in this connection I assign the patient small household tasks or leisure activities to try out.

Some people expect everything will be fine when they return home and therefore refuse to make use of the opportunities for practising. Frequently

(continued)

these are people who do not have a realistic attitude about their state of health or who belittle the reason they are in the hospital. Or else they are afraid that participating in the activities will make their functional disorder painfully clear. It is important to discuss the motives for this resistance to the program; sometimes it may be a reason to advise intensive after-care (e.g., home helps, meals on wheels, regular visits from a psychiatric nurse).

Often people lack the self-confidence and energy to take care of themselves because of conflicts and tensions at a former time or in their present home situation. Positive experiences in safe surroundings (e.g., this 'experimental' situation, in which the patient can ask for help) can lessen the insecurity and thus stimulate a person to tackle things independently.

The level of independence is decisive in determining future living arrangements; can a person manage to live on their own, without becoming lonesome, and take adequate care of themselves? Or does someone need to have the possibilities for contact and assistance (a hot meal, help with the housework) in order to hold their own?

These are the most important aspects in the treatment of our patients in the resocialization group; in my opinion, they involve specific tasks for an OT.

Besides the work with the two groups of patients I have described, I recommend—and if necessary—make—aids for patients, in collaboration with the physical therapist. Usually these are to help with eating and dressing. Further, the teamwork in our unit demands that each staff member participate in the organization, policy and methodology of the unit, take part in the consultations between disciplines and give lectures to student nurses at the center.

Work concerning my own profession is also important: regular meetings with other OTs, giving information to OT students and providing them with possibilities for practical training.

I hope I have made clear what possibilities there are for an OT in psycho-geriatrics; I believe we should pay more attention to the development of our profession in this field of work. The care of the elderly has become more and more important in our society in the past years, and at the same time the demand for OTs in institutions for psycho-geriatrics has grown. Therefore I think OTs in this sector should keep in touch with one another and exchange experiences. All too often geriatrics still evokes the image of senile, incontinent fuddy-duddies. My experience has been that there is considerable scope for OT in psycho-geriatrics.

Gerontology
Special Interest Section Newsletter; Vol. 5, No. 1, 1982

Writings from Israel: Occupational Therapy in a Geriatric Milieu

Of the many professionals in the medical field of rehabilitation, it is primarily the occupational therapist who is concerned with the individual's ability to be independent. No matter the sex, age, religion, or culture, if a person is physically, mentally, or socially disabled, the occupational therapist is the one who will help and guide him to become as independent as possible.

Independence touches all parts of a person's life. It includes the ability to get up out of bed in the morning, to shower, shave, toilet, apply make-up, dress, sit down at the table and eat; to get to work, hold down a job, do housework, raise the children, shop, pay bills, learn; to make decisions, adjust to change, prepare for the future, to think in the abstract and concrete; to carry on a conversation, enjoy a movie, to participate in sports, take a trip, knit, attend a party, enjoy sex.

In order to help the patient be as independent as possible, the occupational therapist has to identify the limits of the disability and determine whether these limits can or should be changed. With this information, a treatment program can be established that is functional, realistic, and comfortable to the needs of the individual. The process of evaluation and treatment varies from setting to setting and this variation is most apparent when the occupational therapist is identifying limits.

Limits can be anywhere. They can even be imposed on the treatment program itself. In the geriatric setting, the occupational therapist is limited by the age, the disability, the duration of illness, the attitudes of the disabled and his family toward his illness, and by the lifestyle imposed on him.

The problems posed because the individual is past the age of 65 are subtle. Close family members and friends have died. Children have moved away. Businesses are closed, jobs are gone. Apartments once full of noise and activity are now silent and empty. Life has lost much of its meaning.

Disability does not help. Often, one has difficulty getting out of bed, going to the bathroom, or reaching his feet in order to dress himself. Movement can be slow and uncoordinated. There can be dizziness, or an inability to walk or to sit down at the table for meals. Eyesight and hearing might begin to fail. There will be difficulty in reading the newspaper or listening to the radio. There can be a loss of energy, an inability to participate in lengthy conversations. Sometimes there is incontinence. Often there is confusion, an inability to do simple tasks that were once done without thought. And there can be constant pain.

Disability and old age are magnified for those in an institution. There, the setting is foreign. Those who are caring for a person's intimate needs are strangers. The freedom once taken for granted: to be able to drink when thirsty, grab a bite to eat when hungry,

(continued)

take a nap when tired, go for a walk, look at a television or read a book—patient's privacy is constantly invaded by therapists, nurses, social workers, and doctors. His time is regulated. He no longer has control over his own self.

These changes in the individual's everyday life are usually gradual. By the time the disabled elderly person arrives in the institution, he has been ill for many years. Usually his long-time suffering has him convinced that he is useless, to be pitied, and must be attended to for all his needs. This conviction is proof enough to him that he will fail completely in any occupational therapy treatment. Fearful of failure, more times than not he refuses to cooperate. All of this poses limits toward a successful occupational therapy treatment program. It affects one's attitudes toward the disabled elderly and their willingness or unwillingness to receive help, to perform, or to make a new life for themselves.

The disabled person still living at home usually has not been ill long enough to be so convinced of hopelessness. Nonetheless there are limits imposed on a treatment program here. These include the patient's behavior at home before his illness, changes that have come about because of his illness, and whether these changes are viewed by all as positive or negative. Did the family administer to him before the illness, and, if so, is it now advisable for him to be independent? Would family members encourage independence after the therapist leaves? Would they be willing to rearrange the physical properties of the house as necessary to help the disabled be more independent in his own home? These are some of the limits that must be considered before a treatment program can be initiated.

Within the institution, when the patient overcomes feelings of inadequacy and agrees to participate in occupational therapy, then mutual cooperation is needed with the other people that come in contact with him daily. The nursing staff might have to agree to wait for the disabled person to put on his sweater, to wash himself, to

shave. Family members who feed him when they visit, or the caregiver they employ might have to change their behavior and attitudes in order to help the occupational therapist achieve treatment goals.

Finally, limits can be imposed on occupational therapy services because of lack of proper facilities, space, equipment, material, time and qualified help. Each institution is different, each has its own finances, guidelines, and priorities. So each OT department differs from institution to institution.

Once limitations have been established from such variable probabilities within the disabled person's environment, the occupational therapist is then ready to approach the limitations imposed by the disease itself. Is there adequate range of motion and strength in both hands to pull the shirt over the shoulders? Is there ability to pinch and grasp? Is there enough sight to see the clothing? Is there enough coordination to get the soup to the mouth without spilling? Is there enough control over the muscles to chew, swallow, and speak? Is memory intact? Are similarities in color, shape and size recognizable? Does he understand directions? Is he aware that the person is sitting on his left and talking to him? Can he carry on a conversation, think in abstract or concrete terms? How long is his attention span? Does he have patience, understanding, and tolerance?

There can be so many limits to which a person is subjected due to an illness. They, along with those from the disabled's environment, are carefully evaluated for indications of change and changeability. Often changes can be made that reduce the limitations imposed by disease. With the help of activities the occupational therapist can increase range of motion and strength, stabilize coordination, improve visual and tactile perception, cognition, communication skills, memory, and attention span.

Unfortunately, changes are not always possible due to the disease process, an irreversible deficiency, or unbearable pain. If so, the therapist will train the disabled to function in spite

of his disability. He can learn to dress with one hand, eat without sight, or shave without feeling. When indicated, adaptive equipment can be provided that will enable him to put on his socks without bending over, or not to spill soup from a spoon in his unsteady, shaking hand. A splint could be designed to help his fingers and hand be more functional, or to prevent further contractures and deformity. New habits can be introduced to help with memory, perception, or cognitive problems.

The environment, too, might suggest the possibility of change. Replacing buttons with zippers or Velcro might be advisable. Raising the bed to an easily maneuverable level can be suggested. The flush lever on the toilet might need to be changed. The numbers on the telephone might need to be changed to Braille numbers.

Sometimes these changes are unrealistic or uncomfortable to the individual. Splinting an already deformed hand that is not expected to function again might cause more pain and discomfort than the resulting cosmetic improvement would be worth to the patient. Laboring to relearn to read, write, or do math, might not be realistic to the institutionalized patient who has no more needs for such skills. Facing constant failure with perceptual motor and cognitive tasks might be realistically unbearable.

All these possibilities the occupational therapist will consider when deciding on a treatment program suitable for the patient. The therapist knows that not any two individuals are the same. The treatment goals that suit one patient would not necessarily be indicated for another patient with the same disability. Yet, whether one is physically, mentally, or socially disabled, the occupational therapist will evaluate him—his disability, his capabilities, his environment, his needs; his prognosis—in order to help him be as independent as possible.

—*Miriam Barzilay, OTR*
Rehovot, Israel

Standards of Practice—What Do They Mean? Why Do We Need Them?

A professional association is an organization of practitioners who judge one another as professionally competent and who have banded together to perform social functions which they cannot perform in their separate capacity as individuals (1, p. 50).

Standards of practice provide a **ruler** for judging the quality of occupational therapy services, regardless of whether the service is provided by an occupational therapist, an occupational therapy assistant or an aide. Standards define OT by delineating the scope of the variables relevant to occupational performance. The scope of practice is reflected in the variable that the therapist evaluates and treats. Standards also delineate the characteristics of high quality care, by specifying the criteria that can be used to determine whether quality care has been provided.

The types of standards used most often are: **process, outcome,** and **content** (2). **Process** standards are concerned with the implementation of the OT process in regard to intervention and the treatment plan. Standards for the plan as a whole address major client needs, such as, "To increase independence in activities of daily living." Standards for intervention address a single client need, such as, "Teach the client how to use a rocker knife."

Outcome standards define the change that is expected to occur in the client's occupational performance as a result of the OT process (2). Examples of outcome standards are: "Improved orientation to surroundings," "Increased functional mobility," and "Maintenance of shoulder range of motion."

The term **content** standards refers to the content that is shared with others, about the OT process. Thus, the concern is with the quality of communication (oral and written) between the therapist and the client, the family, significant others, and other health professionals (2).

Content standards cover the substance of what needs to be recorded or reported concerning OT intervention and the client's reaction to it, as well as the steps that should be followed in teaching the client, his family, or significant others.

Content standards also refer to the decisions that are made in regard to OT intervention. They govern practice in regard to questions such as: What should be done when a knife is missing from an OT clinic in a psychiatric facility? What should be done to decide on a particular intervention modality or a combination of modalities for a client? What should be done to determine that OT intervention should be discontinued?

Two methods are available for establishing standards of practice (2). The first method involves systematic study of practice and leads to the formulation of validated standards. The second involves the study of practice in a particular health care setting or within a special unit. This leads to the formulation of consensual standards. Consensual standards require validation.

Standards of practice are the means through which OT fulfills its professional responsibility to guarantee the consumer quality services. Standards must be formulated, maintained, and revised in accordance with the theoretical basis and scope of OT practice. The membership must be aware of the standards and educated to comply with them. Standards may be used as a basis for peer review, for self-assessment, and to evaluate the effects of staff development programs. The public must be protected from therapists who fail to comply with the standards. Without such accountability, consumers will lack confidence in the services provided by occupational therapy, which could lead to the extinction of OT.

The AOTA unit responsible for establishing standards of practice is the Commission on Practice (COP). COP is currently chaired by John Farace (California). The Special Interest Sections assist the COP by identifying areas in which standards are needed and in reviewing proposed standards. The Special Interest Sections have direct representation on COP through a liaison position which I currently hold. Mr. Farace is assisted in carrying out the functions of COP by a Steering Committee, comprised of Mary Foto, OTR (California); Diane Hawkins, COTA (Maryland), Jim Hinojosa, OTR (New York), Linda McGourty, OTR (Washington), Doris Shriver, OTR (Colorado), and Jeanette Parkin, OTR (National Office Staff). COP has also developed an extensive liaison network to assist in setting member feedback concerning standards.

1. Merton RK. The functions of the professional association. *American Journal of Nursing*, 58, 1958.
2. Mason EJ. *How To Write Meaningful Nursing Standards*, New York: John Wiley & Sons, 1978.

Gerontology
Special Interest Section Newsletter; Vol. 4, No. 3, 1981

Initiating Occupational Therapy Services

Susan Orloff is the chief occupational therapist at Crafts-Farrow State Hospital in Columbia, SC.

Occupational therapy services are provided to 1,500 geriatric residents of the facility. Occupational therapy (OT), since its introduction to Crafts-Farrow hospital eleven years ago has been an adjunct of the Activity Department, staffed only by COTAs. As of March 27th of this year, the OT Department was established as a separate department under Medical Services.

The goals of the program started by Susan were to establish OT as a rehabilitative rather than recreational/diversional service, to train COTAs to do new evaluation and program procedures, to meet with each department head to establish what their priorities were for OT Services vis-a-vis patients, and to set up administrative procedures of a new OT Department.

Patients are now referred for specific rehabilitative purposes and assigned to a group or individual therapy program. Existing programming consists of reality orientation, grooming, hygiene, ADL, feeding, post-stroke mobility, remotivation, socialization, and environmental awareness (sensory-motor activities). Referrals must be signed by the attending physician. It is then up to the OT staff to evaluate the patient and determine in conjunction with the supervising OTR, appropriate therapy and/or to refer the patient to another treatment service.

In addition to the Activity Department, Crafts-Farrow also offers horticultural and music therapy, full on-campus chaplaincy, social services, psychology, dietary, and speech and hearing departments. It is one of the goals of the OT Department to involve as many other services in the programs as possible. Doing joint patient programs with Activities was easy, but the interest and enthusiasm from other services was both unexpected and welcomed.

One of the OT programs for a group of very confused patients involves the use of hot/cold food temperatures to help differentiate between morning and afternoon. In the morning the patients' meet for hot buttered toast and hot coffee, in the afternoon the same group meets for cold juice and cookies. In addition, tasks of serving, clean-up and familiar object recognition and use are given to the patients. Although the group has only been operating for 5 weeks, it is exciting to see patients who may still not know the exact date, waiting by the door refusing to go elsewhere because it's "OT time." Having this reality orientation group supported and reinforced by other services has helped to speed the patients progress.

Irrespective of the group or individual assignment, it is the goal of the OT Department to enhance each individual's ability to make choices within his environment; choices that will expand his life-space, increase his self-awareness, and promote his rehabilitative process so that placement in alternative settings and/or a return home will be personally rewarding and successful for all those involved.

Any therapists interested in finding out more about this exciting program can contact Susan Orloff at the address below.

Submitted by Susan Orloff, OTR
  Chief, OT Services
  Craft's Farrow State Hospital
  7901 Farrow Rd.,
  Columbia, SC 29203

Gerontology
Special Interest Section Newsletter; Vol. 4, No. 2, 1981

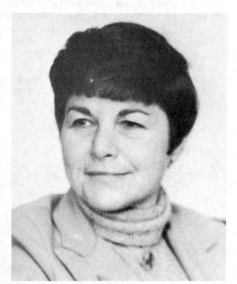

Recommendations from the Mini–White House Conference on Aging

**Organized and Conducted By
Cynthia Epstien, MA, OTR, FAOTA**

Thirty-five therapists met in San Antonio, Texas, during the national AOTA Conference to provide testimony and recommendations for the White House Conference on Aging (WHCoA) regional hearings. The results of the mini-WHCoA have been gathered into a preliminary report for an AOTA position statement to be presented to delegates of the WHCoA. The recommendations were formulated from concerns raised by the participants in the mini-WHCoA. These recommendations are as follows:

1. *Maximal functional independence of the elderly as a health policy goal.* This should include: more programs that promote health and prevent disease; an expansion of services in the long-term care continuum such as day care programs, congregate housing, meals centers, short-term care, respite care, and community living; more efficient delivery of services and better coordination of all health care services for the elderly with more emphasis on the interdisciplinary team approach;

(continued)

more research aimed at affirming the cost effectiveness of such approaches; and more ease in mobilizing the elderly from one care setting to another as changes in functional status occur.

2. *Optimal quality of life for the elderly and their families regardless of environmental setting.* U.S. health policy should develop programs that preserve the individual's quality of life whether in community settings or in institutions; should develop improved understanding and diminish the abuse of the elderly in the media, the community, the institutions, and the family; and should encourage the creation of an age-integrated society.

It should also endeavor to improve the training of all health care providers to optimize the benefits of such care for the elderly.

3. *Provision of physical and mental activity and social involvement for older individuals in all living situations.* This should include: flexible retirement policies based on functional capabilities rather than age; more volunteer programs that use the skills and knowledge of the elderly to promote the well-being of others; more information and referral sources for the elderly in the community for appropriate activity programs; the development of appropriate activity programs in institutions and in communities to meet the varied needs of older individuals; and more research on the effectiveness of such programs in maintaining the health and well-being of the elderly.

4. *Improvement of financial security for the elderly on fixed incomes.* Strengthening the Social Security system and improving the Medicare system to more adequately cover the needs of the elderly is essential. More encouragement, without economic retribution, is needed to continue part-time or desired employment. Protection from the loss of housing due to catastrophic illness or slow recovery is needed to prevent unnecessary continuation of institutionalization.

5. *Reinforce and strengthen family and community supports.* U.S. health policy should focus on developing social, economic, and psychological support systems to enable families and communities to assist older persons. This should include: tax credits for families maintaining the elderly within the home; training for families on the care of the at-risk and ill elderly; expansion of home health and community based services; more community awareness and support for programs serving the elderly, and more community and family involvement with the institutionalized elderly.

6. *Identification of the roles and functions of all health care professions and para-professionals in the care of the elderly and the provision of appropriate referrals and services for older persons and their families.* U.S. health policy should delineate the roles and functions of health care professions and establish centralized referral mechanisms for providing the necessary services to the elderly and their families or caregivers.

7. *Improve the training and education of individuals working with the gerontological population.* There should be additional reseach and training programs to produce knowledgeable practitioners in all health and social service professions for work with the elderly.

These recommendations will be studied further and a statement will be formulated and presented to the AOTA Executive Board for approval for use as a position statement for our organization.

Submitted by Cynthia Epstein, OTR, and Teepa Snow, OTR

Gerontology
Special Interest Section Newsletter; Vol. 3, No. 3, 1980

Home Services Extend Independence

Project Independence is a community health program designed to maximize the older adults' potential for independent living. Utilizing a team approach that often includes other community health care providers, the project's occupational therapists and dieticians address both the physical and psychosocial needs of their clients through programs and services encompassing components of prevention, intervention, and referral. Funded by the Northwest Area Foundation and administered through United Hospitals, Inc., services are provided free to the senior residents of 16 Public Housing Agency high rise apartments in St. Paul, MN.

Clients may be referred by any community health care provider, they may refer themselves, or they may receive services after an outreach visit by project staff. Nutrition and general health assessments and the ADL evaluation provide a data base for the problem list and program plan. If deemed necessary, a referral is made to another agency or health care provider, usually Meals-On-Wheels or a social service agency. Doctor's orders are obtained for therapeutic diet counseling, for functional occupational therapy, etc. Because Project Independence clients often have two or more chronic medical problems, the occupational therapy focus is on prevention and maintenance, ADL evaluation and instruction, provision of adaptive aids, instruction in joint protection and work simplification. Social support for the frail elderly at high-risk is also important, and regular visits are the shared responsibility of occupational therapy and nutrition staff.

Group sessions are important for the socialization they provide. The groups that have been formed are exercise groups, weight loss groups, nutrition education classes, volunteer groups, arthritis self-help groups, and walking groups.

Exercise groups meet regularly at 4 highrise apartments. The enthusiastic participants often wear their yellow T-shirts with the slogan, "Join the Active People Over 60." If the resident has been told to restrict activity or if any question arises regarding ability to participate, the resident's physician is consulted. Everyone in the weight loss groups receives individualized counseling and follow-up or "reinforcement" visits, and they are encouraged to join the exercise group or the walking group.

The outdoor walking groups function independently at most high rises after the first-time walk with the COTA. The COTA observes the walkers for potential difficulties, sets the pace, and determines the route. It is especially important to eliminate routes with uneven sidewalks!

The volunteer group makes a variety of items for Ramsey County Welfare Department: mittens, scarves, moccasins, and toys. The group was organized to be independent, but, like most groups, needs the enthusiastic support and the presence of the staff to keep motivation high.

Perhaps the most challenging aspect of the project is prevention via health education and promotion of preventive health care behaviors. Included are the traditional work simplification, energy conservation, and joint protection techniques. However, problems arise because health, for many of the older clients, remains an abstract concept, and many perceive little benefit to be gained at this time from a change in habits. The

(continued)

Home Services

staff must use a variety of approaches and methods to promote the belief that knowledge and application of good health practices does provide tangible benefits at any age.

Examples of our "promotion" are afternoon socials that entice attendance with nutritious refreshments and a Victor Borge film extolling fitness for seniors. The exercise classes discuss various aspects of health and refer people to the nutrition classes, which similarly relate regular exercise to good health. The project distributes newsletters, informational booklets, and individual instructions, all typed in large print to compensate for possible visual deficits. This information is often modified to enhance comprehension and acceptance because over fifty percent of our clients have had less than a ninth grade education.

Although it is difficult to measure the results of prevention programs, there is evidence that we are achieving the project's goal, i.e., maximizing the elderly clients' independence. We can observe immediate results when we intervene directly by modifying the environment or by providing adaptive equipment to increase functional independence. The on-going ADL evaluations demonstrate that our clients increase their level of independence and maintain those gains. Further, we expect to demonstrate a decreased rate of institutionalization for our clients after two years of services.— *Dixie Hayday, coordinator; Mary Ann Salvato, OTR; Shirleen Hokkanen, COTA; Lynn Ferguson, COTA; and Judy Phernetton, COTA*

Gerontology
Special Interest Section Newsletter; Vol. 3, No. 1, 1980

Professional Development: Writing a Grant Proposal

By Marlys M. Mitchell, PhD, OTR

Write a grant proposal? Who, me? Perhaps you, the reader, have thought about writing a proposal but quickly or reluctantly rejected the idea because you had no support system to guide you through the process and no ideas regarding how to start the task. This article will describe types of proposals, types of funding agencies, a format for writing a proposal; give general hints and suggestions; and discuss evaluation.

Perusal of any newspaper, regardless of size of circulation, shows that grants are awarded everywhere. Stories about million dollar foundation grants and government grants abound. The figures are staggering. It is natural to assume it is easy to obtain some of this vast pool of funding. This is especially true when the sums you are seeking are relatively small.

Success rates for getting a proposal funded are small, often as low as 10%, as the number of applications usually far exceeds the funds available. Then why try? Because there is a need for new and innovative programs; because there are consumers in need of what is to be "marketed."

Types of Proposals. Proposals may be distinguished in several ways. The first distinction is type of proposal. Types of proposals are: *program proposals*—to make identified services available to individuals, families, groups, or communities; *research proposals*—to evaluate or study a problem, group, organization, or service; *planning proposals*—to permit planning and coordination concerning a problem, group, organization, agency, or set of services; *training proposals*—to provide training and preservice or inservice education to individuals, groups, and organizations; and *technical assistance proposals*—to provide assistance to agencies, groups, organizations, and communities in establishing, implementing, and evaluating programs. Most proposals submitted by health and human service groups are program proposals, but many proposals contain a combination of two or more types.

A second kind of distinction is whether a proposal is made for an ongoing project or for a demonstration progect. The funding source typically indicates the nature of the available funds and specifies the regulations to be applied. Third, proposals may be solicited or unsolicited. A solicited proposal is publicized through written requests for proposals (RFP) made available to a wide group of individuals, agencies, and organizations. An unsolicited proposal is sent to a funding source without specification by that source of timeliness, type of proposal, or type of project.

Types of Funding Agencies. Three general types of funding agencies are the government, foundations, and corporations. Government sources fund projects for teaching/training, service, and research. RFPs specify priorities for funding to be given to proposals submitted. Careful reading of RFPs is important in finding the appropriate agency to which to submit a proposal. Government sources, as well as foundations consider special projects for funding. These projects permit great flexibility and creativity in development and implementation.

Identification of foundations can be done through reference works such as *The Foundation Directory, The Foundation Grants Index,* or the *Annual Register of Grant Support.* Government granting agencies can be located in the *Federal Register,* the *Catalog of Federal Domestic Assistance,* or the *U.S. Government Manual.* Corporations can be identified through *Forbes Market 500, Fortune Double 500 Directory, Dun and Bradstreet's Million Dollar Directory* or *Standard and Poor's Register of Corporations, Directors, and Executives.*

Grantsmanship. Marketing your project to a funding source makes your proposal more attractive than selling it. The difference is in the approach. In selling a project, you develop an idea, write a proposal, find a funding source, and submit a proposal. In marketing a project, you discover and act on the needs and desires of funding source, rather than on your needs. Success in grant funding depends on focusing systematically on the manner in which your project fulfills the needs of the granting agency, not on the manner in which it fills your needs.

Some steps to follow in developing a proposal include learning about the sources of funding, evaluating your attitude toward grantsmanship, developing grant ideas, determining your odds for funding, determining your most likely source of support, making an initial contact with the funding source, and writing the proposal (1).

Writing the Proposal

Funding agencies usually have their own forms and format for completion of proposals. These are obtained directly from the grant source.

The items of information include:
abstract,
statement of the problem, justification or need,
review of relevant literature,
objectives to be accomplished,

(continued)

Grant Proposal

procedures or methodolgy to achieve the objective,

evaluation techniques,

recommended dissemination procedures,

staffing needs,

budget requirements,

appendix materials, and

time line (2).

The Format

The GNOME chart is adapted from a model developed by Lefferts (1). GNOME stands for Goals, Needs, Objectives, Methods, and Evaluation. Developing answers for the various aspects of the chart leads one to structure a logical flow in conceptualizing the proposed project. The adapted model is shown below:

Goal	Need	Objective	Activity	Method/ Evaluation	Time Line

The *goals* are broad, general statements of your proposed program. Typically, a proposal has two or three goals. The *need* presents documentation of data from a review of literature or community/client survey to support your goal. *Objectives* are measureable actions which obviate the need and help you achieve your goals. Often two or three objectives are necessary to achieve a goal. Bloom's Taxonomy (3) is helpful in formulating objectives. *Methods* are enabling activities, the actions of the project which aid in fulfilling the objectives which meet the goal. Several activities are usually proposed to accomplish an objective. *Evaluation* is designed to determine whether an objective has been met. Evaluation procedures should ensure assessment of methods and/or objectives. Finally, a *time line* is useful in formulating an overall plan for the conduct of the project.

Intellectual discipline and attention to the above factors facilitates writing a grant proposal. The format and factors of the model compel the writer to envision the entie project from conceptualization to the implementation and evaluation.

A Sample

An illustrative chart is shown to demonstrate the model used to develop a grant proposal. (See below)

Tips on Writing Grant Proposals

The following tips will not ensure funding, but they will facilitate the writing process and make the final document readable and attractive.

- The project innovator should write the document, with planning meetings prior to writing, and review by others after the first draft is written. Writing by a committee is cumbersome and fragmented.
- Write in the third person—they, not I, or in the impersonal.
- Use a short title, ten words or less. If you've thought of a cute title, don't use it.
- A table of contents helps the reader if the proposal is long.
- Underline key words in the textual material to emphasize important concepts.
- Make your point as clearly and as quickly as possible. You're trying to make a point, not obscure it.
- Make positive statements, such as, "the program *will*," rather than, "*plan* to" or "*hope* to".
- Allow twice as much time as you think is needed to write the proposal.
- If you don't know how to start, complete the adapted GNOME chart, and then plan the budget. With those two accomplishments, writing has purpose, focus and direction.
- Keep it Short and Simple (KISS).

Evaluation

When the proposal is written and submitted, an unknown "they" will review the proposal, along with dozens or hundreds of other proposals. What are the questions to be asked or the criteria by which your proposal will be judged? All granting agencies have their own criteria, which may or may not be available to the applicant.

One set of questions to be asked concerns the framework, the methods, and the results. Framework questions will examine the problem statement, the definitions, the literature review, and the documentation. Methodology questions will detect omissions, evaluate measurement instruments and their reliability, evaluate control measures, identify populations, and examine procedures to be employed. Questions related to expected results will evaluate feasibility of methods to obtain results, importance of results, and dissemination of information.

Another set of criteria used to analyze fundability include: proven project workability, staff credentials, uniqueness, and appeal to funder (4).

Summary

Grant writing takes time, effort, and practice. Believe it or not, it can be an enjoyable experience. It takes almost as long to write a proposal for $100 as it does to write one for $100,000 and the rewards in terms of satisfaction are almost equal. Following the suggestions, guidelines, and procedures given in this article will not assure funding, but it will systematize your approach to the task of writing a proposal.

GNOME CHART — OT IN GERONTOLOGY

GOAL	NEED	OBJECTIVE	METHOD/ ACTIVITIES	EVALUATION	TIME LINE
1. To increase public awareness of services provided by OT	1. OT is a new service to be provided by Well County Hospital with a rehab wing with 100 beds	1-1 To deliver formal presentation about OT to all professional groups in Well County Hospital within one year	1-1-1 Prepare lecture 1-1-2 Prepare slide tape presentation	1-1 Keep records of presentation 1-2 Feedback from viewers, peers 1-3 Record breadth of speaking requests	July, Aug, Sept
		1-2 To prepare a brochure regarding OT	1-2-1 Contact hospital administration regarding distribution of brochure	1-4 Distribution of brochures (number) 1-5 Types of agencies or professionals distributed	Sept, Oct
2. To increase utilization of OT services	2. Data from National Rehabilitation Association show that 75% of patients in rehab centers have potential for return to work	2-1 To plan treatment programs for 50 patients within one year	2-1-1 Schedule and provide OT service in room, clinic 2-1-2 Transitional care visit to home	2-1 Assess progress via treatment notes 2-2 Record number of visits by OT in center and in home	Nov–June
	2-2 To participate in weekly patient case conferences		2-1-3 Home and community follow up visits 2-2-1 Present OT activity treatment program 2-2-2 Follow up with patients and professionals	2-3 Record number of community contacts and visits 2-4 Assess number of referrals for OT	Nov–June

References

1. Lefferts, R: *Getting a Grant.* Englewood Cliffs, N.J.: Prentice-Hall, Inc. 1978.
2. Orlich, DC, Orlich PR: *The Art of Writing Successful R & D Proposals.* Pleasantville, NY: Redgrave Pub. Co., 1977.
3. Bloom, B (Ed): *Taxonomy of Educational Objectives,* Handbook I: Cognitive Domain. NY: Longman, 1956.
4. Conrad, DL: *The Grants Planner,* San Francisco, CA: Institute for Fund Raising, 1978.

Gerontology
Special Interest Section Newsletter; Vol. 3, No. 1, 1980

A Group Approach to the Rehabilitation of Stroke Patients

By Noelle Berry, OTR, and Julie Garrity, MS, Licensed Speech Pathologist, Lakeside Nursing Home, Ithaca, NY

A year ago a Stroke Group was formed at Lakeside Nursing Home to bring together residents with similar problems. Factors contributing to the formation of this group were:

— the observation that among residents with cerebral vascular accident there appeared to be a lack of understanding of stroke, its causes, and associated disabilities.

— a need to practice skills learned in therapy in a natural setting.

— the observation that these residents needed ongoing support in coping with their disability-related anxieties, frustrations, and fears.

— the awareness that knowledge about a medical condition facilitates its acceptance.

— the need for a mechanism to facilitate meeting others with similar problems to alleviate isolation and loneliness.

Group members were selected from those receiving occupational therapy and speech therapy. Residents from both the Health Related Facility and the Skilled Nursing Facility were eligible. Participants were required to be able to function in a group setting. To provide an optimum level of interaction and individual participation, group size was limited to five.

Individual treatment goals are developed from the occupational therapy and speech therapy evaluations. Performance in fine motor coordination, speech and language, group participation, perceptual-motor functioning, and psychological functioning is assessed. Progress is documented monthly. Goals are reviewed every three months at a patient care conference.

The group meets once a week for approximately one hour. Each week's activity is determined jointly by the residents and the therapists. A monthly calendar of scheduled activities is given to each member.

Some examples of the goals and the activities used to reach them follow:

A. Express experiences and feelings related to their stroke.
1. View stroke film series (Concept Media Series)
2. Discuss newspaper article — "A Family Works a Miracle," by D.H. Mel.em, *The New York Times Magazine,* March 11, 1979, Section C.
B. Increase independence in activities of daily living
1. Cook, bake, and clean up
2. Participate in community activities
a. Ride a bus
b. Perform car transfers
c. Go to a restaurant
3. Plant and care for the garden
4. Role-play life situations
C. Communicate in a small group
1. Participate in games such as story telling, lotto
2. Discuss topics of interest
D. Stimulate leisure interests
1. Carve pumpkins for the Special Children's Center
2. Bake for other residents and staff
3. Compile a cookbook of kitchen-tested recipes; compile suggestions for one-handed cooking

The original group formed one year ago is still meeting regularly. Referrals to the program have increased and a second group will be formed in the near future.

Gerontology
Special Interest Section Newsletter; Vol. 2, No. 4, 1979

Directions in Long-Term Care: Cracker Barrel Session, 1979 Conference

By Cynthia F. Epstein, MA, OTR, FAOTA

The issue from my viewpoint is not that our day may come, in fact, it has arrived! Our concern should be today's total health care system and its responsiveness to the needs of our expanding older population.

Statistics tell us that our older citizens who are categorized as *at risk of institutionalization* tend to be more than 75 years of age. Given our understanding of the aging process, we are aware that sensory and motor systems in this segment of the population operate with gradually decreasing efficiency. Most of our seniors, however, are unaware of these subtle changes, and use minimal compensatory techniques to continue functional independence within their home environments. No one bothers to further educate them or increase their awareness of how to cope more successfully with their deficits.

Eventually, lack of appropriate coping skills may lead to trauma, such as a fractured hip and then a necessary hospitalization.

We are all familiar with the acute health care system and its focus on assuring maximum recovery of the patient through immobilization and elimination of all decision-making tasks. This unfamiliar and controlling environment, while medically necessary, encourages complete dependency on the part of the frail and impaired senior who is in a crisis state. Should we then be surprised that the hospitalized older person suddenly begins to demonstrate increasing signs of *organicity, senility,* and *confusion* along with the presenting physical problem? Upon discharge, the patient may go home with supportive homecare services, or to a nursing home if coping skills and the home environment are not stable enough. In either case, treatment plans tend to focus on improving physical capacities, with little emphasis on helping the individual deal with their sudden awareness of a diminished ability to live independently.

How many of our seniors faced with this type of life crisis have the skills of an occupational therapist to call upon? It is through our intervention that this *at risk senior* can best develop the adaptive skills necessary to remain in or return to home. Our philosophy and perspective regarding the importance of maintaining health through self-directed activity is critical to this senior's survival in the community.

Not only must we assure that the senior has the benefit of our service and perspec-

(continued)

Cracker Barrel Session

tive, but equally important, we must educate and engage those around the senior of the treatment process. It is *not the patient alone* whom we treat. The system or environment which supports and interacts with the individual requires equal intervention from the occupational therapist.

Using a comprehensive evaluation, we should all be comfortable developing a treatment plan for the frail, impaired senior previously described. Whether at home or in a long-term care facility, we will provide tasks which will incorporate sensory and motor components, independent living skills, cognitive and psychosocial skills and necessary adaptations. In their nuturing and supportive role, we can comfortably deal with our clients, encouraging and facilitating their progress.

What we tend to overlook, however, is that this client is only part of our treatment concern, The environment in which the client exists must have equal weight in our treatment plan. It is here that our comfort level tends to diminish. In order to treat the supporting environment we must change our treatment process and the type of role we assume. We must be willing to assume a more directive and perhaps controlling role, understanding how to use power as a positive force for change.

Just as we use primary keys in our patient evaluation, we must identify primary keys in our system evaluation. We need to identify and assess those who are the power people, how they view occupational therapy intervention in their system, and what the most effective strategies would be to effect positive change for our client. Given our expertise in analysis, we can view the total environment through our "OT Glasses" and identify the less functional portions of the system which would affect the client's potential for successful independent living. The treatment plan would then require use

of more directive techniques and change agent skills, modified by our understanding of behavior and group dynamics. Our goal, facilitating maximum independent functioning for individual consumer in their environment, then becomes achievable through this dual focus. Without this perspective, the necessary carryover and implementation of independent activities will be lost, taking place solely in the occupational therapy treatment milieu.

If we are to accept this challenge, and treat the environment or system with equal skill, we must become more comfortable with this role, and more knowledgeable in how to effect change in a system. Through our evaluation we can identify interests and needs in the system which fit mutually with our occupational therapy perspective. These then, are our starting points. It is ncesssary for us to find appropriate areas of mutual concern, for only in this way will we be able to generate support and enthusiasm for the change we wish to effect.

Where do we start? Which is the most appropriate area to impact? Long-term care is a continuum. It does not begin in the institution. It has its roots in the community.

Since we, as occupational therapists, are concerned with the continuum of care as it influences and affects the older person, we must develop a preventative focus. Therefore, we must address the issues through primary, secondary, and tertiary prevention programs.

In primary prevention we must educate the older consumers regarding the aging process. We must facilitate their understanding through a program of health education that identifies some of the universal functional problems faced in old age and alerts the consumer to possible adaptive behaviors or mechanisms. This type of intervention is possible through our involvement in adult education programs and in

senior citizen centers. Other health care providers in the community need to be educated regarding occupational therapy services so that they will refer clients to us who need our expertise, and ask us to be part of community health education programs.

In secondary prevention, we can address the needs of the consumer whose coping skills have been diminished by the aging process. Accidents in the home, such as hip fracture, can possibly be prevented with occupational therapy services to assist the older person in developing increased awareness of the need for adequate lighting, traction surfaces, work simplification techniques, adaptive equipment, appropriate leisure skills, and regular activity. Therapists involved in senior citizen centers, nutritional sites, home health programs, congregate living situations, retirement villages, adult day care centers and crisis intervention centers can deliver this service.

In tertiary prevention, the area with which we are most familiar, we attempt to reduce dysfunction through the provision of rehabilitative services. Nursing homes, extended care facilities, home health programs, and adult day care centers may be the setting. Whatever the setting, we must focus not only on the direct treatment need, but on the need for health education of staff, client, and the client's support system in the community. We must also be prepared to assume a more direct and visible role to facilitate change in our client's environment and life support system.

It is my belief that we can no longer hide ourselves by staying quietly within the confines of our clinics, or inside a patient's room or home, dealing with the client alone. We are remiss in our application of the concepts of occupational therapy if we consider our sphere of influence in the arena of long-term care as the microcosm instead of the macrocosm.

Gerontology
Special Interest Section Newsletter; Vol. 2, No. 4, 1979

Test Review: Human Development Inventory

By Teepa Snow, BS, OTS

Description: The Human Development Inventory (HDI) was developed by gerontological researchers to assess the psychosocial functioning of elderly residents in long-term care facilities.

Items to be evaluated were generated by a review of the literature in gerontology and psychology, and input from the staff at Ebenezer Center for Aging, Minneapolis, MI. Criteria used for formulating the HDI

were that it: 1) be based on a whole-person model, 2) promote adaptation by systematically assessing strengths as well as needs, 3) be easily translated in individualized care plans, 4) be useful to practitioners and researchers, 5) be able to be studied for reliability and validity, 6) be sensitive to change over time, and 7) be simple enough to be administered by facility personnel.

The HDI evaluates 27 components of

psychosocial function. These items fall into the areas of sensory capabilities, communication skills, alertness, satisfaction, socialization, and inner peace. Responses to each item are rated on a six-point Likert-type scale, assessing the extent as well as the existence of need.

The HDI evaluation follows the format of a semi-structured conversational interview.

(continued)

Human Development

Open-ended questions are asked during the course of casual conversation to avoid a testing/evaluation atmosphere. The objectives of interviewing and observing the resident are to gain some objective and subjective information about psychosocial functional abilities. *Alertness* is assessed from the information about recent and remote memory, orientation to time and place, self-reliance, decision-making ability, and tendency to wander. Satisfaction is assessed via data on adjustment to present residence, satisfaction with the facility and present life, interaction with family and staff, and ability to accept changes in scheduling. *Inner Peace* is assessed by the interviewer's perceptions of the resident's self concept, life review skills, and concern with death and dying for one and others. *Socialization* abilities are assessed via conversation with the residents about the quantity and quality of their interactions, their participation in individual and group activities, and their tendency to remain in their rooms alone. Observations are made of the client in routine daily activities to clarify social information. *Communication* ability is evaluated in terms of verbal, nonverbal, and overall communication skills, and the ability to sustain a conversation. Information on changes in vision, hearing, smell, taste, and tactile sensitivity is obtained during the interview as it relates to their effect on daily living tasks.

The entire interview process takes approximately three hours per resident. This time frame includes actual interview time, medical chart review, write-up time, and time for observing the resident in daily activities. Once the HDI is administered, taking perhaps several sessions to complete, the information gleaned is used to identify strengths and areas of need for the resident. A total care plan is then formulated for the resident which is to be implemented by the entire staff of the facility.

Development: Validity of the HDI was measured by comparing it to other available assessments that measure the same dimensions. Preliminary studies of the scales indicate that the HDI is as least as valid as other instruments in measuring the given areas of psychosocial functioning. Further investigations of the tool's validity are currently in process.

Coefficients of internal consistency are within acceptable limits—between .72-.91 depending on the specific area. Overall inter-rater reliability is .66, which is lower than desirable.

The HDI can be used in a variety of ways in practice and in research. Some of the reasons for using the evaluation are to:

1) obtain an accurate profile of the psychosocial function of a resident in a long-term care facility;
2) gather information on strengths of individuals;
3) identify salient group charactertistics to place residents appropriately into groups that are compatible and complementary;
4) plan individualized treatment intervention and establish a treatment program that can best meet the needs and use the strengths of the resident;
5) assess the progress of the individual in meeting objectives;
6) educate the long-term care staff about the whole-person approach to treatment; and
7) evaluate the resident's ability to plan and execute his own treatment program.

The HDI is contained in a booklet entitled *Human Development Assessment and Care Planning* by Janine Pyrek, Lorraine Snyder, Kathy Carroll, and Lou Ann Mattson. This is available from: Ebenezer Center for Aging and Human Development, Minneapolis, MN 55407. Portions of this test review were taken from this booklet.

Gerontology
Special Interest Section Newsletter; Vol. 2, No. 4, 1979

Self-Assessment: The Aging Neurosensory Systems

1. All the following statements about vision and the elderly are true, **except:**
   a. a mild degree of loss in visual acuity is an intrinsic effect of aging;
   b. a large number of older individuals experience a loss of ability to discriminate colors;
   c. the ability of the lens to accommodate and form a clear image on the retina remains fairly constant throughout adult life;
   d. presbyopia is a chronic condition which occurs in older persons and results in an inability to see objects at close proximity.

2. Reasons for the reduction of visual acuity in the elderly include all, **except:**
   a. a smaller pupil area.
   b. less absorption and scattering of the light into the lens and vitreous.
   c. the presence of cataracts.
   d. increased intra-ocular pressure.

3. Of the following visual disorders, which occurs most commonly in the elderly?
   a. chronic glaucoma
   b. acute glaucoma
   c. senile macular degeneration
   d. cataracts

4. Senile macular degeneration results in:
   a. reduction of peripheral vision.
   b. a disability that can be surgically treated.
   c. a condition that is not helped by the use of magnifying devices.
   d. loss of ability to discriminate detail.

5. All the following aids may help the visually impaired older individual **except:**
   a. increased illumination for the person with cataracts.
   b. night lights to reduce the amount of adjustment from the dark to a lighted room.
   c. positioning your face within the reduced field of vision for the person with glaucoma.
   d. encoding various medicine bottles with colors and/or textures.

6. All the following changes in the structures of the ear lead to impairment of hearing, **except:**
   a. an increase in primary degeneration of the organ of Corti.
   b. an increase in elasticity of the basilar membrane of the cochlea and eardrum.
   c. a reduction of the number of nerve fibers in the sensory cells of the cochlea.
   d. a loss of epithelial nerve cells.
   e. a decrease in the blood supply to the neurosensory receptors.

7. The most common type of hearing impairment in the elderly is:
   a. tinnitus.
   b. hypersensitivity to loud noises.
   c. presbycusis.
   d. impairment of sound localization.

8. What is the percentage of hearing impaired individuals in the elderly population?
   a. 75-85%
   b. 55-65%
   c. 2-5%
   d. 20-30%

(continued)

Neurosensory Systems

9. All the following methods may prove useful in improving audition for hearing-impaired individuals, **except:**
   a. removing the excess wax from the outer ear.
   b. instituting a drug regime to control presbycusis.
   c. providing a hearing aid.
   d. speaking into the least affected ear.

10. In general, the sensitivity to smell:
    a. is the main reason elderly subjects are incorrect in identifying food odors.
    b. is only a minor problem in identifying foods compared to the loss of taste discrimination.
    c. will decline with age if it is used continuously over a person's life span.

11. Associated with the decline in the number of basic functioning neurons is:
    a. the maintained capacity for sending nerve impulses to and from the brain.
    b. a decrease in conduction velocity of nerve impulses.
    c. the maintained speed of voluntary motor movements.

d. a decrease in reflex time for skeletal muscles.

12. The following statements concerning tactile sensitivity are all true, **except:**
    a. vibration sensitivity diminishes after age 50.
    b. defects in vibratory perception occur in about 50% of those over 60.
    c. paresthesia is common among the elderly.
    d. pain threshold decreases among the elderly.

13. The tendency for the elderly to stand with flexed hips and knees is due to:
    a. altered neuromuscular control.
    b. impaired musle power
    c. impaired vestibular function.
    d. degenerative changes in joints.
    e. all of the above.

14. Decubitus ulcers:
    a. cannot be prevented whan a person becomes immobile.
    b. can occur within the first two weeks of institutionalization.
    c. indicate that a person's protein intake has been too high.

References

Brocklehurst, J.C. ed. (1978) *Textbook of Geriatric Medicine and Gerontology.* New York: Churchill Livingstone (pp. 227-289).

Brocklehurst, J.C. and Hanley, T. (1976) *Geriatric Medicine for Students.* New York: Churchill Livingstone (pp. 56-57, 94-105, 196-204).

Elipoulos, C. (1979) *Gerontological Nursing.* New York: Harper and Row, Publishers (pp. 258-273).

Gunter, L.M. and Ryan, J.E. (1976) *Self-Assessment of Current Knowledge in Geriatric Nursing.* Flushing, NY: Medical Examination Publishing Co., Inc. (pp 134-136).

Kart, C.S., Metress, E., and Metress, J. (1978) *Aging and Health: Biologic and Social Perspectives.* Reading, MA: Addison-Wesley Publishing Co. (pp. 60-73).

Lewis, S.C. (1979) *The Mature Years: A Geriatric Occupational Therapy Text.* Thorofare, NJ: Charles B. Slack, Inc. (pp. 26-29)

U.S. Dept of Health, Education, and Welfare, Public Health Service, National Institutes on Health. (1979) *Special Report on Aging: 1979.* NIH Publication No. 79-1907 (pp. 15-16).

Correct answers to Self-Assessment

1.c, 2.b, 3.d, 4.d, 5.a, 6.b, 7.c, 8.d, 9.b, 10.a, 11.a, 12.d, 13.e, 14.b.

Gerontology
Special Interest Section Newsletter; Vol. 2, No. 3, 1979

The Multidimensional Functional Assessment Questionnaire

by Teepa Snow, BS, OTS

Description: The Duke University Center for the Study of Aging and Human Development has devised a procedure for measuring the functional status of individuals and for identifying the health and social services they are receiving. It is part of the Older Americans Resources and Services (OARS) Methodology. The Multidimensional Functional Assessment Questionnaire (MFAQ) consists of two parts. Part A concentrates on function in five dimensions: physical health, mental health, social resources, economic resources, and activities of daily living. Part B focuses on the individual's perceptions of services that area available, needed, and used. The instrument follows the format of a structured interview. It requires about 45 minutes to administer.

Part A consists of seven major sections: demonographic information, social resources, economic resources, mental health, physical health, activities of daily living, and informant's impressions. The *demographic* data requested are: the client's name, address, telephone number, sex, education, location of the interview, and race. The *social resources* category assesses martial status, live-in companions, extent and type of contact with others, availability of a confidante, perceptions of loneliness, and sources and availablility of help. Information on *economic resources* includes employment status, major occupation, source of income, number of dependents, type and costs of housing, adequacy of financial resources, health insurance, and spouse's employment. *Mental health* is the fourth category explored. The Short Portable Mental Status Questionnaire (SPMSQ) and the Short Psychiatric Evaluation Schedule developed by Pfeiffer are used. Specific questions are asked concerning the extent of worry, satisfaction, and interest in life, current mental status, and the change over the last five years in that status. Indices used to assess *physical health* are information on visits to physicians, days sick, days institutionalized, current medications, current illnesses, life style, physical impairments and disabilities, and self-assessment of health. The individual's capabilities in performing *activities of daily living* such as telephoning, cooking, bathing, controlling bowel and bladder, and shopping, and the presence of another person to assist in these activities

are assessed in this section of Part A.

Another individual who is very familiar with the client is then interviewed concerning all the above areas in order to improve perspective on the client's abilities. A final part of the first half of the interview is completed by the interviewer after the formal evaluation. Impressions concerning the client's current status and the reliability of information gathered are recorded. At this time the interviewer also rates the individual's functional status in each of the five areas on a six-point scale. The scale ranges from 0 to 6, with 0 being equivalent to no impairment and 6 indicating total impairment. Each of the responses to interview questions is coded and the combination of answers produces a score indicative of the overall level of functional ability.

Part B of the MFAQ addresses the availability, need, and use of a wide variety of services. The client is asked the extent to which he has used those services in the past six months, the intensity of current use, the perceived need for the services, and the name of the service provider. Examples of services are mental health, financial assist-

(continued)

Functional Assessment Questionnaire

ance, physical therapy, supportive services, and sheltered employment.

Development: The MFAQ was developed by a team of clinicians from a variety of disciplines (occupationl therapy was not included) and research investigators. Validity was assessed by comparing the functional status assigned on the basis of questionnaire responses and the functional status assigned after extensive examination by clinical experts in each of the behavioral areas. The MFAQ results on the activities of daily living category were higher than the results obtained by the physical therapist and nurses. In other areas, there was high agreement between the MFAQ and the clinicians' results.

The MFAQ appropriately discriminates among groups whose functional status one would expect to differ, for instance, nursing home residents versus elderly individuals living in the community.

Interrater reliability coefficients were obtained. In this case, reliability refers to the probability that the same results will be obtained if the same subject is interviewed by another examiner. The reliability coefficients (Kendall's coefficient of concordence) were acceptable (.77-.88 depending on the specific behavioral area assessed).

A soft-covered book is available from the Duke University Center for the Study of Aging and Human Development (Box 2914, Duke University Medical Center, Durham, NC 27710) entitled *Multidimensional Functional Assessment: The OARS Methodology*. It provides background on the development of the instrument, summaries of studies conducted using the instrument, information on the proper use of the instrument, a sample of the questionnaire, and additional information on the rating scales and their use.

Uses of the MFAQ include: initial evaluation prior to (or at the time of) admission to a facility, documentation of treatment, evaluation of the needs of older persons living in the community, and population surveys.

3

Mental Health
Special Interest Section

Mental Health
Special Interest Section Newsletter; Vol. 6, No. 2, 1983

Starting a Stress Management Program

By Sharon Mueller, RN, and Melinda Suto, OT, Adult Day Programme #1, Burnaby Mental Health Centre, Canada

Within the last few years, stress management has become the subject of numerous lectures and workshops. They are sponsored by educational institutions, health care agencies and the business community. What precisely is meant by the phrase "stress management" as it relates to (mental) health care services? For our purposes, we have defined stress management as the "coping behaviors that are learned to reduce the effects of over-stress resulting from the environment, the social and cultural milieu, and specific life events." The purpose of this paper is to convey general knowledge of stress and how it affects people, and to explore individuals' stresses and find effective ways to cope with them.

Although most people could benefit from learning skills with which to cope with life stresses, there exists a high-risk population that we will focus on in this paper. Specifically, these people are: patients (and their families) with a psychiatric disorder, patients who are chronically ill (e.g., diabetes, rheumatoid arthritis), the elderly and the physically handicapped.

People chosen for this group had a variety of psychiatric diagnoses (except those currently psychotic or suicidal), but it was more useful to judge their degree of maladaptive coping behavior than to rely solely on medical diagnoses. Referrals were accepted from the local Community Care Teams, and for people currently in the Day Programme. Those clients who attended the Day Programme and the stress management group had increased opportunities to practice their new skills within a supportive setting and receive feedback on their attempts.

In developing this program, material was used from books by Hans Selye[2,3] and Friedman & Rosenman[1], and prevailing theories on subjects such as nutrition, yoga, balancing exercise, work and play, etc. The treatment program used an educational model and allowed for group discussion. This format encouraged group support, problem-solving and a sharing of personal experiences. During the two and one half hour, once-weekly meetings, homework was discussed, new information presented, and the final half hour involved application of relaxation techniques (i.e., yoga, progressive relaxation, etc.). A handout covering the day's material was also available to participants during this five-week period. Specific outlines for each stress management session are summarized below, followed by a detailed discussion of selected topics.

Session one dealt with the aims of the group, confidentiality, participants' responsibility, and outlined the following four sessions. The topics covered in the first session were defining stress, sources of stress, psychological signs of stress, physiological signs of stress, finding one's optimum stress level, the importance of paying attention to signs of overstress, a personal evaluation that included client goals and individual stressors, and relaxation exercises.

Session two discussed the correlation between stress and illness, reducing negative effects of stress, replacing maladaptive coping behaviors, and changing attitudes toward situations.

Session three included an examination of attitude changes, healthy life-styles, more relaxation techniques, and analyzing individual work/play/sleep patterns.

Session four covered specific stresses inherent in the following life periods: childhood, adolescence, young adulthood, middle age, and aged. Also, we elaborated on the handling of over-stress arising from home, work and social situations.

Session five included a discussion of physical exercises to use when faced with stressful situations, listing in point form of "things to remember" in dealing with stress, role-playing difficult situations using the video, and evaluating of the program to find out whether people achieved their goals.

Defining stress is an important aspect of the program since many people are not aware that they are experiencing a physiological or psychological response to stress. Individual differences are also important. Some people thrive on being busy, whereas others have a much lower tolerance for a busy schedule. Similarly, different people have various methods for handling stress. One person relaxes by doing physical activities, whereas another person prefers to do relaxation exercises or read.

The correlation between stress and illness was also discussed. Emphasis was placed on the ability of the individual to influence his or her health in a positive manner by dealing effectively with stress and by using healthy coping behaviors such as relaxation, yoga, or physical exercise, as opposed to doing such things as overeating and over-smoking. A healthy life style is an important tool in dealing with stress. Such techniques as assertiveness training can be useful, as can attitude change. For example, a person can learn to say "I would like to get this done," instead of "I

must get this done."

Having a balance between work, play and sleep is also important. One exercise used in the course is a "life pie." Clients are asked to divide the pie according to how much time they spend at work, play and sleep over a 24-hour period. These are then divided further into whether these activities are physical or mental. In this way, they can look at how much time is spent in each area and can evaluate where changes are needed to achieve a balanced life style.

The course also deals with the effects of change on stress level. Although Hans Selye's stress scale is outdated, it is discussed briefly, and the importance of not having too much change at one time is emphasized. If, for instance, someone had just changed residences as well as recently married, it might not be a good time to change jobs as well. Even positive events can be stressful when they involve change, and limiting the number of changes occurring at the same time is an important factor in preventing over-stress. It is also important to consider stresses specific to different aspects of life. Home, work and social situations each present certain problems. Stresses arising from home life and social situations are primarily related to skill and comfort in interpersonal relationships. Although work stresses involve these areas, they also involve pressures specific to the job. Stresses arising from any one area can affect the individual's ability to function in another.

The following procedures are used to evaluate how individuals deal with stress. In each instance, clients are asked to identify what they find stressful, and to consider how they are currently dealing with these stresses. Are they doing such things as over-smoking, over-eating, or over-drinking to cope, or are they using more healthy methods? If their usual methods seem inadequate, more useful ways of dealing with stress can be pointed out. Particular attention should be paid to the individual's own stress tolerance. Is he or she a "racehorse" or a "turtle"? What is fun for one person may be stressful for another.

Skills such as diaphragmatic breathing, relaxation exercises and yoga can be taught as alternatives to unhealthy coping behavior. Other behaviors, such as assertiveness training, leading a generally healthy and balanced life style, and using breaks in the day's routine for relaxation and exercise, are useful as well. Limiting change when under stress is also an impor-

(continued)

tant technique, as is being assertive and direct about needs and sharing feelings. A list of specific stresses with possible solutions can then be generated, providing the client with a number of alternatives. The more alternatives the individual has available, the less likely to be overwhelmed by stressful situations.

It is also important to be aware that different life stages give rise to certain specific stresses. A child just starting school, for example, will experience stress as a result of the necessity to leave home, make friends, and function independently, whereas the adolescent will be more concerned with the issues needed to deal with as he or she changes from child to adult. The child or adolescent who is under stress may demonstrate it by stuttering, nail-biting, poor eating and sleeping, or rebellious behavior. If this type of behavior is apparent, it is useful to find out what specific stress is occurring and to look at more positive ways of dealing with it.

Likewise, the young adult, the middle-aged and the elderly have their own set of problems. The young adult will have to make career choices and become emotionally and financially independent. The adult in the middle years will be likely to experience such things as the "empty nest syndrome," accepting the problems of aging and perhaps looking after aging parents. Again, it is important to evaluate the specific stress and to adapt healthy methods of dealing with it. The middle years can be used as a time to re-evaluate life roles and goals and to set new goals for the next thirty years.

Perhaps no age group has more problems of stress than the elderly. Loss of physical or mental ability, loss of friends, power, independence and role in society all contribute to the difficulties of the older citizen. Stresses can be identified and alternate solutions generated for each problem. Planning ahead of time for change of life style can be particularly useful as it enables the individual approaching retirement to cushion the effects of change by developing interests away from work, building a network of friends and developing a variety of interests.

In evaluating techniques for handling stress, several things become apparent. A variety of techniques are needed because specific situations require different skills. In addition, it was evident that different methods work for different people. When clients evaluated the stress management program, no specific technique was seen by the group as being most helpful. Individual groups found different things useful. Some found relaxation exercises and yoga most helpful, whereas others found sharing feelings, being assertive and leading a more balanced life-style most important.

A number of stress management techniques can be adapted for use in the general hospital setting. Health care teaching needn't take a great deal of staff time and can pay off in extra dividends for the patient. First, he needs to evaluate his life-style. Get him to do a "life pie" to assist him in his evaluation. Is his life balanced between work, play and sleep? Does he get adequate exercise and rest? What stresses is he presently under and what is he doing about it? What changes are happening in his life and can some of these be postponed? Will there be any long-term effects of illness and what stress management techniques can he use in view of this illness? The person with coronary difficulties, or the patient with a permanent physical disability, who formerly used vigorous physical exercise as a form of relaxation, will need to look at alternate methods of coping with stress. Relaxation exercises and yoga can be taught and patients could be given cassette tapes to listen to and follow. Teaching the patient to cope with the physical aspects of illness is also important. Talk to the patient and try to ascertain how he or she views that illness. Keeping the stresses of different life periods in mind and helping to evaluate the patient's life style can be useful in identifying the stresses a patient may be under, and can help in planning the nursing care.

In summary then, there are certain general principles in stress management. These are as follows:

1. We need to re-evaluate our life patterns and to take control over our lives.

2. Stress weakens psychological resistance as well as immunological response.

3. Be aware that your emotional and physical health affect each other.

4. Avoid excessive simultaneous life changes. Be aware of which pace of life is appropriate for you and pay attention to yourself.

5. If feeling uncomfortable, stop to consider why and make any appropriate changes.

6. Maintain a steady pace at work and play. Avoid great swings in activity levels. Pace yourself.

7. Remember to equalize stress through variety in daily activities.

8. Live at a tempo and direction best suited to yourself. Remember, "One man's work is another man's play."

9. Adopt a healthy life-style and a positive attitude.

10. Work on clear communication to decrease tension in interpersonal situations. Don't be afraid to make your needs known.

11. Learn a variety of coping techniques so that if one doesn't work you can use another.

12. Note those around you who cope well and try mimicking their behaviors.

13. Remember, it's not stress in itself that is harmful but rather, what you do or don't do to deal with it.

REFERENCES

1. Rosenman, R., and Friedman, M., *Type A Behaviour and Your Heart* Fawcett Crest 1978.
2. Selye, Hans, *The Stress of Life,* McGraw-Hill, 1976.
3. Selye, Hans, *Stress Without Distress,* New American Library 1974.
4. Pelletier, Kenneth, *Mind as healer, mind as layer: a Wholistic approach to preventing stress disorders,* Dell Publishers, 1977.
5. Holmes, T., and Rahe, *"The Social Readjustment Rating Scale"* Journal of Psychosomatic Research 2, (1967)

Mental Health
Special Interest Section Newsletter; Vol. 6, No. 1, 1983

From the Chair, Ann Conway: Occupational Therapy Directions in Mental Health, Task Force Report I

In August 1982, AOTA President Carolyn Baum and the Executive Board charged the Mental Health Special Interest Section (MHSIS) to form a Task Force on OT Directions in Mental Health (MH). I was requested to chair the task force, and other members appointed were: Gail Fidler, OTR, FAOTA; Susan B. Fine, MA, OTR, FAOTA; Linda Kohlman McGourty, MOT, OTR; and Elizabeth Tiffany, MED, OTR. The task force met on November 5, 1982, in Rockville, MD, and this is my first of two reports on its outcome. I am very pleased to report on this task force, since current practice issues and concerns of OTs in mental health were addressed and recommendations for future activities in the Association were developed to resolve these problems. These recommendations already have been communicated to the Executive Board.

Before I outline the recommendations and subsequent outcome of the task force, I want to summarize the process of the meeting. First, the task force reviewed all previous task forces on OT in mental health. Second, the task force addressed the following current professional issues of OT practice in mental health:

- reimbursement of services
- legislation
- the trend of decreasing numbers of OTs working in MH
- OT's relationship to other activity therapy disciplines
- educational preparation of OTs for MH practice
- role blurring
- need for increased visibility of OT in related MH groups, associations, etc.
- need for productivity standards.

These issues have been identified by MHSIS members, the AOTA National Office and the task force.

A special thanks to Mark Rosenfeld, MS, OTR, for his article, "Open Letter To Therapists," in the *MHSIS Newsletter,* Volume 5, No. 2, which delineated some of the above concerns. I also want to thank those of you who wrote letters in response to Mr. Rosenfeld. They were very helpful to the task force.

To proceed to the summary of the specific outcomes of the task force, they are as follows:

1. A role and function paper on OT practice in MH will be developed by AOTA. The Executive Board has charged the Commission on Practice to prepare this paper for the 1984 Representative Assembly. MHSIS members also will be involved in the development of this paper.

2. The task force discussed the importance of having OT recognized as a core profession in MH legislation. The excellent efforts of the AOTA Government and Legal Affairs Division (GLAD) to achieve this goal was commended. The MHSIS will continue to actively support this goal by keeping members abreast of legislation in the *MHSIS Newsletter* and state liaison mailings.

I will be sharing more information about the task force with you in the next *MHSIS Newsletter* and at the MHSIS Annual Meeting in Portland, but if you do have any questions, thoughts, etc., at this point, please let me know. I can be contacted at 3564 Michigan Avenue, Cincinnati, OH 45208.

Mental Health
Special Interest Section Newsletter; Vol. 6, No. 2, 1983

From the Chair, Ann Conway: Occupational Therapy Directions in Mental Health, Task Force Report II

In the last *Mental Health Special Interest Newsletter,* I presented a review of the issues addressed by the Task Force and began outlining recommendations and outcomes to resolve these issues. This report will summarize the remaining activities at this time.

In the future initiatives may be taken by the Association to resolve the practice issues of Occupational Therapy in Mental Health (MH). Past-President Carolyn Baum sent the Task Force Reports to the 1983 Representative Assembly, and I presented the Task Force concerns to the Commission on Education (COE) at their meeting in Portland.

The remaining issues and recommendations identified by the Task Force are:

1. OT needs increased visibility in related MH groups, associations, etc. We need to inform these groups of our knowledge in psychosocial daily living skills and vocational rehabilitation. Consequently, the following projects will be future activities of the MHSIS:

   a. Develop panel presentations to submit to the Hospital and Community Psychiatry (H&CP) and Orthopsychiatry conferences.

   b. Develop a proposal to sponsor a meeting or conference at the H&CP annual conference. This meeting will be held prior to the H&CP Program. In addition, opportunities for members to present to MH groups and conferences are important to achieve this educational goal.

2. A review of some of the activity disciplines will be completed by the Division of Practice, National Office. A matrix of demographic information will be developed to include size, number of members, scope of services, and educational and certification requirements of these disciplines.

3. More information on reimbursement

(continued)

Ann Conway: Task Force Report II

will be available to members. AOTA's Government and Legal Affairs Division (GLAD) devoted the March issue of the *Federal Report* to reimbursement, and specifically refers to mental health practice areas. To obtain a copy, please send $2.50 to GLAD at the AOTA National Office. The check should be made payable to AOTA.

4. Action should be taken to address the shortage of OTs in MH. The number of OTs practicing in MH has increased significantly. As the number of OTs has increased, however, the percentage of OTs working in MH has decreased from 34.6 in 1973 to 26.8 in 1982.

A brochure, *OT in Mental Health*, is currently being developed by the American Occupational Therapy Foundation. Once completed, this brochure will be available to members for recruitment and public relations purposes.

In addition, the issue of the declining number of OTs in MH has been referred to the AOTA Manpower Commission. The Task Force informed the commission that a similar decline of other MH professionals, such as psychiatrists, has been reported. Appropriate study and analysis of this parallel trend was recommended.

5. The educational preparation of OTs for MH practice should be addressed. The following recommendations were presented at the COE meeting held in Portland:

a. *The Revised Education Standards* should be changed to require a Level II Fieldwork placement in a psychosocial setting. This requirement, the Task Force reports, would not only maintain quality practice in MH, but would also be a valuable experience for therapists in all practice areas.*

b. The *Revised Educational Standards* should be more specific so that quality practice is reflected.

c. A quality MH fieldwork center should be identified and used as a model for other centers.

d. The following components should be included in OT curriculums:
- the psychosocial rehabilitation model
- the biological, psychological, and sociological frame of reference
- management/leadership skills
- knowledge of productivity standards

e. A need to have more master's level programs in MH is evident. These curriculums should stress leadership and management skills to prepare OTs for programmatic management.

6. Leadership and management training is needed. As you may know, AOTA's Continuing Education Division is developing a competency-based curriculum in mental health similar in design to the TOTEMS project.

More information concerning the curriculum will be published in the next issue of the *MHSIS Newsletter*.

Mental Health
Special Interest Section Newsletter; Vol. 6, No. 1, 1983

Music for Movement

By Karen J. Miller, MOT, RMT, OTR
The King's Daughter Hospital, Ashland, Kentucky

Music has become a popular addition to movement activities in mental health settings. It is used frequently with calisthenics, sensory integration and for expressive movement. Music is indeed vital to these approaches; therefore, the selection of music should be considered carefully, since it is an essential part of activity analysis and planning.

The purpose of this article is to provide therapists with guidelines for the selection and utilization of music for their various activities. A brief theoretical background will also be provided.

Theory: Why is the selection of music so important? There are certain elements involved in music that are especially significant for any activity involving movement. The first element of music, the tones and notes, functions as an auditory stimulation. Music travels on sound waves that enter the ear and set up vibrations in the tympanic membrane. It moves on into the middle ear as the stapes, incus and malleus bones pick up the vibrations and amplify them so that they will be distinct and more easily interpreted. The vibrations continue to travel on into the inner ear to be received by nerve endings. The CNS translates this information for the brain to tell us what pitches and tones we are hearing. The CNS also transmits information about the other elements of music, rhythm and tempo.

Rhythm and tempo comprise the remaining elements of music relevant to movement. Rhythm is the beat of the music. Tempo is the speed. The sound waves that carry music move in a corresponding manner with the rhythm and tempo. These data are therefore included in the vibrations that enter the ear. The additional stimulation provided by these elements travels via the same route to the CNS. The CNS first interprets it, then relays messages about the rhythm and tempo not only to the brain, but also to the muscles. When the information is received by the musculature, it, in fact, elicits an involuntary motor response. Fine muscle groups will usually respond to these messages before the larger ones. (Discover this yourself the next time you catch yourself tapping your fingers to music you weren't even paying attention to!)

Thus, the musical elements of tone, tempo and rhythm, when combined, enable music to function as a neuromuscular facilitator. This is especially true when it is used to reach a subcortical level. This type of stimulation will make the activity more easily obtained, more fun, because it is easier, and will encourage a spontaneous vs cognitive response. These factors are considera-

(continued)

Music for Movement

tions for sensory integration. Exerting control of the musical selection, or auditory stimulation, is the difference between music as a therapeutic modality and music as just a socially acceptable addition to your sessions.

Guidelines: Music for therapy activities may be chosen from recordings specifically designed for movement, or from classical and contemporary favorites. The following guidelines are suggested:

1. *Tempo*—The tempo or speed should be at a comfortable pace to accomplish the desired motions. Begin with a speed that is at or below the patient's ability to move rhythmically. If patients display psychomotor retardation or poor motor planning, a quick tempo (i.e., the theme from "Rocky") would be inappropriate, since it would cause further confusion and disability. Start with a slow-to-moderate pace. If the participants can do what you ask without too much difficulty, then gradually increase the speed. If you find that the patients have trouble following the tempo and rhythm during the course of a session, you can slow their movements by responding on every other beat of the music or once for every complete measure (i.e., once every four beats). If they can't adapt to that approach, plan to use different music.

2. *Rhythm*—The music should have a steady, unchanging beat that is easily heard and followed. A strong percussion-like background or clapping sound (i.e., "Rise" by Herb Alpert) will be very helpful. There are numerous perceptual-motor records available that were developed with these guidelines in mind, such as "Movin'" by Hap Palmer on Educational Activities, Inc. Many popular or commercial recordings may vary in both tempo and rhythm during one given selection (i.e., theme from "Magnum P.I." can be hard to follow). So, choose pieces that will have a fairly consistent pace. An option is to move only during the segments of the music that are appropriate and take a brief rest during the inappropriate segments. Last, but certainly not least, keep your movements going with the rhythm. This will reinforce the music as a facilitator and will make the movements easier.

3. *Volume*—Music should be easily heard by the entire group, but not so loud that it distracts from the rest of the activity. The leader's voice should be audible without having to shout.

4. *Instrumental vs Vocal*—As a general rule, use instrumental music, especially if your patients are low functioning or distractible. Vocal music adds an additional stimulus. You may find participants focussing on the words and not on the desired movement responses. This can turn their attention to a cortical level. The words could also feed into delusional thoughts or reinforce inappropriate behavior (i.e., preoccupation with sex or drugs, often mentioned in rock music). There certainly are times, however, when vocal music is suitable. It would be fine for many higher functioning groups and for awareness sessions where the words of the song may encourage problem-oriented discussion.

5. *Quality*—Whenever possible, use high quality equipment and recordings. The more realistic the sound waves are, the easier for the CNS to interpret.

6. *Other Considerations*—When selecting music it is important to keep in mind the age, culture and musical tastes of your patient population. You would not want to play music obviously for children when working with adults. Do not rule out all elementary school perceptual-motor records, however; many of the instrumental ones are original music that are not based on children's songs. These can be used successfully with adults.

7. *Leading the Session*—Screen and select your music before using it with patients. You will be far more effective if you take time to become familiar with your selections and experiment a bit with the physical actions you want to present. This will help you maintain the rhythm and pace. A smoothly run session will have a better chance of eliciting spontaneous responses. I have found that patients are more successful doing calisthenic exercises if I don't count the number of repetitions out loud, but stay with the music and change to a new exercise after a few measures or phrases. This seems to diminish cortically controlled movements.

Plan to use the same music for a number of sessions, especially with lower-functioning patients, since repetition has an organizing effect and will help improve responses. Chances are you'll become bored with the music before they do!

8. *Precautions*—As stated earlier, music stimulates and facilitates. Please be aware that you can change behavior just by the music. Apply the same principles you would apply with other forms of stimulation. A slow tempo with a constant, repetitive rhythm can relax or depress. Likewise, quick music with changing or snappy rhythms can excite or elevate. For example, you would not want to use fast disco music with a person in a manic state, but you might want to use a slower, relaxing piece such as "Canon in D" by Pachelbel to calm the person down.

In addition, you may want to avoid very unusual music that may have clashing tones or strange sounds. If it makes you cringe, think of the effect it might have on one of your patients.

The last precaution is to know when not to use music. Extremely confused and distractible patients may require a decrease in stimulation. Adding music to their morning exercises may not be appropriate. However, this needs to be assessed on an individual basis, since music may be so familiar and comforting to certain patients that it may break through some of the confusion.

Summary: Music is a valuable assistant during movement-related activities because it functions as a neuromuscular facilitator. In this role it can act on a subcortical level. This, in turn, encourages the patient to react with a spontaneous, adaptive response.

Specific musical selections have not been given. It is often most convenient and inexpensive to use music from your personal collection or from the public library. However, if you would like a listing of resources of recordings that are especially created for perceptual-motor activities, send a self-addressed, stamped envelope to Karen Miller, Occupational Therapy Department, King's Daughters' Hospital, 2201 Lexington Avenue, Ashland, KY 41101.

A Consultative Program for Children

By Lynn Davis, OTR, Delaware Curative Workshop

The occupational therapist has opportunity to provide a multitude of services to the psychiatrically impaired child. One of the services is treatment of sensory integrative dysfunction. In my contracted services to the day hospital of Terry Children's Psychiatric Center in Wilmington, Delaware, I have found that approximately 60 percent of the clients or students have sensory integrative problems, poor body scheme and body awareness. The sensory integrative dysfunction is often manifested in the following ways:

1. difficulty keeping one's hand to self.
2. poor use of manipulative tools (avoidance of palmar surfaces)
3. bumping and/or hitting into objects in their environment and
4. misinterpretations of touch received by others, i.e., thinks others are hitting him, and/or holds hands too tightly. These manifestations can be changed by improving somatosensory functioning. Thus, specific goal directed consultative services were implemented to enhance the functioning of the clients within their classroom environment.

Initially, these services were implemented to promote improved postural control and body awareness; however, through specifying roles and expectations a number of other needs were met.

A. *Goals of Consultative Services:*
Educator's Goals:

1. Discuss normal growth and development and its effect on movement skills.
2. Gain an awareness of the wide variety of "normal" responses during movement experiences.
3. Become critical in noting a youngster's areas of difficulty.
4. Decrease the use of cognitive clues. (Avoid telling child how to move).
5. Increase knowledge regarding the influence of sensory stimuli including touch, movement and pressure.

Student Client Goals:

1. Increase awareness of body parts and its specific actions.
2. Decrease sensitivity to light touch.
3. Increase repertoire of movement.
4. Foster a positive regard while engaging in a movement experience.
5. Allow student to monitor and adapt his performance with minimal external demands.

B. *Program Description:*
The following three components were developed and implemented to meet the above stated goals.

1. An inservice for educators regarding the theoretical framework of sensation, and the importance of movement. Also, principles of movement education are introduced;
2. Six weekly classroom visits to introduce the students to a variety of movement experiences using balloons and other activities;
3. Written criteria including purpose, activities and clues on how to implement the tasks. This program is carried out through the following week.

C. *Rationale:*
Balloon activities, which were one of the selected treatment activities, were used because they provide an excellent medium to meet both the needs of the educators and their students. The children enjoyed sharing this activity time, and additionally, the activities served to assist change in their skills. Balloons are also inexpensive, portable and provide challenge on a number of different levels. With minimal structure the child can progress at his own pace, recognize success and pursue challenges.

D. *Results:*
This consultative program has been in practice for six weeks. Although, limited in scope, a number of changes have been noted. The educators have gained insight regarding the need to decrease their emphasis on using "cognitive—how to" clues and recognize that there is a wide variance of "normal" movements. The clients have become less rigid in their movements, demonstrate increased awareness of body parts and its actions, and are more explorative by seeking out new movement experiences. Through these consultative services, occupational therapy has provided results which support the benefits of specific, graded movement experiences. Lastly, the specific criteria in the consultation forms have provided this occupational therapist with a definitive role.

If you desire specific information regarding this consultation program, including treatment activities, etc., please feel free to contact me: *Lynn Davis, OTR, Delaware Curative Workshop, Inc., 1600 Washington St., Wilmington, DE 19802*

Mental Health
Special Interest Section Newsletter; Vol. 5, No. 4, 1982

The Borderline Patient and Occupational Therapy Treatment

By Gail Busman Goodman, OTR

Borderline patients are a perplexing and difficult population to treat. Despite current controversy over the criteria for the borderline diagnosis, there is sufficient agreement among professionals to pull together a clinical picture that can be described as typically borderline. Dr. Otto Kernberg and Dr. John Gunderson have done extensive research on borderlines, and their research—Kernberg's theory of object relations and subsequent ego deficits and Gunderson's descriptive behavioral symptoms—can be used to set a foundation for occupational therapy theory for the treatment of borderlines.

Because diagnostic terminology is complex, I have chosen to use Kernberg's structural diagnostic framework. In attempting to understand patients, one can think in terms of ego structures that are stable over time and are the source of observable behavioral symptoms. Differences between borderlines, neurotics and psychotics can be understood through examination of structural diagnosis and developmental milestones of the ego.

Structural Diagnosis

A structural diagnosis defines an organization of the ego that is essentially stable. The critical components are: the defensive mechanisms employed, the ability to maintain reality testing and the presence of identity integration. Differences in these three components will result in either a neurotic, psychotic or borderline structure. Borderline structure occupies an area between psychosis and neurosis, but shares certain structural components with both. It is most easily understood diagramatically. (See diagram number 1.)

The borderline can, at times, present in a neurotic fashion when employing the higher level defenses of intellectualization and rationalization. But he or she can also show a pathological picture when using splitting, denial and projective identification as a means of coping with interpersonal stress. His capacity to shift between these two presentations makes it difficult for others to understand who he is, and perhaps the proverbial "Dr. Jekyll and Mr. Hyde" personality is more descriptive of the borderline and not the schizophrenic

The etiologic basis for the development of the borderline structure is rooted in the separation-individuation phase of development. It is at this stage that the child successfully separates from the mother and begins to internalize positive self-perceptions. At this stage the child begins to substitute higher level defenses for the earlier ones, such as splitting. Those who do not successfully complete this developmental task are essentially "stuck" in toddler-type methods of handling the world and the following ego functions are maintained:
1. splitting—keeping apart opposing views of the same issue
2. increased anxiety when separation from the mother figure is perceived
3. denial of anxiety attached to the act of separation
4. interpersonal relationships that are experienced as all "good" and mothering or all "bad" and rejecting

Relation To Functioning

Borderline patients have multiple dynamic problems related to their inability to function as adults because separating behaviors have been thwarted by the mother and were not supported and rewarded. Unable to fully separate, the borderline patient does not develop functional skills and ego strengths achieved by the child who has separated. All relationships reenact either the clinging, dependent, positive and nurturing aspects of continued symbiosis, or the angry, rejecting and aloof aspects of feeble separation. The patient shifts from feeling himself as omnipotent and powerful and others are to be devalued; or others are idealized and the patient feels he is deservedly rejected. Relationships take on a kind of cat-and-mouse quality—early behaviors aim to create a positive alliance but is followed by demanding and clinging behavior that attempts to sustain a nurturing symbiosis. When positive mothering supplies are not forthcoming, the patient becomes devaluing, angry and grandiose as a way of defending against the anxiety of rejection.

These types of interpersonal behaviors result in frequent chaos between the patient and others, particularly in social relationships that do not tolerate excessive intimacy, such as the work environment. Such situations cause anxiety because the patient cannot fulfill symbiotic needs. Rejections are experienced by the patient and he subsequently employs denial and devaluation as a means of coping. The work environment becomes a stage for the patient to act out his developmental dilemma, but this is both inappropriate and frustrating. A work history of the borderline might reveal several attempts at meaningful employment, all of which were aborted. In-depth questioning might reveal chaotic relationships with bosses and co-workers that escalated to unendurable heights. The borderline patient frequently has a distaste for work.

Another explanation for the patient's marked lack of pleasure and success in work activities can be traced, again, to the developmental phase of separation-individuation. During this time the toddler is using his toys and other nonhuman objects to assist him in his task of separation. They function as projective recipients for those feelings he cannot tolerate. He will disown what he cannot integrate and attribute those qualities to his toys. One sees this process in action when observing a toddler "punish" his toy after being reprimanded himself. A teddy bear is banished to the corner, but then is given forgiving kisses. By manipulating the objects in his play, the child begins to integrate both positive and negative introjects. Eventually the teddy bear is relegated to the top shelf, but he has served an important function.

The borderline patient does not complete this developmental work and main-

(continued)

DIAGRAM NUMBER 1

	Defenses	Reality Testing	Identity Integration
N	higher	maintained	integrated
B	higher and lower	maintained	diffused
P	lower	not maintained	diffused

Borderline Patient

tains projection and projective identification as primary modes of operation. Activities, tasks and nonhuman objects are the recipients of negative feelings and do not provide pleasure. Frequently, borderlines are unable to become involved in a task and simply enjoy doing. They have not graduated to the point of being able to sublimate through doing.

Occupational Therapy Treatment

Occupational therapy treatment typically follows a sequence of events. We begin with an evaluation of the patient's cognitive abilities, physical skills and interpersonal style. We use a concept of graded treatment and we change the environment with the patient's acquisition of skills. We move from simple to complex tasks, gross to fine dexterity, parallel to cooperative group. The therapist's role is to intervene, teach more adaptive ways of functioning, and support and encourage the patient. Our treatment plan focuses on the most intrusive area of dysfunction first; we assist the agitated patient in fostering self-control before concerning ourselves with his ability to conceptualize a complex task. But borderlines require a different perspective on occupational therapy treatment.

Initially, in the OT activities group, the borderline may not present in any pathological or dysfunctional manner. Because there is little intrusion upon his cognitive processes—except under severe stress—he will be able to understand and perform complex tasks. He may appear to work cooperatively with others and in fact, be solicitous to peers. This initial activity style might seem so free of dysfunction that it is perplexing. However, a closer look at the dynamics will reveal several issues.

Remembering the developmental dilemma of separation as the primary issue for the patient, the therapist can interpret superior performance as the initial phase of seduction between herself and the patient. It will probably be followed by escalating needs for attention that will be impossible to satisfy. The relationship will then take a turn and the patient will

become angry, devaluing, perhaps even explosive. Much of this interpersonal drama will be played out through the tasks presented to the patient and other behaviors will surface. The patient may begin to throw out incompleted projects, remain on the periphery of the group, and alternate between seductive and sabotaging behaviors with peers. When these actions are pointed out to him, he may intellectualize them, become coldly condescending or simply deny their existence.

It is important for the therapist to remember what causes the patient's activity style and not counter with equal anger. The therapist must maintain an awareness of the patient's difficulties in functioning autonomously and in being separate. For the borderline, all tasks and groups become his transitional object once again. He will project his negative feelings onto objects, both human and nonhuman, and then devalue the recipient of these feelings as a way of maintaining a pure experience of "I'm good."

The treatment milieu recreates those developmental tasks that are most difficult for him to master. Therefore, the treatment should focus on assisting the patient in owning his split-off projections and integrating them into whole concepts. The role of the therapist is clarification and confrontation of the patient's maladaptive defenses. The treatment aims to first alter the fundamental ego weaknesses; this in turn will affect dysfunctional behaviors.

The treatment plan should include individual projects and group experiences. The individual treatment focus should be a project that is both creative and unique. It will allow for expression of both positive and negative feelings, thereby serving its purpose as a substitute transitional object. By being a projective recipient for the patient's feelings, it will be the source for discussion between therapist and patient.

The group experience can address concrete functional issues and assist the patient in changing his perception of independence as equal to abandonment, anxiety arousal and loss of human connection. The group will dilute the intensity of the

transferential and countertransferential issues that arise between therapist and patient. This will aid the therapist in keeping a perspective on the symbiosis-vs.-separation dynamic. The type of group to which the borderline patient is assigned should challenge his intellectual and creative capacities. Higher level pre-vocational groups that have clear-cut expectations would reproduce the work environment the patient finds difficult. Within this group, the therapist could confront the patient's defensive style with "co-workers" and "supervisors." Discussions among the patients about their capacity to work cooperatively and meet deadlines would help the borderline patient to begin functioning within a work environment. An understanding of why the situation is so difficult would be fruitful as long as verbalization does not become a substitute for doing.

Both the individual task and group experience should maintain the following treatment goals to:

1. provide an expressive modality for discussing and understanding underlying conflicts related to independent functioning
2. help the patient to integrate split-off projections and begin to employ higher defenses within work environments
3. learn appropriate behavior as part of a cooperative group
4. provide corrective intervention in interpersonal relationships
5. aid the patient in transferring new behaviors and skills to the outside (nonhospital) environment.

Borderline patients present a challenge to all psychiatric professionals. By understanding the dynamics that contribute to the dysfunctional patterns these patients present, occupational therapists can provide a treatment milieu that assists the patient in recreating and conquering developmental milestones. Prescribed activities and discussion of the feelings that are aroused during activity will help the patient to move to a higher level of functioning.

Mental Health
Special Interest Section Newsletter; Vol. 5, No. 3, 1982

DSM III: What's in It for Occupational Therapy?

By Barbara Morris Linser, OTR/L, University of Cincinnati Hospital

Based on "Utilization of the DSM III Multi-Axial System by Occupational Therapy" was presented at the 1982, AOTA Annual Conference by Stephen V. Dooley, OTR/L and Barbara Morris Lenser, OTR/L.

Since its publication in 1980, the *Diagnostic and Statistical Manual of Mental Disorders,* third edition, (DSM III)[1] has rapidly become an integral and dynamic tool used by the psychiatric team. Because the DSM III sets forth an entirely new approach to psychiatric diagnosis, it is imperative that occupational therapists understand this new system in order to communicate effectively with the multidisciplinary team and to plan the most appropriate treatment of the psychiatrically diagnosed client. Perhaps the most significant reason for occupational therapists to embrace the DSM III is for research and educational purposes. Through the diagnostic system set forth by the DSM III, a client's level of functioning can be quantified objectively, in a manner understood by all disciplines. Thus, our work as occupational therapists, our research and our theories can be more clearly documented, more easily compiled and better communicated using DSM III terminology.

To understand a DSM III diagnosis, we must first understand the multiaxial system of evaluation. The DSM III sets forth five axes on which an individual should be evaluated. The first three axes form the official diagnosis. Axes four and five provide additional information but are considered optional. These five axes are[2]:

Axis I • Clinical Syndromes
 • Conditions not attributable to a Mental Disorder that are a Focus of Attention or Treatment (V. Codes)
 • Additional Codes
Axis II • Personality Disorders
 • Specific Developmental Disorders
Axis III • Physical Disorders and Conditions
Axis IV • Severity of Psychosocial Stressors
Axis V • Highest Level of Adaptive Functioning Past Year

Axes I and II contain the entire DSM III classification of Mental Disorders.

Each disorder is systematically described, in the DSM III, in terms of current knowledge in the following areas: essential features, associated features, age at onset, course, impairment, complications, predisposing factors, prevalence, sex ratio, familial pattern, and differential diagnosis[3].

"Conditions Not Attributable to a Mental Disorder That Are a Focus of Attention or Treatment" called V. codes. These include such things as occupational problem (V62.20) or uncomplicated bereavement (V62.82) for which a person may seek help but does not constitute a mental disorder.

Axis III refers especially to "Those Physical Disorders and Conditions" that are relevant to the understanding or management of the client. For example, the adolescent with an oppositional disorder who also has diabetes presents a tricky management problem. "Soft neurological signs" may also be recorded on Axis III.

The multiaxial system is a major accomplishment of the DSM III because it asks diagnosticians to respond to more aspects of the client. It is less likely then that important information about a client will be overlooked due to the theoretical orientation of the diagnostician or due to the overwhelming nature of one particular problem the client is experiencing. This system will be helpful to the occupational therapist receiving referrals from a variety of diagnosticians. For example, a patient comes for help because she is having trouble functioning at work and home. Imagine three clinicians diagnosing this patient. The first clinician, a behavioral psychologist, diagnoses the patient's panic attacks. The second clinician, a psychodynamically oriented therapist, notes the patient's Dependent Personality Disorder. The third clinician, a family therapist, notes the patient's recent divorce.[4]

The occupational therapist's initial evaluation and subsequent treatment plan might vary dramatically depending on which clinician referred this patient. A referral from the behavioral psychologist might result in an evaluation of the patient's potential to use relaxation therapy. Were the referral received from the family therapist, the occupational therapist might evaluate ADL and activity configuration changes resulting from the patient's recent divorce.

The DSM III makes an attempt to modify this situation. With the DSM III being used by all three of the above clinicians, the patient's diagnosis would look like this:

Axis I Panic Disorder (300.01)
Axis II Dependent Personality (301.60)
Axis III Deferred (none relevant to this patient's treatment)
Axis IV Extreme (6)
Axis V Fair (4)

The DSM III makes a good attempt to be atheoretical. That is, it uses objective, describable symptoms and not theoretical concepts for diagnostic criteria. To ensure the usefulness of three descriptive diagnostic criteria, field tests were done in a variety of settings. More than 500 clinicians from varying theoretical orientations were involved in these field trials. The results are that each disorder classified in the DSM III is described in terms of symptoms that must be present (inclusion criteria), symptoms that must not be present (exclusion criteria), the amount of time that symptoms are present (duration criteria) and the age of onset of symptoms (age criteria).

The DSM III defines mental disorders as, "a clinically significant behavioral or psychological syndrome, or pattern that occurs in an individual and that is typically associated with either a painful symptom (distress) or impairment in one or more important areas of functioning (disability)"[5].

The rating of the severity of the Psychosocial Stressor (Axis IV) should be based on the clinician's assessment of the stress an "average" person would experience under similar circumstances[6]. "Average" refers to a person

(continued)

DSM III

with similar sociocultural values.

Taking into account the circumstances, one must consider that the average man with five children and a nonworking spouse would experience more stress from losing his job than would a childless man with a working spouse who loses his job.

An individual might react severely to a certain stressor (perhaps an argument with a neighbor); however, the stressor is rated as "mild" because that is how the average person would experience it.

The DSM III states that a person's prognosis is better when a disorder is a result of a severe stressor than when it develops after no stressor or a minimal stressor.

See Table 1 for the codes and terms used in making a rating on Axis IV.

When the psychosocial stressor represents a disruption or change in an occupational role, or represents a potential disruption of the occupational role acquisition process, the occupational therapist should be involved in:

1) adding in-depth evaluative information about Axis IV and,

2) in providing treatment focused on Axis IV.

A rating on Axis V, the highest level of functioning in the past year, takes into consideration three major areas: social relations, occupational functioning, and use of leisure time, according to the DSM III. See Table 2 for the levels of functioning conceptualized by the DSM III for Axis V.

Social relations include all relations with people, with particular emphasis on family and friends.

Occupational functioning refers to functioning as a worker, student or homemaker. The amount, complexity, and quality of work accomplished should be considered along with the person's comfort or discomfort with it.

Use of leisure time includes recreational activities and hobbies. The range and depth of involvement and the pleasure derived should be considered.[7]

Axis V information is considered to have prognostic significance because: "Usually an individual returns to his or her previous level of adaptive functioning after an episode of illness".[8] Occupational therapists must dispute this. An individual's sense of mastery in his or her occupational role can be

(continued)

TABLE 1 Axis IV Severity of Psychosocial Stressors

Code	Term	Adult examples	Child or adolescent examples
1	None	No apparent psychosocial stressor	No apparent psychosocial stressor
2	Minimal	Minor violation of the law; small bank loan	Vacation with family
3	Mild	Argument with neighbor; change in work hours	Change in schoolteacher; new school year
4	Moderate	New career; death of close friend; pregnancy	Chronic parental fighting; change in new school; illness of close relative; birth of sibling
5	Severe	Serious illness in self or family; major financial loss; marital separation; birth of child	Death of peer; divorce of parents; arrest; hospitalization; persistent and harsh parental discipline
6	Extreme	Death of close relative; divorce	Death of parent or sibling; repeated physical or sexual abuse
7	Catastrophic	Concentration camp experience; devastating natural disaster	Multiple family deaths
0	Unspecified	No information, or not applicable	No information, or not applicable

TABLE 2 Axis V Highest Level of Adaptive Functioning Past Year

Levels	Adult examples	Child or adolescent examples
1 SUPERIOR — Unusually effective functioning in social relations, occupational functioning, and use of leisure time.	Single parent living in deteriorating neighborhood takes excellent care of children and home, has warm relations with friends, and finds time for pursuit of hobby.	A 12-year-old girl gets superior grades in school, is extremely popular among her peers, and excels in many sports. She does all of this with apparent ease and comfort.
2 VERY GOOD — Better than average functioning in social relations, occupational functioning, and use of leisure time.	A 65-year-old retired widower does some volunteer work, often sees old friends, and pursues hobbies.	An adolescent boy gets excellent grades, works part-time, has several close friends, and plays banjo in a jazz band. He admits to some distress in "keeping up with everything."
3 GOOD — No more than slight impairment in either social or occupational functioning.	A woman with many friends functions extremely well at a difficult job, but says "the strain is too much."	An 8-year-old boy does well in school, has several friends, but bullies younger children.
4 FAIR — Moderate impairment in either social relations or occupational functioning, or some impairment in both.	A lawyer has trouble carrying through assignments; has several acquaintances, but hardly and close friends.	A 10-year-old girl does poorly in school, but has adequate peer and family relations.
5 POOR — Marked impairment in either social relations or occupational functioning, or moderate impairment in both.	A man with one or two friends has trouble keeping a job for more than a few weeks.	A 14-year-old boy almost fails in school and has trouble getting along with his peers.
6 VERY POOR — Marked impairment in both social relations and occupational functioning.	A woman is unable to do any of her housework and has violent outbursts toward family and neighbors.	A 6-year-old girl needs special help in all subjects and has virtually no peer relationships.
7 GROSSLY IMPAIRED — Gross impairment in virtually all areas of functioning.	An elderly man needs supervision to maintain minimal personal hygiene and is usually incoherent.	A 4-year-old boy needs constant restraint to avoid hurting himself and is almost totally lacking in skills.
0 UNSPECIFIED	No information.	No information.

American Psychiatric Association
Diagnostic and Statistical Manual of Mental Disorders, Third Edition,
Washington, DC, APA. 1980

DSM III

devastated by an illness. The occupational therapy process is needed to address many aspects of functioning: self-esteem, performance anxiety, exploration of skills and limits, acquisition of new, more adaptive skills such as sensory integration, self-assertion, self-expression and balancing work, play and self-care skills, to name a few, are needed to help resolve illness, bring return of function and maintenance of health. Occupational therapists should stress that improving the functional level of an individual is part of the treatment process and not an automatic result of resolution of the illness. The occupational therapist can work in tandem with the psychotherapist to raise the functional level of an individual. This can be done in a step-by-step method or in a parallel method. An example of the step-by-step method would be a patient who is achieving some conflict resolution in 1:1 therapy, is then given activities by the occupational therapist that would ena-

ble the patient to discover new boundaries, which allows the patient to experience mastery, resulting in decreased defenses, which in turn, enables the patient to deal with even more difficult issues in 1:1 therapy. In the parallel mode the interactive component of the two therapies cannot be traced, but is present, and each therapy facilitates the other. By working with psychiatry in this fashion on a case-by-case basis and by providing extensive evaluations of patient's functional levels in diagnostic conferences, occupational therapists can further emphasize the importance of the information presented in Axis V of the DSM III system. The inclusion of Axis V in this diagnostic system validates the work of occupational therapists. However, the optional use of this axis presents a challenge to occupational therapists to communicate the nonoptional nature of "functioning" as a part of the treatment process. As a profession, our knowledge of evaluation and treatment

in this area is much more in-depth than the information presented in the DSM III. The DSM III was written in part by an interdisciplinary task force. Through DSM III, occupational therapy has a mandate to participate in the task force and advisory committees that will write the DSM IV. This participation will allow the DSM IV to further reflect the contributions of occupational therapy in the field of psychiatry.

BIBLIOGRAPHY

[1] Diagnostic and Statistical Manual of Mental Disorders (3rd edition; Washington, DC: American Psychiatric Association, 1980).
[2] DSM III, p. 23.
[3] DSM III, p. 9.
[4] DSM III: A Comprehensive Approach to Diagnosis. Janet B. Williams, Social Work; Volume 2, March 1981, p. 102.
[5] DSM III, p. 6.
[6] DSM III, p. 26.
[7] DSM III, pp. 28, 29.
[8] DSM III, p. 28.

Mental Health
Special Interest Section Newsletter; Vol. 5, No. 2, 1982

An Open Letter to Therapists

I am writing as New York State Mental Health SIG Liaison to seek your input regarding a trend away from OT Departments and toward interdisciplinary departments in psychiatric hospitals in this part of the country. In the past decade, some New York hospitals have administratively combined previously separate OT and recreation therapy departments. In other facilities, OT had been the only activities discipline. Often these OT departments loosened their boundaries to include lines for members of dance, art, music, recreation therapy disciplines and rehabilitation counselors. OTs generally continued as directors of these departments, and often OT staff remained in the majority. However, members of the other disciplines naturally sought to improve their

career ladders, salaries, and employability. As a result, departments gradually shifted their composition so that professions were more equally represented. Role blurring seemed necessary in order to continue to offer a balanced therapeutic program to patients. As the role definition of OTs in these settings became less distinct, and the numbers of practitioners of other disciplines increased, it was less clear to hospital administrators that OTs alone should serve as department directors. In consequence, some directorships have been lost to our profession. OT lines are easily exchanged for those of other "activities therapies," since they are grouped administratively. OT roles have become blurred or narrowly conceived in departments containing such a variety of

resources. The "creative-expressive therapies" (dance, music, and art therapies) have become politically competitive in the struggle for shrinking pieces of the pie in mental health.

I would like to know if the trend I have described is occurring widely outside the New York area. If so, is my perception of this situation congruent with your view? Finally, has AOTA formulated policy or strategy regarding this issue? If you share the concern of some OTs in New York State that this trend in mental health be discussed further, please send your experiences and opinions in writing to Terry Korhorn.

Sincerely, *Mark S. Rosenfeld*, MS, *OTR*, New York State MHSIG Liaison, 1601 Third Avenue, 10C, New York, NY 10028.

In-Service Education

By Kathy L. Kaplan, OTR, Senior Occupational Therapist, George Washington University Hospital-Psychiatry

A frequent role of occupational therapists is to educate various health professionals. I am routinely involved in the orientation of medical students to the role of occupational therapy in an acute care setting. Since I am often asked by occupational therapists for suggestions on successful inservices, I would like to share our format as a springboard for other ideas.

The George Washington University Hospital psychiatric inpatient unit is a 34-bed facility for adolescents and adults in acute distress. In addition to providing service, it is a training program for medical trainees and students from other disciplines. The psychiatric occupational therapy department consists of the supervising senior occupational therapist, another occupational therapist, and a recreational therapist. We evaluate and treat referred patients; train occupational therapy students, other professional students, and staff; and contribute to program development.

Every two months we conduct an inservice on the therapeutic program for the rotating third-year medical students. By contributing to the training mission of the unit, we hope to create a postive experience that will influence the students' understanding, appreciation, and appropriate utilization of our professional services when they are practicing physicians. Because of these aims, our focus is on experiential learning and a conceptual framework, rather than a detailed presentation of the particular program on this unit. The inservice consistently receives high rating and generates enthusiasm and participation among the students during their rotation.

The first day the students are on the unit, I introduce myself and welcome the students to the unit. We review the specific occupational therapy and recreational therapy programs through a hand-out, a "survival sheet," which lists the OT and RT staff, what we do, where and when groups are held, how patients are referred, and briefly why we are organized as we are on this unit. Since the first two weeks are the least busy for the medical students, they are

encouraged to attend as many of our groups as possible.

The second week of their rotation, we meet for one and a half hours for the inservice. We begin with an informal introduction of the staff and the medical students (usually six). Often the students will speak about their previous experience with allied health professionals. We then review the purpose of the inservice and the sequence of events for the experience. Each student is asked to fill out a questionnaire to focus his or her attention and to address common myths. (If they catch the humor, we are off to a good start.)

The administrative aspects of the program are addressed briefly. The difference in training and focus of occupational therapy and recreational therapy are explained. The similarities are also pointed out since the programs are coordinated on this unit to facilitate the effective delivery of patient care.

A chart is used to explain the conceptual model of the department. The overriding concern is human occupation. The balance among work/play/self-care activities is elaborated upon with the roles and habits necessary to maintain health. A patient example is used to elucidate the cognitive, motor, sensory-integrative, psychologic, and social skills needed to perform daily tasks.

In order to give practice in analyzing skills and thinking about the concepts presented in the overview, practical exercises follow. There are three activities presented during the one and a half hours. The first focuses on evaluation and individual treatment, the second on exploratory treatment groups and the concept of levels of arousal, and the third on competence and achievement levels of treatment. Each activity is reviewed after completion in terms of the skills required to perform each activity, similar environmental characteristics of activities in the students' daily lives, and typical patients appropriate for each level.

The activity used to demonstrate components of an individual evaluation or treatment is the "magic

square." Each person is given a paper, pencil, and ruler and is asked not to begin until the sequence of instructions is completed. The instructions describe drawing lines that end up forming a checkerboard. Although the activity is not one we use to evaluate patients, it is effective to use with the medical students because the classroom test-like situation is familiar to them and sets a tone of taking the material seriously.

The activity is discussed in light of the capacities required to perform adequately and the factors which interfere with successful accomplishment. The students are asked to identify which subskills they used. Some of the examples highlighted in the cognitive sphere are previous experience with a ruler, ability to retain four instructions, and the ability to concentrate despite distractions. The task analysis contrasts the concrete step by step approach with abstract problem solving through visualizing the completed form prior to drawing it. Other subskills needed to do the task competently include perception of spatial relations, fine motor coordination, and frustration tolerance.

It is interesting to note how such a structured activity elicits individualized responses. Students report different feelings about competition, response to authority, and anxiety. We relate their experiences to the idea that the meaning each person ascribes to his experience is as important as the way in which the product appears. Then we discuss the structure of the group in terms of demands for socialization. The uses of a parallel type of group with certain types of patients are compared with times in daily life when it is common for an aggregate of persons to do things simultaneously (e.g., in a movie theatre or at a Laundromat). Finally, based on the students' observations on the unit, specific patients who could probably perform this task are predicted and those who could benefit from some other form of individual work are identified.

The next portion of the inservice

(continued)

In-Service Education

takes places in a larger room in order to do parachute activities. A sequence of activities is presented from simple waves, bouncing balls, changing places with someone, to sitting under the parachute like a tent. The students usually enjoy the experience, shown by their laughing, making jokes, and offering suggestions. This environment is designed to be safe and playful in order to explore movements, materials, and interactions. The skills required to perform are analyzed and contrasted to the first activity. Here, fewer cognitive demands are necessary because instructions are given one at a time and the opportunity for imitation is prevalent. The motor involvement is high, although the students are not aware of the amount of exercise during the activity because it is such fun.

After the activity, the exploratory nature of the group is discussed as well as the relevance of play at all ages of normal growth and development. The demands for interaction, skills, and roles are examined, as well as how they can be adapted to increase or decrease complexity. For example, we have a low-level activity-oriented group for psychotic patients in which the

parachute may be used with patients seated and able to focus for only ten minutes. Then there is a task group in which patients, once shown a few examples of the activities, could make up their own variations and maintain their attention for at least thirty minutes.

The last activity, back in the original room, is taken from a leisure awareness group. The group divides into pairs with one person asking his partner three questions: 1) What is one activity you did last summer? 2) What is one activity you enjoyed as a child? and 3) How would you spend your time if you only had three months to live? The partners have about five minutes to answer each question. Then the person in each pair who asked the questions introduces his partner to the group and explains his answers to the three questions. Both partners do not share information because of time constraints.

Some of the skills needed to adequately perform this activity include trust, the ability to communicate, and the ability to decide how much to share about oneself. Memory is also necessary to repeat the information to the

group. The demands for more intimate social interaction are contrasted with the previous two activities. The importance of values and interests in guiding action are made explicit by the exercise. Discussion of work, school, and recreational activities are used to highlight the way in which the skills, habits, and roles required by this treatment level, generalize to other environments. The predominately cognitive, motor, and social aspects of the three activities done during the inservice are commented upon to demonstrate the broad range of occupational activities. Typical patients, on the unit and in the day treatment and outpatient programs, appropriate for the types of groups at this last level are identified.

The inservice ends with a review of the purpose, sequence, and themes of the experiences. The importance of healing through occupation is stressed. Materials are provided concerning the treatment groups, with an open invitation to attend and to work collaboratively with the staff. The students are thanked for their participation and asked to fill out a questionnaire to provide feedback.

Mental Health
Special Interest Section Newsletter; Vol. 4, No. 4, 1981

Day Treatment

By John Gabriel

There is a need for a broad range of community services to assist people with impaired functional level from psychiatric disability. The day treatment center provides a gamut of services in a community-based setting to enhance the lives of its members and support their continued involvement in the community. Various terminology can be applied: day care, day health care, psychiatric day treatment, partial hospitalization and day hospital care.

Philosophy

The general philosophy of community-based mental health treatment is that man is in a large part a being who lives and defines himself in relation to his community. It views man's problems in living as a result of a description in the relationship between self and others. Day treatment has as its goals the treatment of per-

sons in distress in the community wherever possible. The Day Treatment Program is, therefore, established in a non-hospital setting with maximum involvement of self-help and other occupational therapy objectives.

Day treatment is intended to provide persons with a temporary social-emotional structure to facilitate the development or enhancement of daily living skills. Emphasis is placed on assessing and treating the total person by considering his strengths as well as weaknesses, and by productively involving family and/or significant others.

The major emphasis within day treatment is on goal achievement, particularly in developing skills in activities of daily living and social relationships. The client's active involvement in setting positive and realistic goals and in achieving those goals represent a commitment to client involve-

ment and accountability. Goals which foster prolonged and extensive dependency on a program is seen as detrimental.

Program Description

The Mid-Erie Mental Health Services Day Treatment Program of Erie County, New York, is designed to serve as an alternative to, or transitional stage from psychiatric hospitalization. Day treatment occupies an intermediate position within the continuity of the health care system, by functioning as a transitional service in the process of reentering clients within the community after discharge from in-care services and by preventing institutionalization for clients who cannot be maintained adequately by counseling services alone.

Day treatment's overall goal is to bring

(continued)

Day Treatment

each client to his or her highest possible level of independent functioning and self-realization. Emphasis within the program is on goal achievement, particularly in developing skills associated with activities of daily living, use of leisure time, communication and socialization. Group and occupational therapy modalities are geared to assess and develop client work skills, decision-making ability, feeling management and self-acceptance. The program stresses stabilization of clients within the community as socially productive citizens.

Program content is adjusted to meet the needs of individual clients with recognition that clients' needs will change during the course of involvement in the program. Specific packaged, structured programs are developed and maintained to guarantee flexibility and an interesting, challenging program format to meet the needs of the client population. These structured programs are central to the small group learning sessions. These sessions are most beneficial and manageable with 8-12 clients.

The small group learning sessions contain some instruction, some discussion and/or some short-term group or individual activities with each session. These sessions are available in levels, i.e., (1) basic grooming and (2) health issues; (1) basic money skills and (2) budgeting and money management; (1) basic communication skills and (2) listening styles or assertiveness training. While younger clients will require prevocational training programming, clients over the age of 65 can be directed toward recognition of their skills and interests in avocational areas. Similar program elements can be adapted and graded to meet the needs of various populations.

Where feasible, program elements include mechanisms for assessing clients' level of functioning in the area being addressed by the specific elements, as well as opportunities for the client to recognize his own changes and progress. Individual or group paper and pencil tasks, group activity, and individual activities resulting in products to be the source of discussion and feedback are used. Programs are structured in such a way that there are clear performance expectations with a minimum of threat to maintain cooperative involvement with program elements and an acceptance of differing client levels of functioning.

Day Treatment Entry Criteria

Referral to day treatment is from discharge planners from area hospitals or from out-care counselors within the agency. A psychiatrist monitors client's treatment progress and medication regime. Specific entry criteria area:

1. Sixteen or more years old.
2. In need of treatment service because of decreasing social competency.
3. Capable of living independently in the community or in a minimally supportive environment.
4. Need for reality orientation.
5. Need to enhance basic survival skills.
6. Need for social activity to prevent institutionalized behavior patterns.
7. Have a primary diagnosis of mental illness which is known to be treatable and have the expectation of a significant increase in functioning as a result of treatment within six months.
8. Physically able to perfom self-care activities (i.e., feeding, toileting, grooming, dressing, etc.).

Day Treatment Exit Criteria

The program is geared to a here and now framework. Staff conveys to clients a sense of their being on their way to independent living and having control in deciding the quality of that life. Staff and client negotiate treatment goals, therefore, mutually agreeable discharge from day treatment is also discussed. Specific exit criteria area:

1. Achievement of treatment goals.
2. Assessed as functioning in a "moderate" to "high" level on the Mental Health Assessment in all life areas as assessed by the multidisciplinary staff as having reached the maximum level of functioning possible in a particular life area.
3. Ability to maintain a level of functioning in keeping with life demands with a less intensive treatment mode.
4. Decision that level of goal achievement is sufficient and the program is no longer helpful.
5. Significant change in client which requires incare services for a brief interval and cannot be safely dealt with in a day treatment setting.

Summary

Overcrowding of long-term psychiatric hospitals has created a need for community-based mental health. A day treatment program that is occupational therapy oriented has been successful in serving as an alternative to, or transitional stage from, psychiatric hospitalization. Treatment is geared to provide a temporary social-emotional structure to facilitate the development of independent living skills.

Mental Health
Special Interest Section Newsletter; Vol. 4, No. 3, 1981

The Role of Occupational Therapy in the Vocational Rehabilitation of Psychiatric Patients

By Lela A. Llorens, PhD, OTR/L, FAOTA

This paper presents a brief review of the role of occupational therapy with psychiatric clients in vocational rehabilitation. Pre-vocational evaluation, work adjustment skill development and the development of independent living skills are considered within the domain of occupational therapy.

It is believed that patients/clients have "a right to a meaningful life and the right to participate in all aspects of that life. Each individual has the need to learn adaptive, coping techniques to accomplish this goal."(1)

The ability to work is often a measure of a person's adjustment to the environment and with him or herself. Assisting the psychiatric client toward better work adjustment and gainful employment serves all humankind(2).

The advent of short-term psychiatric treatment, chemotherapy, and briefer periods of hospitalization has resulted in more clients being returned to the community. The involvement of state agencies of vocational rehabilitation with psychiatric clients has contributed greatly to the need for methods, techniques and programs in occupational therapy that will

(continued)

Vocational Rehabilitation of Psychiatric Patients

provide useful information to psychiatric team members: the psychiatrist, social worker, recreational therapist, psychiatric nurse, psychologist, and rehabilitation counselor. Each assists in vocational planning for the discharged psychiatric patient.

Pre-vocational evaluation, work adjustment skill development, and independent living skills development provide such services.

To distinguish between vocational and prevocational evaluation, Rosenberg and Wellerson define vocational evaluation as the "accurate appraisal and measurement of skills, dexterity, aptitudes and potentials for work." It is usually required for individuals who are changing occupations or beginning a new occupation. Pre-vocational evaluation on the other hand is "concerned with the development (and appraisal) of work habits, work tolerance, coordination and productive speed." It is usually required for persons who have never worked and, therefore, do not know the meaning of work or those who have not worked for a number of years and need help in developing proper work habits, and productive speed. It may also be required for those who need help in adjusting to a work environment because of lack of confidence, severe anxiety and fearfulness in new situations.

Pre-vocational evaluation for the psychiatric patient is concerned with the evaluation of work habits, work tolerance, the ability to accept supervision, the extent to which the patient can work independently, and his level of productivity (3).

The goal of pre-vocational evaluation is to assess work behavior and vocational potential through the application of practical, reality-based assessment techniques. The strategies include: "testing and evaluating work abilities and retention of skills; evaluating physical, psychological, and social factors such as work tolerance, habits, and interpersonal qualities." (4) Testing objectives can be met through the use of carefully selected media that simulate or closely resemble actual job-related requirements.

Pre-vocational evaluation may involve simulated work tasks or real work tasks. Simulated work tasks are administered and supervised under simulated working conditions. The clients may be selected primarily on the basis of their need for evaluation as demonstrated by past history or present consideration for vocational counseling. Those clients who show chronic maladjustment in the vocational area, either through lack of employment for long periods of through frequent changes of jobs would be considered for evaluation. Clients with good or reasonably good work histories are not usually considered for pre-vocational evaluation.

Work tasks that may be used in such a program can include "sorting and packaging, assembly and production tasks. The sorting and packaging tasks may consist of separating and packaging large quantities of warehouse supplies such as index cards, soap powder, manila envelopes, etc., into smaller amounts. Assembly tasks may consist of cutting, punching, assembling or padding mimeographed materials that are used in various departments throughout the institution. Production tasks may be related to manufacture of items to be used in or by the institution such as custom built bookshelf walls, tie racks, periodical dividers, route slips, furniture, etc."(3)

The clients may be observed and evaluated on characteristics that are believed to be necessary for successful functioning in a work situation. Behaviors such as attendance, punctuality, appearance, motivation, reliability, energy output, attention span, independence, sociability and reaction to authority may be observed. Also affective behaviors may be evaluated such as mood, anxiety, stability, frustration tolerance, reality contact and self-concept may be evaluated. The therapist, in selecting job-sampling techniques, must ensure that the evaluation program provides a realistic measure of abilities and an accurate prediction of work potential. Before the tasks or tests are given, the client may receive an orientation to the purpose of the evaluation and to the specific tests or tasks being used. Throughout the period of test or task administration, the therapist adheres to strict evaluation procedures and closely observes and records the client's performance in each work task, test or each job sample.

A detailed report of evaluation results may be prepared and include "the identification of work samples used; a summary of the client's interest and aptitude to engage in the jobs related to the work samples used; and a recommendation for further work adjustment services, formal vocatinal training or termination from the program".(4)

Pre-vocational work adjustment skills may be developed in an occupational therapy activity program or in a specially designed work adjustment program.

In an occupational therapy activity program, patients may be assigned tasks to progress in a step-wise manner to assist in the development of deficit areas that have been identified in the pre-vocational evaluation. The behaviors of attendance, punctuality, appearance, motivation, reliability, attention span, independence, sociability and response to authority as well as frustration tolerance and self-concept may be enhanced and improved through the application of carefully selected tasks and activities that are monitored with appropriate feedback. Continual observation and periodic re-

evaluation can be used to determine the rate of progress and potential for goal achievement.

An extension of the Pre-vocational/Work Adjustment Services may include work placement, that is, evaluation of the client's readiness for work through placement in a work situation. In some settings, clients may be placed in areas such as the business office, food service, housekeeping, laboratories, maintenance department, occupational therapy, recreational therapy, or the warehouse (3).

Placement in a work setting provides for consistent, structured activity. The value of observing a client in a structured situation in which he or she is assigned a task and where certain standards of work are maintained is that a reliable judgment can be made relative to the patient's ability to perform where motivation may be minimal. Questions such as: "can the client adapt to the situation?" and, "are his or her symptoms under control?" can be answered under such observation. Also, such arrangements do not allow the patient to avoid the stress ordinarily involved in a work situation as is possible in other kinds of activities.

As part of the vocational rehabilitation team, the occupational therapist may, in addition to prevocational evaluation, develop adaptive or assistive devices, assist in designing more effective work situations, provide other services to improve functional performance, and assist the client in developing independent living skills.

Following the development of work adjustment skills, the patient or client may need to develop independent living skills. Independent living skills include interpersonal skills, such as self-advocacy and socialization, and coping skills, such as emotional and financial independence. Independent Living Programs (ILPs) are an essential adjunct to existing services and one of the newest identified services provided by occupational therapists for severely disabled psychiatric patients. To date, ILPs have been effected primarily for the physically disabled. The principles, however, apply to all severely disabled clients.

The OT's ability to evaluate a client using an holistic approach, coupled with knowledge of the methods and equipment that enhance functioning, places the OT in an important position to facilitate the implementation of independent living programs. Independent living in a suitable environment with appropriate coping skills go hand-in-hand with vocational rehabilitation (5).

It has been shown that patients who are prepared for work through work adjustment skill development but who do not

(continued)

Vocational Rehabilitation of Psychiatric Patients

have adequate coping skills with which to function independently within the community will have less chance for adaptation and success in the occupational performance area of work (2). Combined prevocational evaluation services and rehabilitation counseling increase the client's chances for vocational success (6,7).

References

1. Grant, H.K., Clark, T.A., and Duncan, J.K.: *Identification and Description of the Vocational Rehabilitation Content and Instruction Pertinent to Occupational Therapy Educational Programs.* The Ohio State University Research Foundation, 1314 Kinnear Road, Columbus, Ohio 43212. pp. 41-2.
2. Llorens, L.A., Levy, R. and Rubin, E.Z.: "Work adjustment program: a prevocational experience". *Am J Occup Ther* 18:15-19.
3. Llorens, L.A.: Aspects of prevocational evaluation with psychiatric patients, *Can J. Occup Ther.* Spring, 1966.
4. American Occupational Therapy Association. The role of occupational therapy in the vocational rehabilitation process. Official Position Paper. *Am J Occup Ther* 14:881-883.
5. Tylenda, B.: Independent living for the physically disabled, *Dev Dis Spec Sect Newsletter*, 4:1.
6. Ethridge, D.: Prevocational assessment of rehabilitation potential of psychiatric patients. *Am J Occup Ther* 22:161-167.
7. Distefano, M.K. and Pryer, M.W.: Vocational evaluation and successful placement of psychiatric clients in a vocational rehabilitation program, *Am J Occup Ther* 24:205-207.

Mental Health
Special Interest Section Newsletter; Vol. 4, No. 3, 1981

Individualized Psychosocial Assessment of Chronic Psychiatric Patients in a Day Treatment Setting

By Theresa Bocks, RN; Helen Gordon, OTR; Brian A. Brozost, DPA

Preface

The purpose of this paper is to share with our colleagues in Mental Health, who provide day treatment services, an assessment tool we found helpful in (1) assessing the patient's progress and/or regress; (2) assessing the therapeutic value of the established programs; (3) determining areas for staff inservice needs. The form is basically a psychosocial check list on a four-point scale that identifies the weaknesses and strengths of the patient and provides an accurate profile of needs. The profile is established by having each staff member who works with the patient rate the patient in his/her activity.

Background

Our day treatment programs fall into three categories: (1) activities requiring social interaction, i.e., crafts, recreation, art, music; (2) daily survival skills, i.e., nutrition, grooming, current events, community awareness; (3) psychosocial aspects, i.e., assertiveness training, skill training, social readjustment training.

The service functions on the team concept and includes a recreation therapist, occupational therapists, nurse, psychologist, music therapist, art therapist, vocational rehabilitation counselor and assistant, mental health therapy aides, and social worker—all with unique educational backgrounds and with a variety of experience. Each staff member is responsible for a variety of functions that may be outside his/her own area of expertise or discipline.

During the past six months our average daily census has been growing because of

increase of community placements. At the present time 55-60 attend daily. Each patient is referred to the service by a primary therapist within the facility and/or from a community health agency. Each patient has a treatment plan formulated by a multidisciplinary team that includes the day treatment staff. The extent of patient participation is determined by the individual's needs and may vary from one day a week (5 hours) to five days a week (25 hours).

The Bureau of Program Evaluation, Office of Mental Health, requested that we participate in collecting normative data for its pilot study on the "Adult Functioning Index." To give you a picture of the age, educational background and level of functioning of our day treatment population, we include some of the data collected on 76 of our patients.

Adult Function Index General Information

Age	Male	Female
20-30	7	7
31-40	5	7
41-50	6	4
51-60	6	15
61-70	11	6
71-80	0	2
81-90	0	0
TOTAL	35	41

Education	Male	Female
Less than grade school	8	5
Grade School	15	19
High School	12	14
Assoc. Arts. of Science	0	1
Bachelor's	0	1
Master's	0	1
TOTAL	35	41

According to the Global Assessment Scale 241-GAS (R.L. Spitzer, M. Gibbon and J. Endicott), the majority of our patients fall between the 31 to 65 range. This indicates major impairment in several areas, making them most vulnerable for rehospitalization and reinforcing the need for a day program. One of the objectives of our service is to provide an alternative to hospitalization.

After referral to our program, an initial interview and orientation to the service is provided. An individualized schedule is developed for each patient with two basic objectives in mind: (1) activities that enhance the individual's self confidence, self-esteem, body image and social interactions as well as (2) activities of personal interest. Our service encourages an individual to live in the community by building upon his strengths and assets. By doing so, it helps participants to achieve a higher level of social and emotional growth and to increase independence. Under the supervision of our qualified staff, an ongoing assessment of the individual's needs is made. This is done by day-to-day monitoring and supervision and by periodic assessments. Each staff member has input—it is not an isolated observation. The group treatment approach provides a setting for mutual interaction as well as a learning and sharing experience for the individual. The program is highly structured with limited free time during the treatment day. Staff has found that this type of structure has made it easier for the patient to adjust to the service and to gain self-confidence which is so often initially lacking. It also makes it possible for staff observation and appraisal of patient progress and/or re-

(continued)

Psychosocial Assessment

gress. Patients are under minimal or close supervision at all times.

Measurement Tool

After the initial observation period which the patient participates in the program for five visits, an assessment is made by each staff member who leads an activity in which the individual participates. This allows observation of the patient in his scheduled program which varies from day to day (7 to 10 activities per week). These ratings are then entered on an assessment form. This sheet is utilized in an effort to (1) determine the areas of strengths and weaknesses of the patients, (2) to select groups with patients whose needs are similar, (3) to identify patients who need a higher or lower level day program. This form also (4) indicates the areas of weaknesses that Day Treatment Service has to deal with—a weakness inherent in that particular group. This may, in turn, lead to refinement of staff development skills. It should become obvious that this form is a worksheet to be used by staff and is not a part of the patient's record. After the initial assessment the patient is reevaluated six weeks later, in three months and subse-

quently every six months. This timing has been suggested because it is hypothesized that more changes will occur early in a patient's program.

In the past year, we've used this method of evaluating levels of functioning. It has assisted us in recommending patients to the primary therapists for referral to higher level programs. Once transferred those patients have shown little to no difficulty in adjusting to the more flexible programs. This tool has also been a good indication of the success or failure of the patients who have been readied for community placement. It has been our observation that those individual patients who have had difficulty adjusting to the type of program that Day Treatment Service provides have also had difficulty once they have been placed in the community.

Along with the periodic patient assessments we have made an effort to "fine tune" this instrument. As we use this, our staff recognizes the need for change in various areas to give a more reliable profile of patients' level of functioning.

It identifies the items that measure what we are looking for. Even though patients are rated by different staff members in various situations or activities, the scores

have been noted to be consistent overall, giving reliability and objectivity to our tool. The validity of this measurement tool is empirically demonstrated in the behavioral changes noted.

Summary

One of the biggest assets from the staff point of view is the fact that patients are observed immediately as part of the assessment program, eliminating a variety of forms and standardized tools that have been devised. This gives both patients and staff members an opportunity right from the very start to build on the patient's strengths rather than to initially focus in on his/her weaknesses, which generally are results of traditional forms. In this sense we accomplish two things: (1) provision of a satisfying experience, (2) development of self-esteem and confidence, which ultimately overcomes the initial weaknesses. Staff is not taken from group activities to administer any tests. Observations, routinely an integral part of any therapeutic program, are documented on this check list from the very beginning, and require no additional staff training or

(continued)

ROCHESTER PSYCHIATRIC CENTER

DTS PATIENT PROGRESS ASSESSMENT

CSU - DAY TREATMENT SERVICES

NAME:

KEY: 1 = Never; 2 = Sometimes; 3 = Often; 4 = Almost Always; NA = Not Applicable

	PROGRAM
	DATE
COMMITMENT TO PROGRAM:	
Attends DTS	
Follows schedule	
Interested in program	
REALITY ORIENTATION:	
Relates to topic	
Appropriate affect	
Free of delusions/hallucin.	
INTERPERSONAL RELATIONS:	
Initiates conversation	
Appropriate empathy	
Expresses own opinion	
Tolerates divergent opinions	
PROBLEM SOLVING SKILLS:	
Comprehends directions	
Follows directions	
Tolerates frustration	
Good attention span	
Good coordination	
Works without superv'n	
Shows initiative	
Can make decisions	
Neatness	
PHYSICAL APPEARANCE:	
Good personal hygiene	
Appropriate dress	
Attends to hygiene without prompting	
AVERAGE SCORE:	

Psychosocial Assessment

expertise, thus making it useful for a multidisciplinary team.

Acknowledgment

This psychosocial check list represents the efforts of the Community Services Unit—Day Treatment Service staff of the Rochester Psychiatric Center. They helped devise the tool, used it, revised it, and are still fine tuning it.

Related Readings

1. Mosey, A.C.: Activities Therapy. New York: Raven Press, 1973.
2. Fidler, G.; Fidler, J.: Occupational Therapy, A Communication Process in Psychiatry. New York: The Macmillian Company, 1963.
2. Hopkins, H.L.; Smith, H.D.; Willard and Spackman's Occupational Therapy, Fifth Edition. Philadelphia: J.B. Lippincott Co., 1978.
4. Moyer, E.A.: Index of Assessments Used by Occupational Therapists in Mental Health, mimeographed January 30, 1981, by Mental Health Specialty Section of the American Occupational Therapy Association.
5. Spitzer, R.L.; Gibbon, M.; and Endicott,J.: Global Assessment Scale, New York: New York State Department of Mental Hygiene, 1973.

Mental Health
Special Interest Section Newsletter; Vol. 4, No. 2, 1981

A Guide to Helping

By Terry D. Korhorn

Helping communications may be for better or for worse. As a therapist, you have a significant influence on the life of another person. It should be noted, that this influence can, in fact, change the person. It stands to reason then, that this change can be for better or for worse. You must, therefore, be aware of what you are doing and take every precaution to ensure that you are helping and not hurting the person you are communicating with.

As a therapist, you are most effective when you *understand* and *act* upon your understanding. Understanding and action are the *key* ingredients of effective helping communication. As a therapist, you have the responsibility to understand yourself, for it is the therapist who best understands himself/herself, that is most likely to understand others. People seeking help generally do not understand themselves, or are unable to act upon what understanding they do have. It is your job, as a therapist, to assist them in gaining an understanding of themselves. Having gained a mutual understanding of the problem, you can work together to do something about it.

Therapists who are most actively involved with others have the greatest potential for being helpful. *Involvement* with other people leads to an understanding of other people. This understanding is necessary in order to see things the way that other people do and to know how to communicate with them effectively. This understanding stemming from involvement permits you to experience the situation the same way he/she does and thereby begin to act on the situation together.

What You Need to Know to Help

Being an occupational therapist does not guarantee effective helping communica-

tions. Some guidelines that will be of assistance in understanding our goals in a helping relationship are listed below:

1) Get the people you are helping to *explore* their problems. *Remember,* you cannot help a person unless you understand the persons' problem, and you cannot understand their problems unless you know something about them. Sometimes it is necessary for people to share at length their thoughts and feelings before specific problems are readily visible. Limited exploration can result in empty solutions for what you think are the person's problems. When the people explore themselves, they help you understand their problems better.

2) Get the person you are helping to *understand* himself. It is not enough that you understand the person's problems. While the things he relates may have meaning to you, this meaning may not be seen by him. It is, therefore, necessary for you to let him know how you are interpreting what he is saying so that together you can more clearly identify the specific problem situation. It is not enough to have one of you understand the problem. Effective helping communication requires the participation of both of you.

3) Get the person you are helping to *act* upon his understanding. After having thoroughly explored the problem situation to the extent of gaining a mutual understanding, it seems reasonable to assume that each of you may have solutions which could be implemented. *Together,* you can examine these solutions and attempt to find those solutions which appear to be the most workable and have the greatest advantages. When an agreement is made on a course of action, you should assist the person in developing a program for accomplishing his goals and work through the program with him until it is determined whether or not it is successful.

4) The different components of the helping relationship are related to each other.

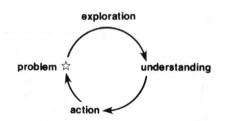

The cycle of exploration, understanding, and action is repeated over and over again. The person you are helping, after acting upon an understanding of his problem, finds out the consequences of his actions. These consequences give him new information which he can use to develop new and deeper explorations of himself, leading to a fuller, richer understanding of his life, resulting in new and more effective courses of action.

Exploration and Understanding

You will be most effective early in a relationship when you respond to the person you are helping.

In the beginning of a helping relationship, you should give your undivided attention to understanding the person, and in so doing, assist him in understanding himself. This requires you to listen objectively and really "hear" what he is trying to say. In addition, you should try to "tune into" his thoughts and feelings. The manner in which you respond to the person is very important in that your responses should involve him in the process of self-exploration, leading to self-understanding. You will also find that the manner in

(continued)

Guide to Helping

which the person responds to you will provide a means for you to check if you are really "tuned in" to what the person is saying. Your response can then let him know that he really is being understood.

In order to "tune into" other persons and get them to talk, to explore their ideas, feelings, and problems, you must respond effectively. This requires some skill on the part of the therapist. Four areas should be developed for maximum effectiveness; they are:

1) *Active Listening*—Give your undivided attention, showing it through your body language and comments. Listen with a purpose—because you want to understand, learn, and help. Listen carefully, going beyond words and into themes and feelings. Avoid giving judgment about what is said.

2) *Empathy*—Keep in tune with the persons' ideas and feelings. Attempt to see things from their eyes and from their perspective. Let them have feedback as to what they see and feel.

3) *Respect*—Let the person know you care for him and that you believe in his ability to help himself. As you get to know the person, you respect him for what he is *capable* of doing and you convey this to him.

4) *Concreteness*—Help the other person to be specific about his own experiences and feelings. Do not allow the person to substitute "thinking" for feeling.

Action

You, as a therapist, will be most effective during the later phases of helping if you initiate action. You have attempted to get the person to understand himself at a deeper level and now you challenge him to act upon that understanding. To get the person to act, you must also act in order to

lead the person to initiate his own ideas. Your action consists of:

1) *Genuineness*—a lack of "phoniness." There should be no discrepancy between what is said and what is done.

2) *Self-disclosure*—sharing personal experience with the person you are helping.

3) *Confrontation*—telling it like it is. Confront the person with the reality of the situation. Once you confront, you need to follow through at working out the differences between you.

4) *Immediacy*—talking about the here and now of the relationship. You act upon what you see going on between yourself and the person you are helping.

Putting It All Together

Now that you have been introduced to some of the fundamentals of effective helping communications, let's put all the considerations together in order to see the whole picture more clearly.

A person comes to you seeking help because he can't help himself. As a helper you first offer him understanding that is interchangeable in terms of the feelings and meaning that he is expressing. This is done in an effort to get him to explore his problems more fully. Once he begins to explore his problems more fully, you offer higher levels of understanding (i.e., adding to and clarifying his expressions). With this higher level of understanding offered by you, he may be able to understand his problems more fully. If he comes to understand his problem more fully you will sense his need to do something about it. Together you and he can develop courses of action that give him the best chance of dealing with his problems.

Remember, the process doesn't end here. The person you are helping learns from acting, and the process of explora-

tion-understanding-action is repeated in many different ways and in many different problem areas. Your task is to always work in such a way as to give the person the best chance of succeeding. At all points, the helping process tries to get the person to act on his understanding. When he acts he learns new things and opens up new areas. When he explores these new areas he comes to new understanding and then acts again in a new and more effective way.

A Final Comment

Being an occupational therapist requires good helping skills. Developing these skills and using them fully is not a simple matter. You may at times feel very unsuccessful and become discouraged. To become effective, however, requires that you endure these unpleasant feelings and continue to practice the helping process by remaining actively involved. Your active involvement with the helping process will ensure continued learning and growing for you and through your own learning and growing you can help others to learn and grow.

Helpful References on Helping
Benjamin, A. *The Helping Interview* (3rd Ed.). Boston: Houghton-Mifflin, 1981.
Carkhuff, R. and Anthony, W. *The Skills of Helping*. Amherst: Human Resources Development, 1979.
Carkhuff, R. *The Art of Helping IV*. Amherst: Human Resources Development, 1980.
Dixon, S. L. *Working With People in Crisis: Theory and Practice*. St. Louis: Mosby, 1979.
Hames, C. and Joseph D. *Basic Concepts of Helping: A Holistic Approach*. New York: Appleton, Century, Crofts, 1980.
Tolbert, E. L. *An Introduction to Guidance*. Boston: Little, Brown, and Company, 1978.

Mental Health
Special Interest Section Newsletter; Vol. 4, No. 1, 1981

Effects of Psychotropic Drugs on the Occupational Therapy Process

By Doris A. Smith, MEd, OTR

Since the late 1950s the majority of mental health clients who have received occupational therapy were also receiving one or more psychotropic drugs. What effect have these drugs had on patients and on the occupational therapy evaluation and treatment process?

Some of these effects will be explored here, along with a brief review of the

therapeutic and side (adverse) effects of the antipsychotic (neuroleptic or major tranquilizer) drugs. A hypothetical group of patients will be described to illustrate some of the behaviors, activities, settings, and media that the occupational therapist should consider as he/she evaluates, plans and carries out treatment with a client (clients) who is (are) taking an anti-

psychotic drug.

Psychotropic drugs include any drug that affects psychic function and behavior. Antipsychotic, antidepressant, antimanic, and antianxiety drugs comprise the four major groups of psychotropic drugs currently in use. Until the introduction of these new drugs in the mid-1950s, there

(continued)

Psychotropic Drugs

had been a steady increase in hospitalized mental patients until there were approximately 560,000 patients in state and local government hospitals in the U.S. in 1955 (Freedman, et al, 1976, pp. 943-4). Twelve years later, in 1967, due mainly to drug therapy, this population had decreased to 426,000 (Freedman, et al, 1976, p. 944) and by 1974 it declined to 216,000 (Ethridge, 1976, p. 624). This decline has continued due to improvements in drug therapy, client's subsequent responsiveness to other therapies (including occupational therapy), increases in community mental health services, new mental health codes, and recent judicial and legislative decisions which have recognized the individual's right to treatment and to the least restrictive environment for treatment.

Although psychotropic drugs rarely produce a cure, they usually benefit the patient by diminishing the symptoms of the disorder. For example, the schizophrenic patient receiving an antipsychotic drug usually shows less of the following symptoms: thought disorder, blunted affect, withdrawal, hallucinations, delusions, hostility and resistiveness, with no loss and usually marked improvement in cognitive functions (Freedman, 1976).

This improvement has enabled the patient who is receiving drug therapy to be more responsive to occupational therapy. This ability to respond has been noted in the literature. Kline and Davis (1973, p. 54) wrote, "Not only did drugs come into widespread use, but such other modalities as psychotherapy and group, family, occupational and recreational therapies were used to a greater extent, mostly because patients on drug therapy were able to take part in and benefit from these therapies." Freedman, et al (1976, p. 943) in their textbook for psychiatrists note that "The fact that clinically significant therapeutic effects could be produced by a drug created an atmosphere that emphasized positive treatment and led to the vigorous application of milieu therapy, psychotherapy, group therapy and occupational therapy."

Despite the positive effects on 70% to 80% of patients who receive psychotropic drugs (Clark, et al; 1979) and the increased demand for occupational therapy and increased ability of patients to respond to our services, there are many disturbing side effects that we observe in our patients who receive drug therapy. What can occupational therapists do when they observe the negative effects of drugs?

Three recent books (Bockar, 1976; Goldsmith, 1977; and Irons, 1978) written for mental health professionals emphasized the need for awareness of side effects of psychotropic drugs so that these can be reported to the physician. Goldsmith (1977, pp. vii-viii) says the mental health worker "... should be prepared to refer a

patient for medication and to monitor drugs' actions between contacts with the prescribing physician." He goes on to say "... their observations may be crucial to the doctor who makes these decisions." Bockar (1976) in her introduction states as the purpose of her book a need for a developing awareness by nonmedical psychotherapists of the effects of drugs, because the M.D. prescribing the drugs rarely sees the patient, and the patient and M.D. need the shared observations of the nonmedical professional to obtain the best treatment. One book, *Occupational Therapy*, refers to psychotropic drugs and that one (Hopkins and Smith, 1978, p. 296) devotes one paragraph and a small inset (listing four major medication groups and possible side effects) to this subject. Tiffany who authored this chapter, says, "The therapist who works with clients who are receiving medication needs to be aware of the possibility of side effects. In addition to the fact that side effects may be extremely troublesome and upsetting to the client, it is essential that they be monitored closely, so that changes in medication will be made when necessary."

Noting and reporting side effects that occur in one's clients is an important contribution that a therapist should and does make, but there are other important considerations for the therapist working with a client or group of clients who are on psychotropic drugs. These center around the following questions. How does this drug affect the person's ability to function in daily activities and in relationships with others? How do specific drugs, such as mellaril, thorazine, haldol, valium, cylert, tofranil, with both the therapeutic and side effects, influence the behaviors and syndromes that the therapist observes during evaluations? How will the drug affect goals for the client, and activities, settings and media that will be selected for treatment? How can the occupational therapist design treatment to capitalize on the therapeutic effects of the drug the client is receiving and diminish the negative side effects?

These questions will be explored here relative only to the antipsychotic drugs, although these are questions that can apply to any of the other psychotropic drugs.

The antipsychotic drugs, also known as neuroleptics, major tranquilizers and antischizophrenic drugs, have the capacity to modify affective states without seriously impairing cognitive function. The major gains from these drugs are noted within the first six weeks, and gains can continue up to 12 to 18 months. Some of the positive effects are a decrease in psychotic thinking; there is a decrease in projection, delusions, suspiciousness, perplexity, ideas of reference, and hallucinations. There is a normalization of psychomotor behavior; the hyperactive client is less active and the retarded, slow patient is more alert. The

client becomes more responsive (with more affect) and cooperative with increased interest in and response to the environment and other people.

The major toxic reactions to these agents are the extrapyramidal syndromes; Parkinsonism, akasthesia, and tardive dyskinesias. According to Sovner (1978, p. 2) recent studies indicate that tardive dyskinesias (abnormal movements of any part of the body) occur in 40 to 55% of patients who have received moderate to high doses of antipsychotic drugs for a year or more. Therefore, tardive dyskinesia is a syndrome that one is likely to observe when working with clients who receive antipsychotic drugs.

In a pamphlet published by Sandoz Pharmaceuticals to alert persons to signs of tardive dyskinesia, Dr. Sovner (1978, p. 3 & 9) states that one may first observe tardive dyskinesia during a drug holiday, since antipsychotic drugs tend to suppress its clinical signs. It is also most apparent when the client is emotionally aroused and is least apparent during sleep. Early detection is crucial since the earlier the drug dose is reduced or discontinued, the more likely there will be a resolution of this syndrome or a decrease in its severity. A simple method called the "AIMS examination procedure" is described in this pamphlet and is a measure that can be used in the occupational therapist's assessment. There is also reference to a 17-minute film (p. 1) produced by Sandoz Pharmaceuticals. This pamphlet has other information that should be useful for therapists who are working with clients on antipsychotic drugs.

Some other side effects observed in clients who are on neuroleptics that could interfere with daily activities and interpersonal interactions are motor retardation, drooling, tremor, akasthesia (restlessness, inability to sit still, and pacing), akinesia (apathy, blunted affect), dry mouth and throat, weight gain, increased appetite, sedation and drowsiness (especially on large doses), visual changes, sensitivity to the sun, orthostatic hypotension, changes in sexual functions, food aspiration and choking, and many others. These effects vary from individual to individual and vary in intensity or occurrence with different types or compositions of antipsychotic drugs. The books referred to above for allied health professionals, those by Bockar, Goldsmith, and Irons, provide assistance in identifying these differences relative to both therapeutic and side effects of individual drugs.

In order to illustrate the effects that psychotropic drugs can have on the occupational therapy process, a hypothetical group of twelve schizophrenic clients will be considered; each is receiving an antip-

(continued)

Psychotropic Drugs

sychotic drug. Not all of the drugs they are receiving are the same, so it is possible that each person will experience different therapeutic and/or side effects. Also, each person potentially can respond in a unique and unusual manner to a drug. Some may not receive any therapeutic benefits or experience any side effects. For purposes of this discussion, generalizations about these drugs will be made. In actual practice, however, it would be advisable to use a drug reference to identify and determine the potentials (reported effects) of each specific, individual drug in order to enhance the therapeutic effects and to alert the therapist to possible side effects. This will enable the therapist to diminish and sometimes avoid the potential side effects of these drugs.

Relative to the group of twelve clients, assessment of each individual indicates that each of them has many characteristics and manifestations that King described in her article "A Sensory Integrative Approach to Schizophrenia" (1973). These include S-curve posture, immobile shoulder girdle, shuffling gait, weak grip, and internally rotated, adducted and flexed extremities. Following King's recommendations for stimulation of the client's vestibular, proprioceptive and tactile systems, parachute and ball activities will be used. It would seem ideal to conduct these activities out-of-doors where there is adequate space and to design the activities so that each person can bend, turn the head, push and pull against objects, lift the arms overhead and do bilateral activities. What should be considered by the therapist relative to these activities and the drugs in the clients are taking?

Because of therapeutic effects of drugs, one might expect that the clients will be able to understand the directions that are given and be receptive to most communication with them. They will probably not be too withdrawn or hostile or involved in their delusions and hallucinations to participate when requested.

Relative to possible side effects of drugs and the activities described above, the therapist should be alerted to some or all of the following considerations:

1) Is the activity near a source of liquid to counteract the dry mouth and throat that so frequently is a side effect? Can water or a low calorie, nonstimulant (non-caffeine) refreshment be provided before and perhaps midway in the activity so that the clients will not be as likely to leave for a coke or coffee or become uncomfortable because they have a need to relieve this dryness?

2) Are any of the clients on neuroleptics that make them more sensitive to the sun? If so, perhaps sunscreen preparations, long sleeves, a hat, or having the activity indoors will be necessary to adapt to or avoid this possible side effect. The therapist can also minimize the time these persons are out in the sun and observe them closely for reactions to the sun.

3) Will clients be required to bend, to turn their heads and lift their arms overhead suddenly as they participate in the parachute and ball activities? These are all activities appropriate to Lorna Jean King's recommendations, but sudden postural changes do occur in them and may result in severe discomfort, dizziness, or even fainting due to orthostatic postural hypotension. This side effect which is a sudden drop in blood pressure can occur in patients on neuroleptics. (It is also a serious side effect in patients who take antidepressive drugs.)

4) Will light, soft balls be used to enable clients who have blurred vision and contracted or dilated pupils (any of these can occur with neuroleptics) to be able to follow the flying object and have a chance to catch or hit or kick the ball? This would enable the client to be successful in meeting the objective of the activity, and would provide the success and fun which can lead to continued participation in activities.

5) Will the activity be short enough or allow enough moving about to accommodate to and perhaps interrupt akasthesia which is restlessness, inability to sit or stand still, and constant pacing? This symptom or side effect often occurs early in drug therapy even before the therapeutic effects occur.

These are only a few of the *many* possible therapeutic and side effects of drugs and adaptations of activity that should be considered in planning an activity for a client or group of clients who are on neuroleptics. It is possible for occupational therapists through careful observation and thorough assessment of their clients to design treatment goals and activities that can enhance the therapeutic effects of psychotropic drugs and to diminish the side effects. Frequently, the therapeutic effects of a drug outweigh the side effects, and the patient will be continued on the drug. When this occurs, it is a challenge to the occupational therapist to enable the client to adapt to these effects and be able to benefit from all forms of therapy and learn to participate more effectively in daily activities and interactions with people.

This article has explored only a few of the effects of the antipsychotic (neuroleptics) drugs that should be considered by the occupational therapist. There are similar and different effects that occur with the other psychotropic drugs—the antidepressive antimanic, antianxiety, and cerebral stimulant drugs that should be considered when the occupational therapist evaluates a client and develops and carries out a plan for treatment.

The author of this article is writing a book which will be a thorough review of all psychotropic drugs, their therapeutic and side effects, and the influence these drugs have on the occupational therapy process, both evaluation and treatment. Any suggestions, questions or comments relative to this topic or information that might be included in this book will be appreciated. Please forward to Doris A. Smith, Associate Professor of Occupational Therapy, Western Michigan University, Kalamazoo, MI 49008.

REFERENCES

Bockar, J. A., *Primer for the Non-medical Psychotherapist*, Spectrum Publications, New York, 1976.

Clark, M. et al, Drugs and Psychiatry: A New Era *Newsweek*, November 12, 1979. p. 98-104.

Ethridge, D. A., The Management View of the Future of Occupational Therapy in Mental Health, *American Journal of Occupational Therapy*, Vol. 30:10, 1976, p. 623-628.

Freedman, A. M., Kaplan, H. I., and **Sadock, B. J.**, *Modern Synopsis of Psychiatry/II*, Williams and Wilkins Company, Baltimore, 1976.

Goldsmith, W., *Psychiatric Drugs for the Non-medical Mental Health Worker*, Charles C. Thomas, Springfield, Illinois, 1977.

Hopkins, H. L. and **Smith, H. D.**, *Willard and Spackman's Occupational Therapy*, (5th ed.), New York: J. B. Lippincott Company, 1978.

Irons, P. D., *Psychotropic Drugs and Nursing Intervention*, New York: McGraw-Hill Book Company, 1978.

King, L. J., A Sensory-integrative Approach to Schizophrenia, *American Journal of Occupational Therapy*, Vol. 28, 1974, p. 529-536.

Kline, N. S. and **Davis, J. M.**, Psychotropic Drugs, *American Journal of Nursing*, Vol. 73:1, 1973, p. 54-62.

Sovner, R., *Tardive Dyskinesia: Diagnosis and Management*, Sandoz Pharmaceuticals, 1978 (pamphlet).

An Activities Approach to Occupational Therapy in a Short-Term Acute Mental Health Unit

By Barbara Burnham Rider and Julie Trapp Gramblin

Introduction

The role of the occupational therapist in the mental health unit of a general hospital is far different from that of therapists who work in state hospitals, community mental health centers or other long-term facilities. The primary differences relate to length of stay and chronicity of pathology. The mental health unit in a general hospital is characterized by short hospitalization and rapid turnover. Patients may be admitted in a severely disorganized state, but they usually reconstitute quite rapidly.

The short stay and rapid changes in the patient's daily status create unique problems for the occupational therapist. Occupational therapy programs tend to focus on one of two extremes. Many are craft based, relying heavily on short-term projects such as pre-poured ceramics and pre-cut kits. In other cases, the occupational therapist has become so much a part of the unit team that he or she is hardly distinguishable from the other unit staff.

These are activities of which we will give examples later. They rely heavily on traditional occupational therapy media and are based on the Task Group Model developed by Fidler and Fidler in the late '50s and expanded by Mosey in *Activities Therapy* in the early '70s. These activities are selected to fit the unique needs of the short-term psychiatric unit in the general hospital. Although many of them are group activities, they may be modified to use in individual treatment sessions as well. Each activity may be easily completed within a 45-minute period; in fact, it is often possible and even desirable to use several activities in one treatment session.

The Task Group

A Task Group is a time-limited group experience in which patients perform a task for a purpose other than the task itself. The purpose of the task may be to enhance group skills or to develop greater self-awareness or awareness of others. The tasks may be completed in one treatment session or may take one week or longer. They may be structured or there may be very little structure other than the basic rules of the institution, such as the task group method, which may be adapted for verbal, well-organized patients or for regressed patients.

On admission units, or in acute mental health units of general hospitals, the com-

position of the group is not stable enough to plan week-long activities. In fact, the therapist usually does not know from one day to the next who will be in the group. For this reason, activities that can be completed in one treatment session are often most successful. Since it is often impossible to assess each patient individually and plan treatment according to his or her individual needs, more general needs frequently encountered with these patients have been identified.

The activities meet broad, global goals. Some of them appear to require a high level of verbal skill and integrated thought processes; however, in our experience, these tasks have been used successfully with groups of widely varied levels of integration. Most of the activities result in some sort of product, such as a collage or drawing—representation of feelings or of self, or a group production such as a group mural. In some cases, the productions made by the patients can be useful to staff in understanding their patients, the levels of integration, and how they see themselves, their problems, and their assets.

Implementation

Use of the activities may present a problem of implementation to the occupational therapist. We do not recommend a sudden or total break with the old. Therefore, it is critical to have the support of the unit staff. We have found that it works best to make only a partial change initially. Our experience has been with programs that were craft based, and we continued the craft program three days a week and initiated the new Activities Program on the remaining two days. At first there was a dwindling of attendance for the new program. However, after a few weeks, the pattern reversed and the patients were skipping the craft sessions and bringing friends and new patients to the activity sessions.

When implementing the new program, the occupational therapist may encounter a lack of understanding among unit personnel. The occupational therapy group does not duplicate or replace group therapy. The mental health team on general hospital mental health units usually includes psychiatrists, psychologists, nurses, social workers, and therapists. Group treatment sessions conducted by these professionals rely almost exclusive-

ly on verbal expression. Occupational therapy is unique in the use of media as the vehicle for expression. The use of media as the primary role of expression has several distinct advantages:

1. The use of media is often less threatening to the patients than direct verbal expression.

2. The use of media is a total patient experience involving physical, mental, social, emotional, and creative qualities of the individual.

3. Learning that occurs through the use of media is often indirect. The patient may not be immediately aware of the therapeutic outcome of the activity because the awareness is integrated at a level other than the cognitive level.

4. Learning that occurs through the use of media is fun, and is, therefore, more powerful than forced learning.

Therapy, using media, can be a partner to verbal therapy, one reinforces the other. Patients on mental health units in general hospitals participate in indepth therapy groups in which they are often confronted with the necessity of making painful and difficult behavioral changes. Changing behavior may often be painful. Occupational therapy provides an opportunity for patients to balance the intensive, often difficult, experiences of group therapy or individual therapy with an enjoyable, creative learning experience that reinforces or supplements the learning that takes place in group therapy. Outcomes vary, depending upon the specific composition of individuals in the group and the ability of the therapist to build upon the experience. No single activity will produce the same outcome with different groups, nor will an activity produce the same results with the same group at different times. The activities listed are not presented to comprise a cookbook of time fillers. The skill of the therapist is critical to the therapeutic effectiveness of these activities. The effectiveness of the activities depends upon the knowledge of the therapist and upon a strong foundation in occupational therapy theory.

Establishing Treatment Goals

As already mentioned, in the mental health unit of a general hospital, the therapist may be unable to establish

(continued)

Activities Approach to Occupational Therapy

individual treatment goals, and it may be necessary to establish goals which are shared by most members of the group. Some commonly shared goals are: 1) building self-esteem, 2) increasing self-awareness, 3) developing group skills, and 4) expressing feelings appropriately.

Many of the activities meet several goals. The therapist might focus on a goal which is a basic treatment goal for most of the patients in the group and select several activities which meet that goal. Or the therapist may select activities that meet a wide range of goals. In any case, it is important to determine the group goal, or goals, first and select activities to meet the goals. It is also important to balance the activities so the patients do not become bored or some patients are not left out.

Determining appropriate treatment goals is critical to the therapeutic effectiveness of any activity. It is essential that the therapist have a thorough knowledge of psychology based on the firm understanding of the various theoretical approaches to occupational therapy. The manner in which the therapist defines goals and presents the activities will vary depending upon the theoretical frame of reference utilized.

Grading Activities

Occupational therapists grade activities. Traditionally, therapists move from structured activities to less structured activities according to the group's ability to handle less structure. Groups may also be graded according to levels; for example, from a parallel group to a cooperative group. Grading group activities in this manner takes time and it is necessary to have 1) some homogeneity in the group, and 2) some assurance the constituency of the group will remain reasonably constant for an established period of time.

In the mental health unit of a general hospital, it is usually impossible to assure either of these criteria. Patients may or may not be formally referred; attendance may or may not be required; a previous evaluation of individual patients may or may not be possible; and patients may be discharged or leave the hospital with little prior notice. These factors, and many others, make traditional grading of activities impossible. While the therapist usually has a general knowledge of who group members will be on any one day, there are usually some new members or some absent members, and the therapist must be able to immediately assess the group and make a judgment about the appropriateness of the activities selected and the level at which they should be presented. In essence, the therapist grades the activity "on the spot."

In some cases, the group itself grades the activity. The activities presented are suitable for a broad range of patient abilities. They can be challenging to well-integrated patients, while at the same time offering an opportunity for participation to very regressed or acutely ill or confused patients. The therapist must be skillful in presenting the activities and guiding the discussion to include each patient at his or her optimal level.

The Importance of Discussion

The critical element in the use of these activities is the therapist. The discussions following the activities are often the most important part of each session and the most valuable therapeutically. The therapist, therefore, must be skillful in leading groups. Since therapists often have not had formal training or experience leading therapy groups, we suggest enlisting as co-therapist a social worker or psychologist or other team members who has had experience leading therapy groups. Another occupational therapist is a good possibility. We support the use of co-therapists because one person always misses something that is going on. It is important to remember that the purpose is to enlist patient discussion, not an opportunity for therapists to lecture or theorize.

And, this raises another point. The therapist must be able to wait and tolerate silence. The group may express resistance to some of the activities—clay projects are a usual one—and be silent and totally uncommunicative when the therapist seeks discussion. The therapist must be cautious not to move in and take over, but rather to guide the group forward.

We have attempted to offer suggestions with each activity to get the discussion started. These are only suggestions and usually something that happened in the group will provide a good starting point for discussion. The therapist must be alert to such incidents.

It is critical to keep the therapeutic goal of the activity in mind and remember that the discussion is part of the activity and also must focus on the goal. Since there are individual goals within a group activity, the needs of each group member must be addressed. Chapter 10 of *Activities Therapy* may be helpful in guiding the therapist to maximize the value of the discussion.

Precautions

As with any form of therapeutic intervention, certain precautions must be observed.

Patients on mental health units are often taking some form of medication which may influence their behavior. In many cases, motor performance and/or perceptions are distorted by drugs. It is important for therapists to understand the possible side effects of psychotropic drugs and to know the medication status of each patient. Patients usually know what medication they are taking and should be routinely asked to tell the therapist of any medication changes.

Occasionally, a patient will refuse to participate. This is more likely to occur in the early stages of the implementation of the program. Usually after the program is well established, informal communication networks serve to inform patients about what to expect, thereby eliminating the anxiety which often accompanies the unknown or the unexpected. If a patient does refuse to participate, the therapist must be able to judge the situation and determine the best action to take in the particular situation. We have found that it is often best to honor the patient's request and allow him or her to return to the unit or work on a project in another area of the clinic.

The occupational therapy group is **not** an intensive, in-depth, probing, analytical form of therapy. Rather, the purpose is to build patients' interaction skills, increase their understanding of themselves and others, and raise their opinion of themselves as valuable individuals and valued group members. It is not merely a diversional, pleasurable experience. The therapist must be skillful in assuring a creative and personally positive experience for each group member.

Summary

The activities presented here are designed for the occupational therapy program in a short-term mental health unit in a general hospital. They require no special equipment or materials and can be completed in one treatment session or less. They are positive, building experiences designed to supplement and reinforce group therapy, and they rely heavily on traditional occupational therapy media. They are not cookbook exercises, but require the expertise and theoretical knowledge of a registered occupational therapist.

A complete packet of activities can be obtained from: Barbara Burnham Rider, MS, OTR, Occupational Therapy Department, Western Michigan University, Kalamazoo, MI 49008, for a nominal re-production fee.

Samples from the Activity Card File include the following:

Creative Circle

Goal: Warm up
Time: Ten minutes
Setting: Room large enough for the group to form a circle
Materials: None
Group: Six or more members

(continued)

Activities Approach to Occupational Therapy

Process: The group forms a circle with arms on each other's shoulders. They are then instructed to "be a creative circle" or "let's do something that no other circle has ever done." The reactions to this kind of freedom vary according to the spontaneity level of the group. There is no set way that the circle must respond. Therefore, creativity, or the lack of it, of the group at the moment is utilized.

Difficult Situation

Goal: Increase interaction skills. Raise self-esteem.
Time: Thirty minutes
Setting: Room for group members to move around freely
Materials: None
Group: Any size
Process: Group members are polled on what kinds of situations are difficult for them to handle. A member volunteers to participate and enacts his situation, using people in the group to role play if necessary. Participants are allowed to experiment with various behaviors if

they desire. As closure, the group shares and offers feedback. Some common scenes are: a) return department merchandise, b) being given a traffic ticket, c) making introductions, and d) aggressive salesman.

Memories

Goal: Increase self-awareness
Time: Fifteen to twenty minutes
Setting: Around a table
Group: Six to ten
Materials: Large paper, crayons
Process: Instruct members to "Draw your earliest memory." Discussion may focus on what memories stand out and why; what memories will stand out about their present lives, etc.
Variation: "Draw the happiest experience of your life." "Draw the saddest experience of your life." Combine the first two variations.

Mirroring Body

Goal: To increase body awareness. Warm up.
Time: Ten minutes

Setting: An area large enough to move around without touching another person
Materials: Music
Group: Any size large enough for discussion.
Process: Break up into pairs facing each other, have one partner imitate the other during music, stop the music and freeze the position. Become aware of how it feels in different positions. Imitate your partner! Share experiences in group discussion.

Sell Yourself!

Goal: Raise self-esteem. Increase self-awareness.
Time: Fifteen to twenty minutes
Setting: Around a table
Materials: Large paper, crayons, marking pens, etc.
Group: Six to ten
Process: Instruct members to "Draw a full page advertisment selling yourself." Keep the discussion on a positive vein.
Variation: Make a collage advertisement.

Mental Health
Special Interest Section Newsletter; Vol. 3, No. 3, 1980

Future Concepts of the COTA Role, Part I

The following is edited from a position paper by Terry D. Brittell, COTA, ROH.

What are the future role concepts of the Certified Occupational Therapy Assistant for the 1990s? What are the future directions for active professional involvement, for continuing education, and for professional competency?

What is in store for the COTA in the coming years ahead? Do you perceive yourself remaining at the entry level or progressing to the optimum level of performance within the profession? The profession of occupational therapy is limited only by the creative imagination of its therapists. Our knowledge of role theory and the relationship of persons to an activity-oriented life makes us well suited for future program development, such as industry, schools, correctional institutions, senior citizen programs, rural health programs, developmental centers, or community counseling. Here are some possible suggestions for meeting these future developments:

1. Find a model program after which you design yours.
2. Find an OTR to team up with you.
3. Get some financial backing.
4. Get the credentials you need.

The first critical responsibility is involvement in our professional organizations. I challenge you to offer a reasonable explanation as to why positions open to COTAs on Affiliate Boards are often occupied by OTRs. Or, at the district level we find ourselves hard pressed to secure COTA nominees for office or even for appointed committee leadership. I am well aware of the anticipated dread of becoming an executive board member. But that's where the action is. Volunteer for COTA representative for your district, run for office, edit the newsletter. Do something! How about writing a "Practice Paper" to share you ideas with your fellow colleagues at your district or state conference? Have you ever thought about writing an article for a magazine, your local newspaper or for other professional journals? This can be very creative and rewarding. Under the AOTA reorganizational plan, a COTA can represent a region in the Representative Assembly. How about it?

We must assume the advocacy model as proposed by Jerry Johnson, AOTA past president and of our current AOTA president, Mae Hightower-Vandamm. Don't just sit there complaining, do something. Become a role model.

Another critical issue for our future is

continuing education. I believe strongly in specialty certification for COTAs. As you know since the reorganization of AOTA, you have an opportunity to enroll in one or more areas of specialization. Continuing competence through education becomes the responsibility of each of us, COTA and OTR. It is consistent with a professional philosophy of growth, continuing to update skill; if not, you will fall behind.

The last major issue is the current role concept of the COTA. By New York State laws, therapists (OTRs) are deemed professionals by virtue of their educational and examination level. The COTAs are *certified, not licensed* according to their educational level. The OTR is a designer of theoretically based treatment programs, highly skilled in program evaluation, assessments, screenings and possesses an indepth educational background in biomedical sciences, whereas the assistant has general knowledge in these areas, but high technical skills. The OTR at the entry level should be a generalist in psychiatry and physical dysfunction, for any age level client, while the COTA tends to specialize at the entry level in psychiatry, gerontology, mental retardation and/or physical dysfunction.

(continued)

Future Concepts—Part I

Much has been verbalized and documented about our image, the conflicts in roles and our place within the profession. The "overlap" in tasks and in the delivery of service has added confusion and misunderstanding. OTRs are expected to be responsible for all tasks performed by COTAs according to AOTA's "Delineation of Roles." *Both* COTAs and OTRs should be responsible for some assessments, planning and treatment—"intervention." What differs is the level of responsibility, of supervision, of academic background, and of the objectives of the treatment.

In an *AJOT* XXII, 5, 1968, article, Ruth Brunyate Wiemer wrote of *Drafting Plans for the Future:* "I submit that the goal of many voices here is to have as the profession's official stand, the fact that the COTA is an occupational therapist and not a subservient assistant to an occupational therapist; that within the profession there are varying avenues of educational preparation, qualifying criteria, just as competence, capacity for judgment and exercise of responsibility vary with the level of preparation, so too do they exist with individual variation with either the professional or technical level. I also infer within the profession there can and do exist COTAs whose competence for a given assigned responsibility exceeds that of a more elaborately educated but less endowed professional, just as there do exist COTAs and OTRs whose individual competence fall below our desired optimum for an assigned task. Yes, there are levels of preparation, qualification and competence. I conclude that you cannot be at a given level unless you are contained with the commodity whose level is being gauged. The COTA is an occupational therapist, certified. Occupational therapists are prepared at two levels, professional and technical, i.e., registered and certified."

If we now can assume our present role as being a mature professional with basic understanding of our respective functions, then we can realize the potential for drafting plans for the future. I would like to focus on the Academy concept, developed by the New York State Occupational Therapy Association in November of 1977, and now being further defined for finalization which delineates three levels of membership as follows:

Generalist—holds competency certification from American Occupational Therapy Association or other recognized certification body and demonstrates professional interest in maintaining and upgrading competence as to current professional levels, e.g., inservice, lectures, conferences, and a variety of special interest group presentations.

Skilled Clinician—requires certification from recognized body (which will be identified—sometime in the future) plus two years of clinical experience to apply. The Skilled Clinician will be recognized for achieving some areas of distinction within a specialty area and demonstrated participation, in continuing education, both in specialty and in continuing education.

Master Clinician—requires certification from a recognized body, demonstrated participation in continuing education, and practice development, education or research, plus achieving recognition in a wide sphere of influence for mastery of an area of distinction within one or more specialty area.

In reviewing AOTA's delineation of roles for the entry-level COTA, one can visualize the use of continuing education, level of competency, supervision and role clarification for delineation of membership levels for COTAs. Therefore, I would like to propose the following levels: *Entry, Skilled Clinician*, and *Master Clinician*.

The next issue of the *Newsletter* will present the proposed levels for the profession from the position paper by Terry D. Brittell.

Mental Health
Special Interest Section Newsletter; Vol. 4, No. 1, 1981

Future Concepts of the COTA Role, Part II

The following is edited from a position paper by Terry P. Brittell, COTA, ROH. Part I of this article was published in the recent Newsletter *(Vol. 3, No. 3, 1980).*

After reviewing AOTA's delineation of roles for the entry level COTA in Part I, I can visualize the use of continuing education, levels of competency, supervision, and role clarification for the establishment of membership levels for COTAs. I would propose the following levels: entry, skilled clinician, and master clinician.

Entry—Technical Position—Level I: May perform the following duties under the clinical supervision of a registered occupational therapist (in some instances, administration supervision may be provided by an occupational therapy assistant—Level III).

Treatment:
—assess occupational performance skills in the areas of activities of daily living (ADL), work and play/leisure.
—carry out treatment plan for health maintenance

—adapt treatment media to meet specific patient/client needs
—member of interdisciplinary treatment team
—document client progress in chart
—participate in discharge planning
—maintain attendance and treatment records.

Unit Maintenance/Management:
—responsible for maintenance of equipment and clinic area
—observe all safety standards
—determine supply needs for clinic
—schedule patient/clinic treatment for OT clinic
—provide input regarding patient/client need to assist with program development.

Supervision
—may provide inservice training in activities to to other staff, sharing skills and technical knowledge.

Skilled Clinician—Level II: Qualified to perform all duties of the occupational therapy assistant (Level I). In addition, may perform the following duties under the supervision of a registered occupational therapist.

Treatment:
—develop treatment plan for specific patient/client in the areas of ADL, work, and play/leisure
—develop and coordinate program for patient follow-up in the community
—develop and coordinate ward activity and/or general activity programs
—serve as consultant to more than one treatment team for activities
—may assist and construct certain adaptive equipment and orthotics
—develop activity programs

Unit Maintenance/Management:
—maintain appropriate records of clinic, equipment and supply use
—provide input regarding budget and space needs for clinic
—provide input for determination of capital equipment needs of clinic

(continued)

Future Concepts—Part II

Supervision:
—coordinate OTA Level I staff in program, as well as other staff assisting in activity programs
—provide inservice training in technical skills to occupational therapy staff and/or other disciplines
—provide supervision for COTA student trainees

Master Clinician—Level III: Qualified to perform all duties of the occupational therapy assistant (Levels I and II). In addition, may perform the following duties under the supervision of a registered occupational therapist.

Supervision:
—will be given as needed, rather than direct.

Treatment:
—responsible for program implementation
—screenings/assessments
—scheduling
—treatment planning
—treatment
—evaluate

Programming:
—planning
—budgeting
—evaluating
—supervision of staff

General Activity Program:
—program development and planning
—inservice
—consultant
—supervision of staff
—supervision of staff—CETA and summer employees
—supervision of volunteers
—supervision of COTA/OTR student (fieldwork supervisor)

Administration:
—participate in program development and/or provide consultant services
—coodinate community activity programs with those of other community agencies, such as ARC and various day treatment centers
—direct community activity program
—may supervise the performance of assigned COTA and paraprofessional staff (human service—social work students, etc.)

—clinical teaching for occupational therapy students
—order supplies and/or equipment
—maintain inventory
—develop assessments
—program evaluation research
—soliciting and management of donations
—community speaker
—client/patient advocate
—liaison with community agencies
—custodian of petty cash funds, donations for program planning
—home visits
—resource/consultant for outside agencies
—crisis intervention
—monthly reports
—inservice multi-discipline staff

Conclusion: The advancement of occupational therapy through a network of professional levels for both therapists and assistants will assure a bright future. However, only if based on proficiency, development of specialization, and continued education, will any levels of professional competency complement each other.

Mental Health
Special Interest Section Newsletter; Vol. 3, No. 3, 1980

Day Treatment Services

Many therapists have called and written indicating a need for a basic format for day treatment services. In an effort to assist in meeting this need, the following program is presented, which has been adapted and edited from a current proposal by Richard Cooper and Terry Korhorn. More complete information can be obtained from the authors.

The program will be a day treatment service through occupational therapy and counseling for emotionally impaired adults who will attend, on site, during part of the day. Services will be provided to clients to remediate psychosocial dysfunction through a structured social environment. The activities and social milieu will form a background for a variety of treatment media which will attempt to change behaviors, attitudes, skills, and coping abilities of the client.

The population served will be adults who are experiencing psychosocial dysfunction and are as a consequence, impaired in their ability to function in a satisfactory manner in their natural environments. Clients will be individually assessed and placed on specific levels of the program based on personal adjustment factors, intelligence, and social

maturity. This will allow for some variation in the ages accepted. Clients served may be referred from the community, community agencies, and community schools.

The goal of the program will be to identify and facilitate individual strengths in order to minimize weaknesses in behaviors, attitudes, skills, and coping abilities that have impaired the client's abilities to function in a satisfactory manner in his/her natural environment. This goal will be met through individualized assessment, individualized treatment planning, and diverse implementation methods. Each client's program will be evaluated periodically to determine programmatic success.

The service goals of the program will follow the clinical treatment model. The program will systematically direct the clinical components of assessment, treatment planning, implementation, and evaluation toward each client and his or her individual problem situation.

Program Components:

1. *Assessment* will include the estimation of the client's potential, what the client has achieved, how the client achieves, and how the client feels about his or her level of achievement. This

will be accomplished through a variety of formal and informal tests with all information being analyzed and interpreted to present the client's strengths, weaknesses, and treatment needs.

2. *Prescription/treatment planning* will use the assessment findings to determine what can be done to facilitate the client's satisfactory functioning in his or her natural environment. Both long- and short-term goals will be established. Objectives will be stated in behavioral terms.

3. *Implementation* of the prescription/treatment plan will be done through diverse social methodology to fulfill the client's specific needs within the reality of the natural environment. The natural environment will include the program, the client's family, and the general community within which the client functions.

4. *Evaluation* of the treatment given will be done to determine the progression of the client toward the goal of making satisfactory adjustments to his or her natural environment. This

(continued)

Day Treatment Services

evaluation will include the communication of client goals and evaluation of his achievements to the client, the client's family, and the referral agency. Adjustments in the prescription/treatment plan will be based on evaluation of programmatic success.

Program Aims

The general aim of the program will be to provide psychiatric day treatment services for the community under the direction of an occupational therapist with supportive counseling services provided by a social worker or psychologist.

The specific aims of the program will include the use of diverse treatment media structured into units in order to maintain the client in his natural environment, including his own work setting, without the need for inpatient services. The treatment units will provide appropriate activities and end-products in a setting which will allow opportunities to practice social adjustment behaviors with immediate feedback. The units will be designed to fill the client's emotional, social, physical, pre-vocational, and avocational needs through a positively oriented program. This approach will provide for positive self-identification. The program will provide the home-family with intervention, and the community with an assessment center as well as a day crisis center.

The program will provide services which will be of value to the client and the community.

The value to the client lies in the provision of a positively oriented program designed to facilitate appropriate adjustments to his or her natural environment. This would mean that the client would not have to leave that natural environment due to mental dysfunction or crisis situations.

The value to the community lies in the provision of day care services to a population within the community which may not have alternative services, with the exception of removal from the natural environment. All of these services can be provided at an appropriate cost factor.

Mental Health

Special Interest Section Newsletter; Vol. 3, No. 2, 1980

Research Results Support Occupational Therapy's Effectiveness

The results of a national Veterans Administration cooperative study were recently published in *The Archives of General Psychiatry* (Vol. 36, September 1979, pp. 1055-1066). Entitled "Day Treatment and Psychotropic Drugs in the After-care of Schizophrenic Patients," the study presented some data that are a big boost for the importance of occupational therapy in working with chronic patients. Ten day centers were studied for four years. Some centers were found to be effective in treating chronic schizophrenic patients and others were not. Significantly more occupational therapy ($p < .05$) was offered at the effective centers. The less effective centers significantly ($p < .001$) offered more family counseling and group-psychotherapy. Factors that were not significantly different between the two types of centers were: special work training groups, educational counseling, recreational therapy, medication, and individual psychotherapy. The more effective day centers were also characterized significantly by specific plans for evaluation, less social workers and psychologists, more part-time staff, and longer treatment.

The authors (who did not include any OTs) concluded "In terms of our findings, it is possible that the less intensively personal and more object focused activity of occupational therapy produced better outcomes than the intensive interpersonal stimulation often encountered in group therapy." If you do not have access to this journal, request a copy from co-author Margaret W. Linn, PhD, VA Hospital, 1201 NW 16th St., Miami, FL 33125. This is a good paper to share with mental health leaders in your state!

Mental Health

Special Interest Section Newsletter; Vol. 3, No. 2, 1980

Human Rights in Research

Do you want to do clinical research but feel bewildered about clearing your Human Rights Committee? Most large institutions have a committee that reviews all research proposals to see that patients' human rights are not violated. Our committee is called the Institutional Review Board (IRB). Many of the concerns of this committee are dictated by federal regulations as well as legal protections for the University. Our student research must clear both the IRB at the University and receive approval from the facility where the research is conducted. Sometimes this may involve just a letter from the administrator or it may involve an approval from the Board or human rights committee at the facility. If the proposal is written with all areas of human rights carefully considered, we have found few problems with getting the needed approval. In a few cases, it became apparent early on that the facility was either inexperienced or unrealistic about the research and it was easier to approach another facility. Areas that must be covered in your proposal include:

— other review committees which might be considering your proposal;

— use of consent forms (Here, these are required only if the subject is "at risk." However, we use these in all studies as a matter of courtesy. Photos and films require consent also.);

— confidentiality protection;

— how the results will be communicated and to what audiences (you should include all possibilities);

— whether the patients will be in a drugged, painful, or stressful condition and how you will overcome the effects of the condition in the consent process;

(continued)

Human Rights

— if a control group is used and the treatment is beneficial, can the control group receive treatment at a later date;
— whether "special groups" such as minors, pregnant women, prisoners, mentally retarded or mentally disabled persons are included and why this population *must* be used. If possible, prior studies showing the effects of the experimental procedure on competent, noninstitutional adults should be cited;
— inclusion of a personal compensation clause indicating that the University will not pay for treatment of injuries which occur as a result of participation in the research, although treatment will be available;
— inclusion of a permission letter from the administrator of the experimental setting if it is outside your work setting and does not have an IRB;

— description of the subjects and actual time each will participate;
— whether your results will be available to the participants;
— what possible risks are involved. What will you do if adverse effects occur (i.e., drop subject, change procedure, terminate research project). What is the benefit-risk ratio? Are negative effects reversible? Will normal treatment be withheld for the participants? Is there alternative treatment?);
— what precautions will be taken to avoid hazards;
— at what point the experiment will be terminated, if hazards materialize, for the individual or the entire study;
— how potential subjects will be screened and factors that will be the basis of screening;
— if the subject must give consent within 48

hours, why it is necessary to give such a short time for decision-making.

The experience of going through the human rights mechanism is somewhat like doing your income tax. You need to start off by getting the proper forms, talk to a local expert and allow yourself plenty of time for changes, especially last minute changes in regulations. Our proposals are actually fairly short since we have a form to complete which we were instructed to complete as briefly as possible with certain phrases described as "more acceptable." It is the 17 copies that kills us! Sample, completed forms and consent letters are available from Elizabeth Moyer if you send a large envelope with 2 stamps and give a brief description of your intended study to: Elizabeth Moyer, c/o O.T. Dept., University Station, Birmingham, AL 35294.

Mental Health
Special Interest Section Newsletter; Vol. 2, No. 4, 1979

Clinical Educator Questionnaire Results

Results of the survey to identify what evaluations students are expected to be knowledgeable upon arrival at their psychiatric field experience are described below. 499 questionnaires were mailed and 137 returned. The respondents included 97% OTRs, 1% ATs, and 2% others. The data represents the percentage of clinical supervisors responding to the category.

Which of the following method/s of evaluation do you expect the student to be proficient in?

Individual Task	70%
Group Task	59%
Interview	63%
Observation	83%
Chart Review	55%

I do not expect the student to know a formal evaluation procedure — 0%

Column I indicates those evaluations in which respondents expected the student to be proficient (a) and those in which they expected the student to be knowedgeable (b).

Column II indicates those evaluation in which the clinicians *ideally* would expect the student to be proficient (a) or to be knowledgeable (b).

	Column I (expected)		Column II (ideally)	
	a %	b %	a %	b %
Mosey				
Survey of task				
Skills	25	41	25	17
Group Interaction	26	42	13	24
Activities of				
Daily Living	26	38	17	24
Child Care Survey	05	29	22	17
Work Survey	08	44	18	21
Recreation Survey	07	46	17	20
Activity Configuration				
(Mosey or Watanabe)	14	42	19	20
Diagnostic Test				
Battery	07	28	11	21
Comprehensive Occupa-				
tional Therapy Evaluation	11	41	05	24
Buck-Magazine Picture				
Collage	11	20	10	23
Lawn and O'Kane	02	15	11	26
Shoemym Battery	04	21	13	25
Fidler Battery	04	40	13	23
Azima Battery	04	37	22	21
Goodman Battery	08	30	12	25
Interest Checklist	33	35	12	25
Moorhead: Occupa-				
tional History	09	24	06	18
Adolescent Role				
Assessment	05	29	09	24
Lafyette Clinic				
Battery	02	17	09	23
Object History	06	21	13	27
Play History	05	25	09	28
Social Adaptability				
Test	06	18	10	20
Occupational Behavior				
Rating Scales (Kimes)	05	24	90	01
Self Puzzle	05	18	0	0

Sixty-six psychological tests were identified as evaluations in which clinical supervisors expect students to be knowledgeable.

For individuals who requested a reference list, the following should be helpful.

Androes, L., Dreyfus, E. and **Bloesch, M.,** "Diagnostic Test Battery for Occupational Therapy" *AJOT,* XIX(2), 1965

Ayres, A., "A Form to Evaluate the Work Behavior of Patients" *AJOT,* VIII(2) 1954

Bendroth, S. and **Southam, M.,** "Objective Evaluation of Projective Material" *AJOT,* XXVII(2), 1973

Black, M., "Adolescent Role Assessment" *AJOT,* XXX(2), 1976

Brayman, S., Kirby, T., Misenheimer, A. and **Short, M.,** "Comprehensive Occupational Therapy Education Scale" *AJOT,* XXX(2), 1976

Buck, R., and **Provancher, M.,** "Magazine Pictures Collages as an Evaluative Technique" *AJOT,* XXVI(1), 1972

Casanova, J., "Comprehensive Evaluation of Basic Living Skills" *AJOT,* XXX(2), 1976

Lawn, E., and **O'Kane, C.,** "Psychosocial Symbols as Communicative Media" *AJOT,* 27(1), 1973

Lerner, C., and **Ross, G.,** "The Magazine Picture Collage" *AJOT,* 31(3), 1977

Matsutsuyu, J., "The Interest Checklist" *AJOT,* 23(4), 1969

Shoemyn, C., "Occupational Therapy Orientation and Evaluation" *AJOT,* XXIV(4), 1970

Wolff, R., "A Behavior Rating Scale" *AJOT,* XV(1), 1961

I want to thank those who took the time to respond. — *Barbara Jo Hemphill, MS, OTR, Cleveland State University.*

Sample Discharge Form

With more and more emphasis on measuring the effectiveness of OT services, therapists are beginning to develop formal discharge procedures and forms. Jacque Bell, MS, OTR (Iowa), sent me one of the best forms I have seen recently. She is willing to share her discharge form with you. (Remember to credit the source if you do adopt it! You only need to say, "Reprinted with permission of Jacque Bell.")

Mercy Hospital
Occupational Therapy Council
Bluffs, IA

Discharge Summary
Developed By Jacque Bell, MS, OTR

Patient: _____

Admission Date: _____

Discharge Date: _____

Patient attended _____ treatment sessions in _____ treatment days.

Case No. _____

Dr. _____

Behavior 1 Week Prior to Discharge

	Present	Absent
Regular attendance, unless excused	___	___
Punctual 4 out of 5 times	___	___
Appropriately dressed and groomed	___	___
Independently begins tasks	___	___
Attends to task full session without constant reassurance or supervision	___	___
Completes task in appropriate length of time	___	___
Makes decisions independently regarding activities	___	___
Demonstrates initiative with tasks	___	___
Initiates conversation	___	___
Demonstrates pride in personal accomplishments	___	___
Discusses feelings and concerns with little anxiety or hostility	___	___
Participates in 3 voluntary activities	___	___
Independent in self-care	___	___
No inappropriate behavior	___	___

Non-Measurable Treatment Objectives

	Improved	No Improvement	Not Applicable
Self concept	___	___	___
Knowledge of basic living skills	___	___	___
Environmental management	___	___	___
Parenting skills	___	___	___
Marital relations	___	___	___
Budgeting	___	___	___
Nutrition	___	___	___
Exercises	___	___	___
Work skills	___	___	___
Time management skills	___	___	___
Leisure interests	___	___	___
Assertiveness	___	___	___
Insight into behavior	___	___	___
Acceptance of responsibility for behavior	___	___	___
Relationship with authority figures (Staff)	___	___	___
Acceptance of structure	___	___	___
Ability to handle frustration	___	___	___

Therapist comments:

Patient's plans for first week after discharge:

Patient's assessment of progress he/she has made:

Patient's concerns at the time of discharge:

Follow-up recommendations:

Signed: _____

Mental Health
Special Interest Section Newsletter; Vol. 2, No. 3, 1979

Adult-Size Equipment Used in Sensory Integration Treatment at Warren State Hospital

By Karen Pettit, MEd, OTR

During the last year and a half at Warren State Hospital we have been struggling with equipment designs and adaptations of children's sensory integration equipment for use with chronic adult psychiatric patients. As patients began to be aware that they had options concerning their treatment, our mission as therapists was to design equipment that would reach a number of patients and that would stimulate movement and growth in both a neurophysiological and emotional sense.

One piece of equipment that we have found valuable and most versatile is the "interchangeable bar".

Description: A pipe 115 inches long and 1½-inches in diameter is suspended from the ceiling via a swivel hook and "D" ring/mountain climbing hook, a carabiner. The swivel hook is connected to the pipe by another "D" ring, which is inserted into two ¾-inch in diameter chains that are attached to the pipe by "D" rings inserted into the set of 1½-inch welded rings on the top of the pipe and directly underneath on the bottom side of the pipe. There are sets of welded rings in order to adapt the equipment for various uses, one set at each end and one set in the middle. The two outside chains are 84 inches long with 1½-inch welded rings inserted at 4-inch intervals and placed approximately half way up the chain to enable the chains to be used for each of the four adaptations. An additional piece of chain is required for the swivel double hammock and for the double bolster swing. This piece of chain is made of 1-inch stock; it is larger in size to permit one to adjust the middle of the pipe to provide extra support and prevents the bar from bending in the middle.

Uses: The "interchangeable bar" can be used as four different pieces of equipment, namely: 1. as a stationary double hammock, 2. as an inner tube crawl through and swing, 3. as a swivel double hammock, and 4. as a double bolster swing. Each of these adaptations will be described together with their sensory integration benefits.

Sensory Integration Benefits: The most frequently used aspect of the apparatus is the *stationary double hammock*. Essentially the bar is suspended approximately one foot to a foot and a half off the ground (after the hammocks are attached and the people are inside them). Usually when we start adults in the double hammocks we have them sit so that their legs are hanging out each side. This position gives some extra security because their feet and hands can touch the

ground and can control the rate of rotation. An advantage to the double hammock is that it allows the therapist to be in constant touch with the amount and kind of stimulation the patient is receiving. Many games and motor activities can be incorporated to help the vestibular stimulation become organizing rather than disorganizing and help the patient who is hypersensitive gradually be able to integrate and tolerate more vestibular stimulation. One activity we use is to arrange the inner tubes around the mats we placed under the bar. After the two people are situated in the hammocks, someone will throw Nerf balls to catch, then the people in the hammocks can place the balls inside the inner tubes or throw the balls at a target.

Often we lower the bar in its closest position to the floor and *suspend 9 to 10 truck inner tubes*. Our patients like to crawl inside most often in prone position and gently swing themselves slowly, their feet usually on the ground and their hands and arms hang through the inner tubes so that they can control their own rate of movement either back and forth or in a rotating manner. Some enjoy lying on their backs and allowing the truck tubes to provide the support which enables the therapist to do the stimulating. Often patients that are posturally insecure feel safe enough because they are so close to the ground that they will allow their head to relax and go backwards providing that stimulation to the otoliths that is so difficult to get.

The other two uses for the "interchangeable bar" are the *double swivel adaptations for hammocks and bolster swings*. Both of these require the additional piece of 1-inch stock chain 38 inches long. This is used to support the middle of the bar so that it does not bend and break the bar or weaken the welded rings to which the chain is connected. Two pieces of 1¼-inch pipe are added to the bar with two sets of rings welded to each end of this 47-inch long pipe. The pipe also has one ring welded on the top of this pipe in the center. Essentially, we have two hammocks or bolster swings that swivel two different ways, one from the ceiling swivel, which rotates the entire long pipe from which the two shorter pipes are suspended, and the other which comes from each individual swivel attached to both the long 115-inch pipe and the shorter 47-inch pipe. The double bolster arrangement can be lowered so that one can climb over it in an obstacle course or hang from underneath to work on antigravity postures. When in this

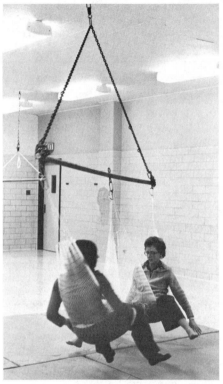

This adaptation was named stationary double hammock because of its ability to rotate in one plane permitted by the swivel hook attached to the I Beam in the ceiling and the two chains supporting each end of the bar. The hammocks are unable to rotate independently of the bar. Both Valerie Dejean, OTR, and Lois Pochert, OTR facing the camera, are working cooperatively to control the amount of rotation and the speed of rotation by their hands and feet.

lower position it is also conducive for hanging supine and prone over the top of the bolster, again promoting stimulation to the otoliths that help improve postural insecurity. The double swivel hammocks are attached similar to the bolster swings with "D" rings connecting at each end of the short pipe. This arrangement not only provides additional variety and interest in the treatment plan, but also, the patient receives rotational stimulation and up and down motion like a teeter totter, causing some co-contraction and proprioceptive stimulation. Each hammock or bolster swing can rotate in two different directions simultaneously from one pivotal point in the ceiling.

Safety Considerations: In order for the "interchangeable bar" to be used effectively, there should be at least 10 square feet of space to allow for rotation and for swinging back and forth. Some very psychotic pa-

(continued)

Adult-Size Equipment

tients, and those who are apraxic, find this piece of equipment initially confusing. It is difficult for them to conceptualize just how it operates, so that the therapist must be acutely aware of the patients when the bar is in motion, and when they are getting in and out of the hammocks. When using this piece of equipment the two people involved must be able to work cooperatively, for if one sits down on the bolster or hammock before the other, the bar is no longer balanced. This can be very frightening. Such an experience in the initial stage of therapist's relationship with a chronic psychotic patient could set things back several sessions. When the apparatus is rotating the chains sometimes will make a sound and one's first response is a fear that it is going to fall; some patients will panic and immediately get up, throwing the bar off balance and send the other person to the floor. We always surround the entire area with mats. Sometimes some people

place inner tubes inside the hammocks, causing them to be raised higher off the ground and increasing the difficulty in getting inside the hammocks. When this occurs, one must be careful while the patients are getting inside the hammocks; occasionally one of them will not have the righting reactions necessary to maintain balance and will fall to the floor. It is important that both people are comparable in their ability to get in and out of the hammocks, and that they have equal tolerance for rotation and movement, or that one is able to adjust to the other's level of slower movement. This is true for every position the apparatus will provide. Maintenance consists of frequent checks of the "D" rings and connecting welds, and checking that the swivels, "D" rings and connections are lubricated to prevent squeaking and friction. The "D" rings must also be checked so that they do not become sprung from the weight of the ap-

paratus and the people inside. We also make periodic checks of the ceiling bolts that are fastened into the steel I Beams and the cotter pin inside the swivel hooks that supports the majority of the weight.

Summary: The "Interchangeable bar" provides four basic adaptations and focuses the sensory integration treatment benefits into two primary areas. First, it assists us in the development of a variety of methods to stimulate postural responses while requiring adaptive responses, particularly climbing and hanging from the bolster swings in antigravity postures, as well as providing some nonthreatening ways to stimulate the otoliths; for example, inside the inner tubes while being totally supported except for one's head. Second, it has provided us with graded levels of vestibular stimulation promoting gradual increased toleration and integration of vestibular stimulation.

Mental Health
Special Interest Section Newsletter; Vol. 2, No. 3, 1979

Progress on MHSS Goals, May 1978 to May 1980

GOAL 1 — *Coordinate with New York and California OT Mental Health Symposiums to increase participation and promote publication of presentations.*

Close communication has been established with the New York liaison and the California planning committee in regard to initiating regional mental health meetings in conjunction with their annual conferences. The chairperson attended the California conference in 1978 to explore possibilities. The California event was well covered in the *MHSS Newsletter* and proposed budget for 1979-80 includes some monies to subsidize two designated regional conferences.

GOAL 2 — *Prepare and begin publishing process for the several potential OT Mental Health Publications.*

Procedures for publishing have been worked out with Betty Cox at AOTA National Office and three persons so far have offered to serve on a MHSS Editorial Board. Four packets of papers to be considered have thus far been received from members. A survey was made at the MHSS Business Meeting in Detroit to determine needs for possible study packet topics. The proposed budget for 1979-80 includes some seed money for publishing. Although not projects of the MHSS, the development of a book on Mental Health OT assessments and a journal on Mental Health OT was probably facilitated by more centralized communication for OTs in mental health.

GOAL 3 — *Prepare for publication or an annual collection of OT Mental Health papers.*

Some of the papers received may be used toward an annual collection of papers; however, thus far no theme for the first publication has been determined.

GOAL 4 — *Establish active study groups in 20 states.*

Thus far MHSS group activity has been reported from 13 states to the standing committee. Only three states have not yet appointed a liaison. State level activities by liaisons have been a strong concern of the standing committee and regional assignments have enabled closer communication and support for some state liaisons. State liaison activities have been highlighted in the *MHSS Newsletter* and shared at the Detroit business meeting.

GOAL 5 — *Publish a newsletter responsive to member's needs.*

Three issues have been published this year with one additional one in progress. Budgeting for 1979-80 continues quarterly newsletters. Issues this year have focused on sensory intergration, daily living skills and creative-expressive programs.

GOAL 6 — *Maintain a resource bank of OTs in mental health which is used frequently by members and outside agencies.*

The resource bank now has 24 categories, most well filled with resource members. This year the resource bank members answered correspondence and some responded to special requests to submit newsletter items and potential publication material. Some were asked to attend special MHSS Task Force meetings in Detroit on the Chronic Patient, the Paradigm and Assessment.

GOAL 7 — *Compile resources for OTs in mental health, including audiovisual materials, bibliographies, non-OT supporters and practice files.*

A survey is currently in progress for audiovisual resources after determining that a listing was not available from AOTA. This survey, which was sent to liaisons and OT schools, also requests non-OT supporters and potential papers for publishing or for the study packets. Several selected bibliographies have already been received (a few brief ones were published in the MHSS Newsletter) and work is in progress to compile a comprehensive mental health OT bibliography including past AOTA conference papers.

GOAL 8 — *Establish a research advisory committee.*

A MHSS Research Resource Bank exists and once a research advisory committee is requested, it will be drawn from this group.

(continued)

MHSS Goals

GOAL 9 — *Gather data on mental health content of OT curricula.*

The first meeting of a few mental health educators was spontaneously held at the Commission of Education meeting in San Diego. This year at Detroit, a COE meeting of these educators was announced ahead of time. Lyn Hill (New York) is coordinating our efforts in education.

GOAL 10 — *Continue analysis of characteristics of OTs in mental health.*

An analysis was completed of members' needs and from the membership survey, much of which has been shared with members via the *MHSS Newsletter*. Additional information which has not been previously gathered will probably be sent to members with renewal of membership.

GOAL 11 — *Provide for OT representation at related conferences including specifically APA Hospital and Community Psychiatry, National Association of Activity Therapy and Rehabilitation Program Directors, and the International Association for Psychosocial Rehabilitation.*

This year occupational therapists attended and shared reports on annual meetings of the NAATRPD, the International Association for Psychosocial Rehabilitation and the American Orthopsychiatric Association. Official representation of the section was not possible since funding was not available. Funding to encourage such representation is included in next year's budget.

GOAL 12 — *With National Office, devise and begin to carry out plan to establish closer communication with the National Institute of Mental Health.*

The chair, a standing committee member, and two other mental health OTs met with AOTA National Office Staff in February to discuss strategies with the NIMH and response to the President's Commission on Mental Health Report, released in 1978. A number of strategies were identified including encouraging mental health OTs to be more political and to develop state level contacts.

GOAL 13 — *Sponsor an Institute on Assessment at the 1979 AOTA Detroit Conference and an institute on theory at the 1980 AOTA Denver Conference.*

An Institute on Assessment was offered at Detroit and was popular in enrollment despite a high fee because of materials included. Planning is continuing for institutes or series at Denver, perhaps on philosophy or the paradigm, as well as chronic patient needs, roles with other creative therapies, and perhaps a follow-up on assessment.

GOAL 14 — *Begin compilation of assessment tools used in OT by mental health practitioners, with descriptions.*

The Assessment Survey is completed with a good response, presented at the Detroit Conference. A publication on the survey results and assessment institute has been outlined and is being considered. The three manuals used in the institute will be available from private sources for a time after the conference. They will be considered for a series of assessment manuals being considered for publishing by the MHSS.

GOAL 15 — *Begin compilation of AOTA research institute mental health presentations.*

Presenters were compiled from the San Diego Conference, but the mental health portion of Detroit's Research Institute was cancelled. (Unfortunately, it conflicted with the Assessment Institute.) — *Elizabeth A. Moyer, MS, OTR, FAOTA, Chair, Mental Health Specialty Section.*

Mental Health
Special Interest Section Newsletter; Vol. 2, No. 1, 1979

Member Survey: Critical Issues Identified

On the 1978 SS yellow sheets members were asked "what do you think are the critical issues the Specialty Section should address?" 715 of the 3500 members replied and an item analysis revealed the following priorities:

		Percent
1)	Our need to adapt to the trend towards *Community* Mental Health including prevention programs, transitional living programs and our roles in community mental health centers	19.6
2)	Developing, standardizing and sharing patient assessment	18.3
3)	Continuing Education	17.9
4)	Research, especially to standardize assessments and to measure the impact of our programs	15.9
5)	Accountability—including PSRO, standards, effective documentation	14.5
6)	Practice: New techniques and program	12.4
7)	Roles/job descriptions of the MH OTR/COTA	11.6
8)	Theoretical base/definition for OT in mental health	9.5
9)	Publications	8.3
10)	Basic education, improve and standardize academic and clinical content	8.1
11)	Communication between therapists	7.4
12)	Sensory integration, validating and increasing use of SI	7.3
13)	Third party reimbursement/funding	7.1
14)	Team functioning	6.4
15)	Boundary problems with creative therapies	6.3
16)	Public relations with clients, psychiatrists, general public	4.9
17)	Short term psychiatric program ideas	4.2
18)	Master's graduate education issues, including developing new OT master's in MH programs and consideration of masters as entry level	3.5
19)	Administration; including working with non OT supervisors and OTs in adequately prepared to be supervisors	2.4
20)	Legislation—changes and implementation	2.4

The rest of the identified issues has been sent to your state liaison.

Mental Health
Special Interest Section Newsletter; Vol. 2, No. 1, 1979

The Working Patient

Therapists in mental health, especially those in institutions can become easily confused by the current fuzzy status of the working patient. Some administrators seem to be too! We sought clarification from Ronald M. Soskin of the National Center for Law and the Handicapped, Inc. (South Bend, IN). This was his helpful reply: "In response to your letter of August 4, 1978 concerning the current status of work as therapy for patients in mental institutions, I must first distinguish between several types of work which patients perform. Patients work can be divided into personal-housekeeping tasks (making one's own bed), institutional maintenance work, and vocational training.

In *Souder v. Brennan*, 367 F. Supp. 808 (D.D.C. 1973), the federal district court for the District of Columbia, interpreting Congressional amendments in 1966 to the Fair Labor Standards Act, held that working patients should be considered to be employees. Thus they must be paid at the federal minimum wage, whether the work performed was therapeutic or not, if the institution derived an economic benefit from the work. Subsequently, the United States Supreme Court in *National League of Cities v. usery*, 426 U.S. 833 (1976) ruled that state employees who perform state functions could not be controlled by the Federal Government for that would entail an encroachment upon state sovereignty. The decision did not involve mental patients but the resultant interpretation has been that the federal minimum wage does not apply to patients and that the *Souder* reasoning is no longer applicable. There have been several subsequent suits to try to clarify what work

is permissible and what work must be compensated but no definitive decisions have been issued.

Basically, the Thirteenth Amendment's prohibition against involuntary servitude should prohibit forced labor. If a patient works, he should be covered by the state minimum wage laws or other state statutes or regulations governing employment. The clearest developing guidelines seem to be that a patient cannot be forced to do work which involves the operation and maintenance of the institution. Personal housekeeping tasks. Work that is claimed to be vocational or therapeutic still lies within a gray area and the burden should rest upon the institution to justify any uncompensated labor as clearly a therapeutic exercise linked to treatment and eventual discharge. Any labor that appears to be benefiting the institution economically would clearly be suspect and thus should be compensated.

Many questions in this area still need to be resolved. No clear definition of therapeutic labor exists. The coerciveness of "voluntary" labor by patients must be scrutinized. The elimination of opportunities to work, if the patient must be compensated (which has been many states' responses), must be questioned. Therefore, at this point we must still await future decisions to clarify these issues."

In addition, Frank Mallon of the AOTA GLAD obtained even more information about the situation via the Mental Health Law Project. This is available from the editor on request. He also pointed out that "In summary, the latest Supreme Court decision affirmed that the Fair Labor Standards

Act, a federal law, cannot be applied to state institutions, unless the state chooses to do so. Therefore, each state is left to determine if and how much payment will be provided to patients who perform work in state institutions. States are also left free to determine for themselves whether any distinction should be made between "therapeutic work" and work which essentially provides an economic benefit to the institution.

The Supreme Court's decision does not affect the application of the Fair Labor Standards Act to private institutions. Therefore, patients in these institutions must receive the minimum wages required by the Act. Moreover, "therapeutic work" does not constitute an exception to the Act, if the institution derives an economic benefit from the work performed by the patient."

If you would like even more information, I suggest you read the Special Report in the February 1977 *Hospital and Psychiatry*.

You might want to order the regulations on Workers in Hospitals and Institutions: Employment of Patients at Subminimum Wages from Division of Special Minimum Wages From the Wage and Hour Division, U.S. Department of Labor, 200 Constitution Ave. Room C 4613, Washington DC 20810. It has more explicit information on patients and money in OT type activities.

At a report on this at the National Association of Activity Therapy and Rehabilitation Program Directors meeting in Kansas City a national survey revealed that most institutions were voluntarily trying to comply with the Fair Labor Standards Act. It seems that the number of working patients has dropped drastically but most are being paid.

Mental Health
Special Interest Section Newsletter; Vol. 1, No. 2, 1978

Sensory Integration Activities

Since there was a very short time beween your receiving the Summer issue and the publishing of the Fall issue it has not been possible to get member's ideas for this newsletter. The editor has scraped together some ideas to get the exchange going and we hope that you will send in *your* ideas for the Winter issue (deadline is December 10).

Parachute

Okay, Okay! Due to popular demand, I will list some ways to use the parachute for those of you lucky enough to have one.

First: Parachute activities (involving tonic muscle groups and extension) for activation of the lethargic patient. Have the group (of at least 5 patients) gather up about 8 inches on the edges of the parachute, then starting from a crouching position with the chute on the grounds, slowly life up in unison until the very height of extension is reached. Release together, allowing the gathers to escape the fingers with the stress of the material. One variation of this is to have half or all the group run across the circle under the parachute, trying to get across before it

drops. The "wind" which can be created by the parachute is very positive tactile input which most patients (and therapists) love. I've only met a few, very few, patients who find parachute activity threatening. I have used it successfully with patients who were highly tactilely defensive. Second: Have the group hold the parachute at shoulder level and bounce balls or balloons on top of it. The objective is to try to keep the ball (it should be a light weight ball) on top of the parachute. This is fun and can be done with a

(continued)

Sensory Integration Activities

blanket if you don't have a chute. Third: Have the group flap the chute on ground level making "waves". Group members may enjoy walking around in bare or stocking feet in the "waves".

Parachute activities for relaxation:

1. Have the group raise the chute and then lie on the floor as the chute drops slowly and softly upon them. You may have staff and students raise and lower the chute on the group.

2. Loosely roll a patient up in the parachute. Have him roll over and over until wrapped in the chute but leave the head free. This is good for achieving Rood's "neutral warmth" which is effective with autistic and hyperactive children. Let him lie in the rolled chute until he wants to unroll.

3. Have a patient sit or stand in the middle of the chute while the group either gently makes "waves" or walks around in a circle slowly winding him up in the material. Unwind in the opposite direction. Another variation is to pretend you are the center of a "flower".

4. Swing or rock the patient in the parachute. This is very effective and sensational as well as a good trust exercise. Just make sure you have a very strong chute and a dependable and strong group.

Always play appropriate music while doing parachute activities.

Evaluation

Dick Jennings, OTR, while at Marcy Psychiatric Center, developed a large graph of expected hand strength (norms from AJOT, 1971; p. 77) for the patient's sex and age, then registered the patient's improvement on the same graph weekly. As the patients improved with their SI program they received dramatic, visual feedback on their grip changes.

Adolescents

Having problems finding activities for sensory integration with adolescents? The following activities were used successfully at March Psychiatric Center, NY, by Ed Cox, OTR and Norma Mahoney, COTA.

1. A version of "King of the Mountain" utilizing two rather shakey balance beams joined with a hinge (can be done on one extra long balance beam but not as much fun)—players approach from opposite ends and beat each other with laundry bags filled with cotton (or dacron) stuffing until one falls off. This was extremely popular with both staff and patients.

2. An "exercise" program was done in self-paced groups of 2 or 3 to earn points. A

daily program to compete was posted and recorded on a separate posted chart. This included traditional situps, etc. plus jump rope, barrel rolls, use of other equipment including a body flexor from Sears (great for vestibular). The boys did surprisingly well with this and after first supervised sessions they would go in sensory integrative room and did well without constant supervision.

3. Bicycling—old bicycles were donated, and parts were donated by local bike manufacturers, and patients repaired bikes and then went on short trips around the grounds (good for top-bottom integration, reciprocal patterns and vestibular especially). The same process was initiated, using a couple of go-carts.

4. Soccer—very popular—this was organized to provide sensory motor experience as well as social skills. Patients played in the mud and became very skillful. This is great for all sorts of SI experiences.

These adolescents were very disturbed, either schziophrenic and regressed or character disorders. Most had extensive learning disabilities.

What activities have you developed that works in your sensory integration programs? Send them in and share them.

Mental Health
Special Interest Section Newsletter; Vol. 1, No. 1, 1978

Initial Development: Report of the Section's First Year

The future of occupational therapy in mental health practice lies in the hands of our practitioners. Effective mobilization of our membership is the key to enriching our professional capacities and resolving the dilemmas confronting us. The dilemmas are many; some transient, and some fundamental. Therapists from across the nation have raised a variety of questions: What is our shifting role in short-term acute-care settings? What must we do to distinguish our expertise from that of other activity therapies? How do we elevate our status in the medical-psychiatric community? How do we increase our availability and impact upon the health services delivery system? How do we deepen our knowledge and understanding of the impact of the activity process upon health and illness? When and how can we fully document the impact of our methods upon our patients?

The preliminary objectives proposed by the National Specialty Section Steering Committee are:

● Define and assess practice

● Increase our public and political visibility and impact

● Develop a resource network of occupational therapists in mental health practice

● Develop a resource network of "friends of OT"

● Identify and provide support for educational needs in basic and continuing education and graduate specialization

● Establish organizational structures for this Specialty Section that facilitates a high level of participation by the Membership

● Evaluate functions and effectiveness of the Specialty Section.

With full appreciation of the need for a rigorous pursuit of ways to resolve the above issues, the first chair and steering committee of this specialty section spent the past eight months identifying a focus and developing strategies for addressing these issues within the context of the seven objectives.

Activities Underway

Much time and preliminary effort was expended in basic organizational tasks: gathering data on mental health practice and our practitioners, identifying priorities of particular importance, setting the wheels in motion for the election of a new chairperson, developing liaison positions from each State, and tackling two of the most frequently mentioned concerns—the paucity of research and the need to standardize patient evaluation procedures. The San Diego Conference launched our official "call to action" on behalf of research and evaluation methodology. Plans were formalized for a major effort in developing an evaluation workshop for the 1979 Detroit conference as well as a longer-term follow-up standardization project.

The tasks confronting us this year were not simple. Our vision of a swell of grass roots activities via local special interest

(continued)

Initial Development

groups was not yet fully visible. We were aware of the watching and waiting attitude of some members, and of an uncertainty on the part of others as to their place in this phase of specialty section activity. It is our firm belief that special interest groups (SIGs) and individual therapists are the backbone of a successful system. Success requires the development, re-activation and continued commitment of SIGs. Priorities and available resources vary from area to area. You are the best advocates from your special interests! State liaison representatives have begun to stimulate the development of local affiliate groups, will continue to keep members informed of relevant issues, and will serve as vehicles for the expression of concerns and ideas to the chair and steering committee. There is work to be done!

Our current internal professional needs must not curtail our public visibility and contributions to State and Federal initiatives. The government's commitment to State and Federal initiatives. The government's commitment to deinstitutionalization and increasing awareness of the need for more relevant community-based services for the chronically mentally ill have been highlighted by the National Institute of Mental Health and the President's Commission on Mental health. This long overdue mandate for effective mental health services for the chronic patient represents an important opportunity for occupational therapists to increase their visibility and take an appropriate leadership role in developing and implementing programs. The need for us to surface as advocates for this group of consumers is critical. With this in mind, the specialty has proposed the formation of a National OT Task Force on the Chronic Patient, which will work in close alliance with consumer advocates, other mental health professionals, and legislators. You will soon hear more about this.

Any statement about our activities and progress requires acknowledgement of the efforts and interest of our first specialty section's steering committee: Carol Nodop, Jenifer Thuell, Diane Shapiro, Carol Shaw, Barbara Smolek, and Columbia University students, Catherine Ahern and Susan Fridie. Their commitment and support has been critical.

The year has been an active one, filled with the crucial and demanding tasks of an infant organization. We tried to do some nuturing of the membership's here-and-now needs, while also attending to the organizational structure that often seems more impersonal, but is important for the section's ultimate well being. To Elizabeth Moyer, newly elected chair, and her steering committee, we extend our best wishes, our continued support, and a Mayflower moving van *filled* with letters, membership data, and more letters! —*Susan B. Fine, MA, OTR. FAOTA*

4

Physical Disabilities
Special Interest Section

ADL and Adaptive Equipment for ALS Patients

Valerie Takai, OTR

The person with amyotropic lateral sclerosis (ALS) presents the occupational therapist with a unique challenge: that of the adult patient with a progressive disability characterized by relentless progression involving only motor impairment. Mentation and sensory function are preserved.

A major function for occupational therapy in the ALS Clinic has been to provide, recommend, and fabricate adaptive equipment as well as upper extremity and cervical orthoses. Ongoing modification and replacement of devices become necessary as the disease progresses. Important parts of the program are teaching techniques of positioning for comfort and function and performing motor assessments for nonvocal communication and other technical aids to assist in arriving at recommendations for equipment.

From the outset, patients and their families are involved in the choice, design, and actual adaptation of equipment. Problem solving is emphasized as a means to prepare constructively for meeting future losses of movement and changes in ability to perform self-care activities.

Whether in the ALS Clinic, the Occupational Therapy Department or in the patient's home, priorities are set with the patient so that those self-care needs most important for the present and future can be met. The time available for each treatment session is fully maximized. Small devices are provided when the patient is seen. The profoundly positive psychological effect of receiving something concrete that can be used immediately to improve function cannot be underestimated.

In performing an ADL evaluation a preliminary motor assessment is made concentrating on, but not limited to, the neck and upper extremities. Due to the varying areas of involvement with no predictable order in the actual progression of symptoms, individual patients present quite different profiles of weakness. Significant variability is also noted in the rate of progression. With rapidly progressive patients, feelings of urgency understandably dominate; plans for management of self-care and equipment recommendations cannot be postponed for a later date. In slowly progressive cases there is time for long-range adaptations such as modifications of home and work-site environments.

The ADL evaluation emphasizes feeding, dressing, washing, and personal hygiene, management of object manipulation such as turning knobs, handles, etc., transfers, communication, and leisure activities. Much time is spent discussing positioning that includes neck, trunk, and upper and lower extremities to prevent future deformities and discomfort. Recommendations are often given for a variety of easy chairs, including recliners, rockers, and wing-back chairs that emphasize full trunk and head support.

Ideas for equipment are derived from several sources. First, devices used by people with severely disabling arthritis and quadriplegia are examined. Another source has been the mass market, which includes a variety of communication devices commonly found in electronic stores such as speaker-phones, alarm systems, and a memowriter with a typewriter keyboard. A third source has been the occupational therapy department, which has contributed ideas for cork-handled utensils, a wide range of soft and molded cervical collars and positioning aids, and a communication cuff. The fourth major source has been ALS patients and their families who have created several ingenious devices. Two such examples are a wheelchair lift which uses heavy duty pulleys and cables and a feeding harness that makes use of strong elbow extensors in one upper extremity to assist weak elbow flexors in the opposite upper extremity.

The majority of ALS patients will eventually require a wheelchair. Since trunk and neck weakness are usually present during the course of the disease, semi-reclining and fully-reclining wheelchairs are generally the wheelchairs of choice. Patients whose insurance enables them to rent equipment may want to consider a lightweight wheelchair when a chair is first indicated if no trunk or cervical weakness is present. Later on they can exchange it for a reclining wheelchair. It has been our experience that even when they can be accommodated in a narrow adult wheelchair, most patients prefer a standard adult size that will afford increased trunk mobility with more sitting space since the narrower chair tends to convey to the patient a sense of confinement that may be both physically and emotionally uncomfortable and disquieting.

Electric hospital beds are the beds of choice because respiratory symptoms may necessitate frequent changes in positioning. This is true whether or not the patient is able to operate the controls.

Padded drop-arm commodes can be used over the toilet while the patient is still ambulatory but has difficulty arising from a standard toilet seat. These can later be used bedside. The padding provides comfort for the marked atrophy present in later stages of the disease.

The most commonly prescribed hand splints are short opponens and cockup splints used in cases with slower progression and commercial wrist supports used in cases with more rapid progression. In patients with very limited atrophy, molded collars are used to improve balance in ambulation in the presence of neck extensor weakness. Soft collars are also often custom-made, using moderately firm foam covered in stockinette. They are used during stages of minimal weakness in a later stages when marked atrophy is present.

Again and again we have found that ALS patients are most comfortable when soft textures are used for items involving physical contact for any length of time. Thus foam cushions, bed pads, and synthetic sheepskin are commonly used.

All ALS patients at some time encounter communication difficulties. These can be problems with writing, operating a regular telephone, speaking, or simply signalling for attention. It is important for ALS patients to be assured that there will always be a means for them to communicate.

(continued)

Adaptive Equipment

Patients are advised concerning different types of telephones to use to compensate for problems such as holding a receiver, dialing, and oral communication. Speaker-phones, automatic dialers, and teletypewriters for the deaf are some of the alternatives. Occupational therapists work with speech pathologists to select and adapt appropriate augmentative devices by providing motor assessments that give input on suitable keyboards, switches, positioning of patient, and choice of movement or movements to operate a paticular aid. Augmentative aids range from letterboards and eye-gaze charts to electronic scanners and personal computers.

By way of summary, the following guidelines are suggested to assist in selecting adaptive equipment for the ALS patient. One must first look at the individual rate of progression, the stage of the disease, and the results of the current motor assessment, especially factors of endurance and positioning.

Another important consideration is whether or not the device can be modified to meet future needs. The weight and texture of the device are extremely important. Devices should be as light and comfortable as possible, preferably with soft textures. They must meet the needs of the patient and with the patient involved in the deci-

sion. The reaction of the family is important, especially when they have to set up and maintain the piece of equipment. It is highly recommended that the patient try each device suggested. I would also like to suggest that a patient be able to obtain a given piece of equipment within a three-week period. This requires that the occupational therapist know of vendors, sources for equipment, and be familiar with the third party payers, equipment pools, and other factors of cost. Time too, must be seriously considered, and decisions made quickly. One literally cannot afford to wait.

Physical Disabilities
Special Interest Section Newsletter; Vol. 6, No. 2, 1983

Classification of Neuromuscular Disorders

The following discussion covers a number of neuromuscular diseases that primarily affect the "motor unit." The "motor unit" encompasses one motor neuron (i.e., anterior horn cell, its axon and all terminal branches) and the muscle fiber it innervates. Neuromuscular diseases may be classified in four categories according to the part of the motor unit affected. They include motor neuron disorders, peripheral neuropathies, disorders of the neuromuscular junction, and myopathies.

Motor neuron disorders. Some examples of lower motor neuron conditions include poliomyelitis, acute and chronic infantile spinal muscular atrophy (acute and chronic Werdnig-Hoffman disease, spinal muscular atrophy type 1, 2, and intermediate), juvenile

spinal muscular atrophy (Kugelberg-Welander disease, spinal muscular atrophy type 3), and progressure muscular atrophy. In amyotrophic lateral sclerosis (ALS), both upper motor neuron as well as lower motor neuron involvement coexist.

Peripheral Neuropathies (axonal, Schwann cell and myelin sheath involvement). These consist of toxic neuropathies, Charcot-Marie-Tooth disease and other heredofamilial peripheral neuropathies, diabetic neuropathies, and Guillain-Barre syndrome.

Disorders of the neuromuscular junction. Some examples include myasthenia gravis, myasthenic syndrome (Eaton-Lambert), and botulism.

Myopathic disorders (muscle fiber and cell membrane involvement). Associated progressive muscular dystrophies include Duchenne, fascioscapulohumeral, limb girdle, and myotonic dystrophy. Polymyositis and dermatomyositis are inflammatory myopathies. Other muscle diseases include metabolic and congenital conditions.

Neurological disorders such as multiple sclerosis and Parkinson's disease are not included in this classification of neuromuscular ("motor unit") disorders because their pathology lies within the central nervous system. The motor unit itself is primarily considered a peripheral structure versus a CNS structure.

Physical Disabilities
Special Interest Section Newsletter; Vol. 6, No. 1, 1983

Perspectives in the Treatment of Parkinsonism

By Evelyn Fernandez, OTR, and Ivanette Goodrich, OTR, University of Miami, Dept. of Neurological Surgery, Miami, FL

The National Parkinson Foundation in Miami was established as a research and outpatient rehabilitation center for individuals with Parkinsonism. Within the last three years, the Foundation has formed an association with the University of Miami, Departments of Neurological Surgery and Neurology.

The professional team available for the patient includes, QT, ST, PT, psychologist and behavioral assistant.

A psychiatrist refers the patient for OT treatment. Major problem areas for Parkinson patients are rigidity, bradykinesia and tremors, which result in difficulties with fine and gross motor coordination and decreased mobility that affect ADL functioning. For the patient, stooped posture, poor balance, and a lack of righting reactions will decrease the ability to maintain independence. In turn, this gradual decrease in function affects their self image and self-confidence.

The goal of treatment is to restore or maintain optimum functioning.

Once evaluation is completed, the individual participates in OT as a member of a group that meets for one hour, two to three times weekly. A group consists of three-to-eight members who work as a team for the first 30 minutes of the session. During this time, the aim of therapy is to increase endurance, coordination, balance and range of motion as well as to encourage socialization and communication.

The program includes an upper extremity, trunk and neck exercise routine, both with and without the use of a dowel stick. Grasping an object helps to decrease the tremor. Breathing techniques, facial exercises and dynamic and static balance activities including ball throwing, catching and kicking are also done. During this time, patients are encouraged to take turns and lead the group activities as well as participate in various games to promote mentation.

For the remaining one-half hour all group members are seated at the same table to work on individual craft activities. The goal of treatment, in this instance, is to increase fine motor and perceptual skills, encourage self-esteem, and promote and increase productivity. The patient's ability to follow instructions, solve problems, and work independently as well as the level of frustration are all noted. Individual treatment is used as a method to encourage communication and motivation. This also allows for individual needs to be met, i.e., increasing attention span and instructing in ADL including use of adaptive aids and techniques of energy conservation.

At holiday time, special activities are planned to include spouses and promote a community holiday spirit.

Parkinson patients experience abulia (loss of will power) and feelings of shame, and a sense of not being accepted by society; as a result, this places a great burden on the spouse who feels a responsibility to take the initiative, thus creating a more dependent relationship. A

(continued)

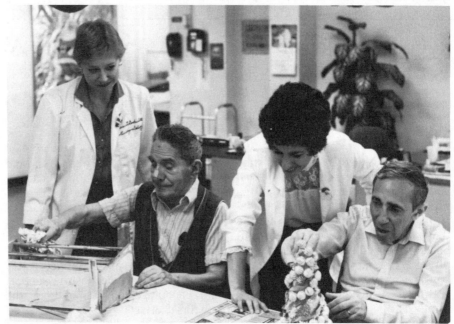

Ivanette Goodrich, OTR (left) and Evelyn Fernandez, OTR, help Parkinson patients increase fine motor skills while creating Christmas gifts. The patients are participating in an eight-member group.

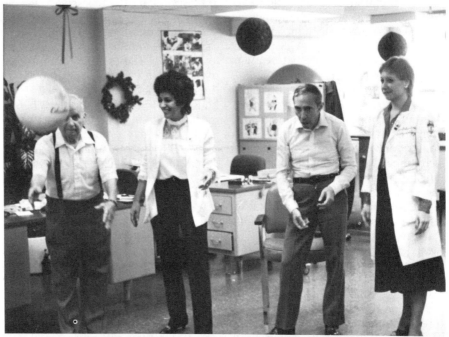

Evelyn Fernandez, OTR (left), and Ivanette Goodrich, OTR, help patients improve gross motor skills with a group ball toss activity.

Parkinsonism

multidisciplinary self-help group was established three years ago to provide a supportive atmosphere where both spouses and patients come to realize that the patients must take some responsibility for themselves through participation in ADL including leisure activities. This social group setting has been successful as an adjunct to other therapies and as a therapy in itself. This is demonstrated by a change in the attitude of the spouses who now have a place to share their concerns and by patients whose barriers of isolation and embarrassment are being broken down.

BIBLIOGRAPHY

Brumlik, J.: Disorders of motion. *American Journal of Physical Medicine*, 1967, *46*, 536 - 543

Davis, J.C.: Team management of Parkinson's disease. *American Journal of Occupational Therapy*, 1977, *31*, 300 - 308

Trombly, C.A. and Scott, A.D.: *Occupational Therapy for Physical Dysfunction*. Baltimore: Williams & Wilkins Co., 1977.

Physical Disabilities
Special Interest Section Newsletter; Vol. 6, No. 2, 1983

Recommended Exercises and Ambulation Aids for People With ALS

Janet Zawodniak, RPT, PT Consultant,
Neuromuscular And ALS Clinics, Mount Sinai Hospital, NY

Physical therapy focuses on assisting ALS patients with attaining optimal and realistic physical function during progressive neuromuscular degeneration. Primary measures include therapeutic exercise, combating ambulation difficulties, and pulmonary physical therapy. Other areas encourage using body compensation techniques and involving patients' family and supportive health personnel whenever possible.

Therapeutic exercise programs must be individualized, continually modified to accommodate ensuing weakness, and are generally implemented during early stages. Since the muscular response to exercise in ALS patients (as compared to normals) is unknown, programs are largely empirical, with patient feedback essential for determining exercise tolerance. In all cases, overfatigue must be avoided. Suggested programs range from general conditioning or endurance training (e.g., swimming, cycling, walking) to passive range of motion. Progressive resistive exercises are not recommended since patients commonly complain of subsequent intense cramping and fatigue. Patients with physically active lifestyles may be advised against exercising to conserve energy for daily activities.

Common major goals include the prevention of disuse atrophy, contractures, and the reduction of spasticity if it limits function. Key design parameters include daily activity level, pattern and extent of weakness, and general physical condition (including coexisting medical problems and age). Despite exercise performance, progressive muscular weakness inevitably occurs, which creates feelings of hopelessness, discouragement, and despair. To perpetuate continued active exercise performance, positive support and encouragement as well as, the beneficial effects of exercise must be emphasized throughout the course of the disease.

Ambulation difficulties arise not only secondary to progessive lower extremity weakness, but commonly occur as a result of varying combinations of lower extremity trunk, and upper extremity weakness. To promote and prolong safe and efficient ambulatory function, assessment of total body muscular function is critical before selecting the most suitable ambulatory aids and body compensation maneuvers. Early complaints may include impairment of balance or slowing of limb motion in activities requiring rapid alternating movements such as when running or making quick turns. With progressive weakness and/or spasticity, commonly used ambulation aids include canes and rolling walkers (progressive upper extremity weakness precludes lifting standard walkers) with forearm or platform crutches intervening in rates of slower progression. Foot drop is a common initial feature that causes ankle instability and falling. Custom and pre-fabricated ankle-foot orthoses are then employed to compensate, the fromer in slower progression. Wrist and intrinsic hand supports are occasionally needed to control devices. Ambulation aids may necessitate adaptation to best suit individual needs. If posterior cervical weakness arises, collars are essential to prevent mechanical neck injuries and to sustain balance and equilibrium during ambulation.

All ambulatory devices and orthoses function to support and/or substitute weakened muscles and joints, reduce excess stress on compensatory muscles, reduce total energy expenditure, and must be lightweight, comfortable, and stable for optimal safety and function.

RESOURCES

The following organizations are devoted to a specific neuromuscular disease or syndrome with the exception of the Muscular Dystrophy Association (MDA), which encompasses more than 40 neuromuscular disorders.

All of these institutions listed below provide information to patients, their families, professionals, and the public.

Amyotrophic Lateral Sclerosis Society of America, PO Box 5951, 153000 Ventura Blvd., Suite 315, Sherman Oaks, CA 91403

MDA, National Office, 810 Seventh Ave., New York, NY 10019

The Myasthenia Gravis Foundation, 15 East 26th St., New York, NY 10010

The National ALS Foundation, 185 Madison Ave., New York, NY 10016

Multiple Sclerosis: Factors that Affect Activity Performance— A Patient Survey

By Kate Beisel, OTR, Whitting, IN

As an occupational therapist who has multiple sclerosis (MS), I have both personal and professional concerns about the role occupational therapists can have in helping people with MS engage in and complete functional activities. This article describes a survey conducted to gain greater knowledge about factors that can limit functional performance for the person with MS.

Multiple sclerosis is one of the most common organic diseases affecting the nervous system. MS and closely related diseases affect an estimated 500,000 people in this country. It is important because it is frequently encountered and almost invariably affects young people.[1] MS does not follow a typical pattern; the nature of the disease is "up and down," usually characterized by various degrees of weakness, fatigue, incoordination, visual disturbance, and difficulties in breathing, speech or swallowing.[2]

Long considered to be a progressive disease, MS information in recent years increasingly has pointed to a benign course in many patients.[3] Thus, it is possible for MS patients to live fairly normal lives and to retain complete or partial working capacity for many years after the initial manifestation of clinical signs and symptoms. This makes functional and vocational rehabilitation a socio-economically sound consideration for many people with MS.[4]

A survey to determine factors that limit or help patient performance was conducted through the *Indiana Multiple Sclerosis Newsletter* in order to reach as many people with MS in Indiana as possible. Two hundred fifty persons with MS responded, representing cities in each division of the state. Twelve questions were posed in the survey. Of these, five were considered to be of specific importance to occupational therapists treating MS patients in the clinic or home. The response to these questions is as follows:

1. *Peak time for activity?* 60% indicated morning, 22% afternoon and 12% evening.
2. *Endurance for activity is hampered if the weather is . . .?* 43% indicated hot weather, 34% cold weather, 13% humid, 10% rainy. Everyone indicated that weather was a factor.
3. *With an "energy high," how do you find yourself (carrying out) activities?* 50% indicated "rushing to complete tasks," 32% "paced themselves," 18% were inconsistent between rushing and pacing.

4. *Amount of rest needed at night?* 42% indicated 8 hours, 21% needed 10 hrs.
5. *When patients are tired, what symptoms interfered first?* 42% indicated lower extremity symptoms, 26% indicated fatigue.

Since the majority indicated their peak time for activity to be in the morning, it appears this time of day would be the ideal time for OT. However, variance exists on this issue. Therapists should determine each patient's peak time and treat accordingly.

Hot and humid weather seemed to cause the most problems. Respondents also indicated breathing difficulties in this weather. To facilitate endurance, it is recommended that air conditioners and dehumidifiers be used to control these weather factors.

Dealing with energy levels is another major concern. Pushing to complete tasks was the most frequent response. It is possible this was chosen due to a concern for energy depletion versus task completion. Poor energy management by the MS patient may lead to greater fatigue and less achievement. It is recommended that a pattern of work or play then rest be introduced to the patient, which would be adjusted to the individual's needs.

Total rest needed per night was included to indicate that in dealing with a disease with symptoms of fatigue a certain amount of rest is required. The occupational therapist should be alerted to the effect lack of sleep may have on performance. Assessment of the patient's sleeping patterns may unveil limitations that can be corrected; for example, back spasms may interfere with sleep and adjustment of medication may be helpful. The attending physician should be notified that this problem is interfering with the patient's functional ability.

Lower extremity pain or weakness becomes a limiting factor, as a direct response to fatigue. It is important to determine if these symptoms are responsive to energy conservation measures. Once again the attending physician should be notified if symptoms are interfering with function.

Total fatigue and weakness are other major factors requiring consideration. It is possible that these two factors may be prodromal to further difficulties such as tremors, slurred speech and incoordination. Rest periods interspersed throughout the day are often beneficial.

The findings of this informal survey suggest that occupational therapists can

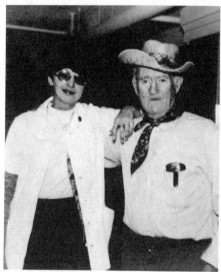

Kate Beisel, OTR, with resident Jack Coats after working in The Residents Garden at Sugar Creek Convalescent Center, Greenfield, IN.

help MS patients by identifying and reducing systemic, behavioral and environmental factors that limit function and performance. Adapted activities, adaptive devices, immediate environment alterations, energy conservation techniques, and ADL skills training can be effective methods for helping the person with MS.

REFERENCES

1. DeJong, Russell, N., M.D., *Enemy of Young Adults,* National Multiple Sclerosis Society, New York, 1978.
2. Braunel, M., James, C.A., Stoval, M.D.: *M.S. Is A Family Affair,* The National Easter Seal Society for Crippled Children and Adults, Chicago, Illinois, 1972.
3. Brown, J.R.: *Recent Studies in Multiple Sclerosis,* National Multiple Sclerosis Society, New York, 1979.
4. Bauer, H.J.: A Manual on Multiple Sclerosis Federation of Multiple Sclerosis Societies, pp 34-36, 1980.

RELATED READINGS

1. Kahana, E., Leiboeitz, U., Alter, M.: *Cerebral Multiple Sclerosis,* New York, Lancet Publications, Inc., Vol. 21, No. 12, 1971.
2. Tourtellotte, W.: *Therapeutics of Multiple Sclerosis,* New York, Raven Press, Vol. 2, 1977.
3. Weinstein, A: Behavioral Aspects of Multiple Sclerosis, New York, Harper and Row, Vol. 7, No. 5, 1970.

ACKNOWLEDGMENTS

Appreciation is expressed to Sheree Farber, MS., OTR., FAOTA; Dottie Weeks, MS., OTR., FAOTA; Tony Kuchta, MBA; and Casey Howell, director, MS Society, Indiana Chapter, for their cooperation and assistance.

Physical Disabilities
Special Interest Section Newsletter; Vol. 6, No. 1, 1983

Therapeutic Issues for the Guillain-Barre Patient

By Karen Kovich, OTR, Rehab. Institute of Chicago, IL

Guillain-Barre (GB) is an acute demyelinating disease of the peripheral nervous system, involving spinal nerve roots, peripheral and cranial nerves. It is characterized by motor weakness or paralysis of two or more extremities. In severe cases, facial and respiratory muscles are involved. It is widely accepted that in response to viral infection or immunization, nerve tissue becomes infiltrated with inflammatory cells and macrophages. This causes subsequent destruction of circumscribed areas of myelin and the axonal fibers lying within. The nature of this sequential relationship is not well understood, but raises important therapeutic issues regarding treatment approach.

The majority of patients with GB begin to recover spontaneously as damaged nerves gradually become remyelinated. The course of the recovery varies greatly, so that therapy must be carefully adjusted to the individual recovery rate.

Physicians and therapists alike take various approaches to the therapeutic treatment of the GB patient, ranging from aggressive to conservative. At present, there exists little or no published research on the methods of treatment and its physiological implications. We must therefore rely on experience, observation and physicians' guidance to determine those forms of therapy best for the patient.

Through extensive work with GB patients, a conservative approach has been most successful in facilitating continuous recovery without exacerbation. On several occasions, when a more aggressive approach was taken, patients consistently complained of increased muscle belly pain. Subsequently, they exhibited a decrease in motor power, at times accompanied by edematous, reddened joints. Following these exacerbations, recovery to a previous grade of muscle strength occurred at a slower rate than it had initially. Some physicians have hypothesized that fatigue interrupts the remyelination process causing further demyelination. Since this occurs repeatedly, the myelin that is laid down becomes nonconcentric or tangled, permanently slowing the nerve conduction rate.

Rehabilitation goals in a conservative approach begin with maintenance of joint range of motion. Splinting distal extremities is done in neutral positions to avoid overstretching muscle groups. Passive range of motion is done gently to the point of pain, keeping in mind the inflammation already present.

Exercise begins in gravity eliminated planes with the assistance of balanced forearm orthoses and slings. The patient may only be able to complete relatively few repetitions of any given movement before fatiguing. It is vital that the therapist know the patient's endurance so that she/he is able to stop activity before the fatigue point is reached, and never push a patient beyond it. Resistance should not be used until all muscles around a given joint are of a fair+ grade and are free from muscle belly tenderness during palpation. Even at this point tolerance must be carefully monitored.

Self-care activities must be restricted un-

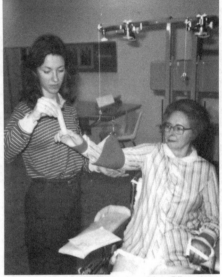

Karen Kovich, OTR, works with a GB patient to increase proximal VE strength and ability for arm placement. The patient is four months post-onset of GB.

til the patient can perform them without fatigue. Problems arise when patients become anxious to regain independence and function, and therapists who are accustomed to being more aggressive with other disabilities, may become frustrated by the slowness of recovery. For this reason, patients and therapists alike must come to understand the limitations to aggressive rehabilitation inherent in the disease. A carefully planned and slowly monitored treatment regime to assure maximal recovery in a safe manner can then follow.

Physical Disabilities
Special Interest Section Newsletter; Vol. 5, No. 4, 1982

The Splinting Controversy in Rheumatoid Arthritis

By Denise Wilkins Hanten, OTR, Rancho Los Amigos Hospital, Downey, CA

Occupational therapists are concerned with helping people with rheumatoid arthritis attain or maintain their highest functional level. In doing so, therapists are often faced with progressive hand problems of pain, weakness, decreased range of motion, and deformities that may lead to decreased functional abilities. For years physicians and therapists have used hand

splints in an attempt to control inflammation, deformities and to aid in maintaining function.

In order to augment clinical impressions, available literature on rationale of splinting and on studies of its effectiveness was explored. Various authors have proposed explanations of the pathomechanics of deformities and have offered differing

opinions on the effectiveness of splinting to help these problems. However, few studies on the effectiveness of splinting in rheumatoid arthritis were found in the literature.

Most of the literature on splinting was published in the 1960s. Few studies have been done recently taking newer splinting

(continued)

Rheumatoid Arthritis

concepts and materials into account. It is hoped that findings from this literature search will aid therapists in developing a personal rationale for splinting and in developing awareness of the need for studies that will document the effectiveness of splints.

The traditional uses of splinting in rheumatoid arthritis have been to decrease inflammation and pain, to prevent or correct deformities, and to increase function. Passive immobilization is used to provide rest to the affected joints, thus reducing pain. Static and dynamic splints have been used to maintain or restore alignment in order to prevent or correct deformity. Functional splints have been used to improve hand use. Each of these areas will be discussed.

Joint immobilization through the use of handsplints has been advocated by many physicians when joints are inflamed. Studies have shown the benefits of joint immobilization such as relief of pain, decreased muscle spasm and inflammation (7,9,14,17,20,25). Dr. Rotstein, Flatt and Shalet have all described the value of splints for decreasing inflammation, reducing stress to the joints and thus improving mobility and function (2,7,17,26). Patients subjectively report reduction in pain from immobilization (19,26). In 1969, Zoeckler (26) found that, out of 59 patients, 85% wore their (prenyl) splint four nights per week during a 12-month follow-up, 22 out of 35 reported moderate or great relief of pain and 21 indicated that morning stiffness in their hands was greatly or moderately relieved. (These statistics might be improved in a study using newer splint materials.)

Many people fear that immobilization will result in decreased range of motion, decreased muscle strength and atrophy, and ultimately, in ankylosis. A study by Gault and Spyker (8) showed this not to be the case. They found that, in patients with low to moderate levels of joint involvement, three weeks of immobilization was beneficial for the affected joints. They found less active joint involvement with no long-lasting decrease in range of motion or muscle strength in patients with early stages (I, II and early III) of rheumatoid arthritis. They also found that the immobilized joints did not flare. The effects of this technique on late stage joint disease (stage IV) have not been determined However, should ankylosis occur, it would most likely be in the position of function.

Controversy also exists concerning the degree of immobilization necessary for improvement. Partridge and Duthie (15) compared the effects on function and disease activity of a four-week program of complete bed rest with continuous splinting versus a program of intermittent splinting (splints were removed and hand

exercises done twice daily). Results showed no permanent range of motion loss in either group. The resulting decrease in power was regained in both groups and improved significantly in the complete rest group. An increase in functional capacity and a decrease in disease activity was found in both groups. It was the authors' impression that the complete rest group had more significant changes than the intermittent rest group. However, statistical significance was not obtained, possibly due to the small sample size. The authors conclude that it is unnecessary to insist on daily active movement in painful joints to prevent ankylosis.

On the other hand, Harris and Copp (10) showed that both techniques, intermittent and complete immobilization, showed essentially no significant difference in range of motion in patients with rheumatoid arthritis.

Thus, it appears that joint immobilization whether continuous or intermittent does reduce the active disease process at the joint. It follows that any splinting that promotes reduction in the inflammatory process at a joint will be beneficial for determining deformity. Hand splinting for the purpose of pain relief and decreasing inflammation seems to be accepted and effective in rheumatoid arthritis.

Many clinicians recommend splinting in rheumatoid arthritis to prevent or correct deformities such as flexion contractures at the wrist and metacarpophalangeal joints, ulnar deviation, boutonniere and swan neck deformities and various thumb deformities (1,4,11,12,14,21,22). However, the rationale and indications for splinting vary from author to author. In addition, few studies have been done to look objectively at the benefits of hand splinting for the prevention or correction of deformity.

Czap (4), Bennett (1) and other proponents of splinting feel that faulty positioning, which may lead to deformities, often results from pain or muscle spasm. This faulty positioning may lead to overstretching or contractures of ligamentous tissue, intrinsic and extrinsic hand muscles. Czap proposes that through correct placement of counter-pressures in the hand from dynamic and static splints that an equilibrium or balance in the hand can be restored (4). (However, splinting to reverse dynamic deformities has not been demonstrated.) He describes the benefits of handsplints to be that they maintain good skeletal alignment, support segmental mass, prevent overstretching and allow hand function in order to maintain the physiologic integrity of structures.

Bennett (1) describes two changes that occur in bones and joints and lead to deformity. The first change is a loss of the normal resiliency in periarticular tissue, making it not possible to correctly align the

structures of the hand. This change in ligamentous tissue is the primary mechanism in deformity. Muscle weakness is secondary to the resulting misuse (disuse, overstretching or shortening). The second change that occurs in joints is faulty "grooving" of the subchrondral bone underlying the degenerating articular cartilage. Since the bones are not aligned, due to faulty mechanical forces, distortion of the subchrondral bone occurs. Therefore, according to Bennett, the ideal splint is one that would permit motion in the normal planes necessary for function and block faulty planes, thereby lessening the degree of ligamentous malalignment and preventing faulty grooving of subchrondral bone.

Smith, Juvinall, Bender and Pearson (22) propose another theory of metacarpophalangeal joint deformity. They feel that the forces exerted by the flexor tendons during pinch and grasp are responsible for subluxation and ulnar deviations at the metacarpophalangeal joint. In arthritis, the normal orientation of the flexor tendons changes due to weakened collateral and volar metacarpophalangeal ligaments. The tendons no longer exert force on the joint, but distal to it, thus subluxing the proximal phalanx volarly during finger flexion. Since the normal direction of pull of the flexor tendons is ulnar, these weakened ligaments also allow ulnar deviation at the metacarpophalangeal joint. An ideal splint would protect the volar ligaments. These authors feel that splinting may lead to prevention of deformities, by altering these specific dynamic flexor forces. Once deformity has occurred, splinting will not correct deformity or restore the structural integrity of joints and tissues (3).

One author, however, does discuss the use of splints to correct deformity (7). Flatt recommends what he terms "remedial splints" in certain cases of rheumatoid arthritis. He proposes that a contracture in a muscle results in a lack of use of the muscle. This leads to more stiffness, setting up a deforming cycle. He feels that hand use should be encouraged by changing hand position from nonfunctional to functional. Flatt uses dynamic splints that provide a gentle, persistent force so that scar tissue will yield. He identifies three conditions in which this type of splinting could be used: adduction contractures of the thumb, stiffness of the interphalangeal joints, and flexion contractures of the metacarpophalangeal joints. However, only if the joint surfaces are congruous should this be used. It is not indicated for subluxed or dislocated joints.

The various rationales for splinting described seem logical, yet confusion remains about the benefits of splinting.

Many therapists find preventive or cor-

(continued)

119

Rheumatoid Arthritis

rective splints effective. Yet, there is a great lack of research substantiating the benefits of splinting to prevent or correct dynamic deformity. (Splinting is clearly effective for preventing positional deformities such as wrist flexion contractures.) In fact, only one controlled study in this area demonstrating the effects of splinting could be found. (3) Convery, Conaty and Nickel (3) studied 51 patients who had been fitted with a functional splint to assess the effect on deformity. This splint was designed according to the principles of Bennett. It allowed motion only in functional planes. This dorsal splint had an action wrist, action metacarpophalangeal joints, with MCP extension assists, which could be adapted to correct the ulnar drift. The results of this study suggested the following: 1. Function was reduced in many patients who wore the splint. Those patients with less deformity disliked the splint most. 2. Progressive deformity as not consistently prevented by wearing the splint. 3. The splint was not effective in correcting deformity. 4. There were more range of motion limitations in the splinted patients than would be expected without splinting. The authors did not suggest that the rheumatoid hand would not be benefitted by other splint designs; only that hand splinting techniques and designs at the time of the study were inadequate for rheumatoid arthritis of the hand (3).

The effects of hand splinting to prevent or correct dynamic deformities in rheumatoid arthritis is still unclear. As the etiology of deformity becomes more clear and design and research in splinting progress, the actual effects of splinting will also, it is hoped, become more clear.

One last aspect of handsplinting to be discussed is its effect on function. The purpose of splinting in this instance is to protect weak muscles (7), substitute for a loss of power (7), and to stabilize a part for a more functional grasp or pinch (5, 16). Splints that support the wrist and finger flexors at a mechanical advantage, and that decrease pain will result in a more functional hand. Quest and Cordery (16)

have developed a functional splint designed to prevent ulnar deviation on active flexion or under external pressure. Their splint provides ulnar support at the proximal phalanges. They do not use this splint on those patients with active disease or on those who need immobilization. They apply it to hands with ulnar deviation and subluxation to aid function and decrease pain. In their report, the splint had been applied favorably to eight patients, all housewives, with no gross deformity. One patient reported that she was able to lift more weight with less pain and no longer needed to be continually aware of injuring her hands.

Functional splints must be individualized for each patient in order to fulfill specific needs without causing further damage elsewhere.

In conclusion, handsplinting in rheumatoid arthritis has traditionally been used for three reasons: 1) to decrease acute joint inflammation and relieve pain, 2) to prevent or correct deformities, and 3) to provide function. Studies have shown the benefits of joint immobilization to decrease inflammation. The benefits of splinting to prevent or correct dynamic deformity are not yet substantiated by research. And finally, functional splints may be very helpful for many people with rheumatoid arthritis.

REFERENCES

1. Bennett, Robert L.: Orthotic Devices to Prevent Deformities of the Hand in Rheumatoid Arthritis. *Arthritis Rheum.*, 8:5: 1006-1018, October, 1965.
2. Clark, William S.: Arthritis and Rehabilitation. *J. Rehab.*, 31: 5: 10-12, Sept.-Oct., 1965.
3. Convery, F.R., J.P. Conaty, and V.L. Nickel: Dynamic Splinting of the Rheumatoid Hand. *Orthotics and Prosthetics*, 21: 249-254, Dec., 1967. (Addendum, *Orthotics and Prosthetics*, 22: 41-45, March, 1968.)
4. Czap, L.: Orthotic Management of the Rheumatoid Hand. *Southern Medical Journal*, 59: 115-117, Sept., 1966.
5. Ehrlich, G.E.: Splinting for Arthritis. *Med. Times*, 96: 485-489, May, 1968.
6. Feinberg, J. and Brandt, K.: Use of Resting Splints by Patients with Rheumatoid Arthritis. *AJOT*, 35: 173-178, March, 1981.
7. Flatt, Adrian: *The Care of the Rheumatoid Hand.* St. Louis: C.V. Mosby Co., 1963.
8. Gault, Sarah J. and Joan Spyker: Beneficial Effect of Immobilization of Joints in Rheumatoid and Related Arthritides: A Splint Study Using Sequential Analysis. *Arthritis Rheum.*, 12: 1: 34-43, Feb., 1969.
9. Granger, Carl et al: Laminated Plaster-Plastic Bandage Splints, *Prosthetics, Orthotics and Devices*, 585-590, August, 1965.
10. Harris, R. and E.P. Copp: Immobilization of the Knee Joint in Rheumatoid Arthritis. *Ann. Rheum. Dis.*, 21: 353-359, 1962.
11. Marmor, Leonard: *Surgery of Rheumatoid Arthritis.* Philadelphia: Lea and Febiger, 1967.
12. Marmor, L., et al: Physical Therapy in Rheumatoid Arthritis of the Hand. *J. Amer. Phys. Ther. Ass.*, 44: 729-733, Aug., 1964.
13. Melvin, J.L.: *Rheumatic Disease: Occupational Therapy and Rehabilitation.* Philadelphia: F.A. Davis Co., 1977.
14. Overton, J. and L.E. Wolcott: The Role of Splints in the Prevention of Deformity in the Rheumatoid Hand and Wrist. *Missouri Med.*, 63: 423-427, June, 1966.
15. Partridge, R.E. and J.J., Duthie: Controlled Trial of the Effect of Complete Immobilization of the Joints in Rheumatoid Arthritis. *Ann. Rheum. Dis.*, 22: 91-99, March, 1963.
16. Quest, I.M. and J. Cordery: A Functional Ulnar Deformity Cuff for the Rheumatoid Deformity. *AJOT*, 25(1): 32-40, Jan.-Feb., 1971.
17. Rotstein, J.: Simple Splinting—Use of Light Splints and Related Conservative Therapy in Joint Disease. Philadelphia: W.B. Saunders, 1965.
18. Rotstein, J.: Use of Splints in Conservative Management of Acutely Inflamed Joints in Rheumatoid Arthritis. *Arch. Phys. Med.*, 46: 198-199, Feb., 1965.
19. Salvanelli, M.: Functional Wrist Splint for Patients with Rheumatoid Arthritis. *Phys. Ther.*, 44: 743-744, August, 1964.
20. Shalit, I.S. and J.L. Decker: Silicone Foam Resting Splints for Rheumatoid Arthritis. *Lancet*, 1: 142-144, Jan. 16, 1965.
21. Spelbring, L.A.: Splinting the Arthritic Hand. *Amer. J. Occup. Ther.*, 20: 40-41, Jan.-Feb., 1966.
22. Smith, E.M., et al: Role of the Finger Flexors in Rheumatoid Deformities of the Metacarpophalangeal Joints. *Arth. and Rheum.*, 7: 467-480, Oct., 1964.
23. Swezey, R.L.: *Arthritis: Rational Therapy and Rehabilitation.* Philadelphia: W.B. Saunders Co., 1978.
24. Swanson, A.B. and J.D. Coleman: Corrective Bracing Needs of the Rheumatoid Arthritic Wrist. *Amer. J. Occup. Ther.*, 20: 38-40, Jan.-Feb., 1966.
25. Van Brocklin, J.D.: Splinting the Rheumatoid Hand. *Arch. Phys. Med.*, 47: 262-265, April, 1966.
26. Zoeckler, A.A. and J.J. Nicholas: Prenyl Hand Splint for Rheumatoid Arthritis. *Phys. Ther.*, 49: 377-379, April, 1969.

Physical Disabilities
Special Interest Section Newsletter; Vol. 5, No. 4, 1982

The ROM Dance Program

By Diane Harlowe, MS, OTR, Director Occupational Therapy and Speech Services, St. Marys Hospital Medical Center, Madison, Wisconsin

One of the most basic recommendations given to patients with rheumatoid arthritis is to establish a good balance of rest and exercise. Rheumatologists frequently prescribe regular periods of rest, and patients often receive instructions for performing general range of motion exercises on a daily basis. Unfortunately, these recommendations are given more frequently than they are carried out. Studies have shown that compliance to home exercise

(continued)

ROM Dance Program

programs is lower than other forms of self-administered treatments. It is not uncommon for patients to describe range of motion exercise as boring, and to resist regular periods of rest. The ROM Dance Program employs nontraditional approaches to address these problems, and this unique program has been met with considerable enthusiasm.

The ROM Dance Program is composed of two main elements: relaxation techniques to be used during regular periods of rest, and the ROM Dance (pronounced ram which stands for range of motion). The ROM Dance is a seven-minute sequence of expressive movements that is performed while listening to, or reciting, a poem. The verse serves to cue specific movements that dramatize the poetic images. The exercise is based on the principles of T'ai-Chi Ch'uan[41-42] and incorporate joint motion in all ranges usually recommended for rheumatoid arthritis.

T'ai-Chi is an ancient Chinese exercise form that is the most delicate of the oriental martial arts. Like T'ai-Chi, the graceful, slow movements of the ROM Dance are performed in a relaxed manner. The gestures of T'ai-Chi symbolizes defense and attack movements, but the ROM Dance employs pleasureable images of warm water, sunshine and friendship.

Touches of Eastern mediation techniques appear in the relaxation component of the ROM Dance Program. A wide variety of methods are introduced, starting with deep breathing, postural and environmental awareness, auto-suggestion, the respiratory one method, and progressive relaxation. Advanced techniques include the use of fantasy, imaginative transformation, visualization and energy alignment.[10-40]

The ROM Dance Program is taught in a series of eight weekly classes at "The Health Works," which is St. Marys Hospital Medical Center's community health education and wellness center in Madison, Wisconsin. The present charge for enrollment is $20.00, and participants are asked to obtain approval from their physicians to attend the program. Course announcements are placed in newspapers and mailed directly to arthritis patients, and the maximum enrollment for each class is 25. The course is presently taught by the health educator and T'ai-Chi expert who played a primary role in program development.

The goals of the ROM Dance Program are to promote an experience of well being; increase frequency, enjoyment and perceived benefit from involvement in daily exercise and rest; and to enhance the individual's ability to cope with pain through the use of nonpharmacological pain management techniques. Each session includes execution of the ROM Dance, guided relaxation, group sharing and health education. Educational components include audiovisual, such as "Helping Hands—Splints for Early Rheumatoid Arthritis,"[44] slides of adaptive equipment[45] and experimental data on the use of relaxation as a pain management technique.[10-40]

While performing the ROM Dance, emphasis is placed on posture, deep breathing and proper execution of movements. Instructions are given to focus attention on body parts to achieve conscious relaxation while moving joints through maximum available ranges. Participants are asked to practice the ROM Dance each day, and to continue involvement in any home exercise routine recommended by a physician or therapist.

Relaxation techniques are presented each week in a specific sequence of graded categories. Participants are asked to practice the techniques during daily rest periods, and to identify or create forms that work best for them. Mini hand-held thermometers may be used as an inexpensive biofeedback device,[36] and audio cassette tapes of the ROM Dance Poem and relaxation techniques may be purchased for home use.[45]

The ROM Dance Program was developed by Diane Harlowe, MS, OTR, Director of Occupational Therapy at St. Marys Hospital Medical Center, and Patricia Yu, MS, Health Education Consultant at The Health Works. Contributors were Nancy Walker, OTR, Marion Higby, PT, and Deborah Dennis, PT. The development and pilot study of the program was financed in part through a grant from the Arthritis Foundation, Wisconsin Chapter.

Initial results of the pilot study on 17 participants showed an increase in the frequency of exercise, rest and perceived benefit. The group reported that involvement in the program was beneficial in increasing the ability to cope with arthritis. The pilot study was presented at the 16th Annual Meeting of the Arthritis Health Professions Association in June of 1981.

The ROM Dance has received considerable press coverage on a national level. Articles have appeared in the National Arthritis News, Health Magazine, The Wall Street Journal, The National Enquirer, T'ai-Chi Magazine and the Wisconsin State Journal; and television spots were aired on the Midday, Over Easy and Cable Network News programs. Requests for information have been overwhelming, and we are presently working with WHA-TV to develop a ROM Dance Program instructional media package that will include audio, video and written materials.

REFERENCES

RELAXATION AND PAIN MANAGEMENT

10. Assagioli, R.: *Psychosynthesis—A Manual of Principles and Techniques.* New York: Viking Press, 1971.
11. Bandler, R., Grinder, J.: *Frogs Into Princes.* Real People Press, Moab, Utah, 1979.
12. Benson, H.: *The Relaxation Response.* Morrow, New York, 1977.
13. Blitz, B., and Dinnerstein, A.: Role of Attentional Focus in Pain Perception: Manipulation of Response to Noxious Stimulation by Instructions, *J. Abnorm. Psychol.,* 77: 24-25, 1971.
14. Bresler, D., Trubo, D.: *Free Yourself From Pain.* Simon and Schuster, New York, 1979.
15. Carrington, P.: *Clinical Standardized Meditation (CSM) Instructors Kit.* Pace Educational Systems, New Jersey, 1978.
16. Carrington, P. et al: "The Use of Meditation-Relaxation Techniques for the Management of Stress in a Working Population", *Journal of Occupational Medicine,* 22:4 221-231, 1980.
17. Chaves, J., & Barber, T.: Cognitive Strategies, Experimenter Modeling, and Expectation in the Attention of Pain. *J. Abnorm. Psychol.,* 83: 356-363, 1974.
18. Coue, E.: *How to Practice Suggestion and Auto Suggestion.* American Library Service, New York, 1923.
19. Davis, M. et al: *Relaxation and Stress Reduction Workbook.* New Harbinger Publication, Richmond, CA, 1980.
20. DiGiusto, E.L., Bond, N.W.: Imagery and the Autonomic Nervous System: Some Methodological Issues. *Percept. Mot. Skills,* 48(2): 427-38, 1979.
21. Goldfried, M., and Trier, C.: Effectiveness of Relaxation as an Active Coping Skill. *J. Abnorm. Psychol.,* 83: 348-355, 1974.
22. Jacobson, E.: *Progressive Relaxation.* University of Chicago Press, Chicago, 1929, 1938. (Midway Reprint, 1974.)
23. Jacobson, E.: *Progressive Relaxation: A Physiological Approach.* J.B. Lippincott, Philadelphia, 1964.
24. *Journal of Mental Imagery.* Brandon House, Inc., P.O. Box 240, Bronx, N.Y.
25. Levendusky, P., & Pankratz, L.: Self-Control Techniques as an Alternative to Pain Medication, *J. Abnorm. Psychol.,* 84: 165-169, 1975.
26. Luthe, W.: "Autogenic Training, Method, Research and Application in Medicine", *American Journal of Psychotherapy,* Vol. 17, 174-195, 1963.
27. Luthe, W., Schultz, J.H.: Autogenic Therapy. Grune and Stratton, NY, 1969.
28. McGlynn, D., et. al.: Graded Imagination and Relaxation as Components of Experimental Desensitization: a psychological evaluation, *Journal of Clinical Psychology,* 35: 542-546, 1979.
29. Meichenbaum, D.: An Overview of Pain Treatment Literature. *Cognitive-Behavior Modification.* Plenum Press, NY, 1969-293, 1977.
30. Neufeld, R., & Davidson, P.: The Effects of Vicarious and Cognitive Rehearsal on Pain Tolerance. *Journal of Psychosomatic Research,* 15: 319-325, 1971.
31. Nisbet, R., & Schachter, W.: Cognitive Manipulation of Pain. *Journal of Experimental Social Psychology,* 2: 227-236, 1966.
32. Paul, G.L.: Physiological Effects of Relaxation Training and Hypnotic Suggestion. *J. Abnorm. Psychol,* 74: 425-437, 1979.
33. Seyle, H.: *Physiology and Pathology of Exposure to Stress.* Acta, Inc., Montreal, 1950.
34. Seyle, H.: *Stress Without Distress.* J.B. Lippincott and Co., Philadelphia, 1974.
35. Shealy, N.: *Biogenics Health Maintenance.* Self-Health Systems, Rt. 2, LaCrosse, WI, 1980.
36. Shealy, N.: *The Pain Game.* Celestial Arts: Millbrae, CA, 1976.
37. Simonton, C., and S.M.: *Getting Well Again.* J.P. Tarcher, NY, 1978.
38. Singer, J., Pipe K.: *The Power of Human Imagination.* Plenum Press, NY, 1978.
39. Spanos, N. Horton, C., & Chaves, J.: The Effect of Two Cognitive Strategies on Pain Threshold. *J. Abnorm. Psychol.,* 84: 677-681, 1975.
40. Wolff, B., & Horland, A.: Effect of Suggestion Upon Experimental Pain: A validation study. *J. Abnorm. Psychol.,* 72: 402-407, 1967.

(continued)

ROM Dance Program

T'AI-CHI CH'UAN

41. Horowitz, T. et al: *T'ai-Chi Ch'uan: A Technique of Power.* Chicago Review Press, Chicago, 1976.
42. Huang, W.S.: *Fundamentals of T'si-Chi Ch'uan.* South Sky Book Co., Hong Kong, 1974.
43. Maisel, E.: *T'ai-Chi for Health.* Delta, NY, 1974.

MEDIA

44. Harlowe, D., Black, B.: *Helping Hands: Splints for Early Rheumatoid Arthritis.* 19 min. slide-tape, Arthritis Foundation, Wisconsin Chapter, 1442 N. Farwell Ave., Milwaukee, WI 53202.
45. Occupational Therapy Department, St. Marys Hospital Medical Center, 707 S. Mills St., Madison, WI 53715 (ROM Dance and Relaxation Experiences, I-IV audio cassettes; Adaptive Equipment Slides).
46. Center for Integral Medicine, P.O. Box 967, Pacific Palisades, CA 90272 (Bresler materials used at UCLA Pain Unit).
47. Environmental SEMS, Syntonic Research Inc., 175 Fifth Ave., NY (Relxation and Environmental Sounds Records and Tapes).
48. Self-Health Systems of Brindebella Farms, Rt. 2, LaCrosse, WI (relxation and pain management tapes).
49. Echo Inc., P.O. Box 87, 2755 Columbus Ave., Springfield, OH 45003 (hand held thermometers).

Physical Disabilities
Special Interest Section Newsletter; Vol. 5, No. 3, 1982

Hand Rehabilitation—A Comprehensive Approach

By Janet Waylett, OTR, Supervising Therapist, Hand Rehabilitation Center, Loma Linda University Medical Center, Loma Linda, CA

Comprehensive hand therapy requires a program that takes the whole person into account, including psychological and vocational needs as well as physical management of the injured hand. The Hand Rehabilitation Center at Loma Linda University Medical Center strives to achieve this by using group process as a therapeutic mode along with physical activities and using a full team approach in patient care.

A complete assessment of the patient at our center includes specific and objective measurements of range of motion, sensibility, strength, edema, condition of the skin or wound, dexterity and functional use of the involved extremity. To complete the evaluation, the patient's ADL status, work and avocational goals are discussed and evaluated as needed. Emotional status and family interaction is observed and recorded. When the services of a psychologist or a social worker are required, this is also provided.

With the information gleaned from the initial evaluation, an individualized treatment program is then initiated. Conventional modalities may be utilized such as Jobst compression or ice packs for edema control, whirlpool for debridement and paraffin bath or hot packs to soften scar tissue prior to exercises or activity.

The use of heat and cold modalities has been taught to our OT staff by the Department of Physical Therapy here at Loma Linda University. We do not believe in shuffling the patient back and forth between OT and PT departments when a more comprehensive, well coordinated and closely supervised program can be provided by one department. We do take physical therapy student affiliates and graduate level PTs for CEU in Hand Rehabilitation and interdepartmental relations are excellent.

Biofeedback is employed as a muscle reeducation device for those patients with extreme weakness or muscle transfers. Classic muscle re-education is used for slightly stronger muscles. Biofeedback may also be used for relaxation in such cases as reflex sympathetic dystrophy. Where venous congestion with obvious edema is the overriding problem, biofeedback may be used with a thermistor instead of the surface EMG electrodes. When muscle grades are F+ and above, patients begin progressive resistive exer-

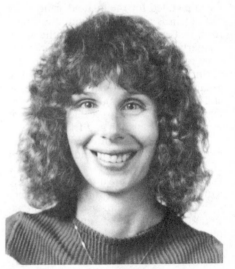

Janet Waylett

cises (PRE). We use the DeLorme method of isotonic exercise to incorporate full range of motion along with muscle strengthening. The extremely versatile "Weight Well" is an excellent exercise for fingers, thumb, wrist and forearm (see photo). Reciprocal pulleys, skateboard, wand exercises, shoulder wheel and finger ladder are utilized for shoulder and elbow injuries.

Craft projects are an integral part of the patients' treatment program. Employing existing range of motion, strength, endurance and dexterity in a goal-directed activity can demonstrate to the patient the skill and use that remains in the hand. When possible, work simulation is included as part of the craft program and consideration is given to adapting avocational equip-

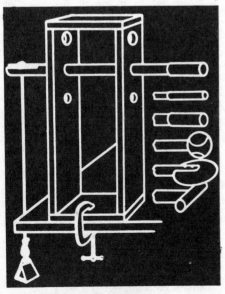

The Weight Well

(continued)

Hand Rehabilitation—Comprehensive Approach

ment—such as golf clubs. A productive goal-oriented activity can increase motivation and emotional well-being.

The social interaction process that occurs during the three hours the patients are in treatment at the center assists in increasing awareness of others with hand injuries and in facilitating patient attempts to regain function and be productive again.

Splinting is one of the most important aspects of our treatment since splinting maintains or increases range of motion obtained during clinic treatment. Dynamic splinting is preferred over static splinting for day wear since it will constantly apply gentle dynamic force on the joint to increase range of motion. Dynamic splints also allow for motion to occur during hand use which permits "muslce pumping" to decrease edema from the area. Static splinting is

used most frequently at night since it is less likely to interfere with sleep. The patient has full responsibility for the splints and is to bring them in for recheck as indicated.

Splinting is part of every patient's treatment and is started on the first day of treatment. In addition to splinting, the home program may include Theraplast exercises, gripper, home "Weight Well", wand exercises, reciprocal pulleys, and selected crafts.

All phases of care are coordinated when patients are seen at Hand Center Rounds by their physician. Treatment goals and modalities are reviewed with the physician at this time and change in range of motion, strength, sensibility or edema is reported. Should the patient require special procedures, such as those provided by pain clinic, EMG or X-ray, the patient is referred

as indicated. The rehabilitation nurse, vocational counselor, or insurance representative coordinating the patient's care is invited to attend Rounds and clarify functional or equipment needs prohibiting eventual return to gainful employment. When the patient is ready for discharge, usually after one to three months of treatment depending on the injury, a visit can be made to the job site if necessary to determine constraints, if any, to be placed on the patient and the need for adaptive equipment.

The goal of the Hand Center is to provide quality care for the whole patient through a comprehensive treatment program. It is our hope that at discharge patients with adaptive behavior or equipment can resume as full and productive lives as they enjoyed prior to the hand injury.

Physical Disabilities
Special Interest Section Newsletter; Vol. 5, No. 3, 1982

A Physician's Viewpoint on Hand Therapy

By Gary K. Frykman, M.D., Medical Director, Hand Rehabilitation Center, Loma Linda University Medical Center, Loma Linda, CA

The Hand Rehabilitation Center concept has made a major contribution to rehabilitating hand-injured patients. The Hand Rehabilitation Center provides concentrated effort to help patients fully integrate the use of their hands in their work, avocations and activities of daily living. Occupational therapists who specialize in hand therapy provide patients with improved care with their knowledge of upper extremity anatomy, physiology, psychology, biomechanics and an understanding of hand function. Patients treated at the Hand Rehabilitation Center return to work earlier than patients without this specialized care of occupational therapists. Therapists save the physician an enormous amount of time by explaining to patients the details of their therapy program and the methods of accomplishing their rehabilitation.

The initial prescription provides a foundation for the treatment program for a particular patient. It must describe the patient's diagnosis, time

from injury or surgery, the specific treatment modalities requested and the limitations or precautions and goals for each patient. If the initial prescription is not clear the occupational therapist should contact the physician to clarify the treatment program requested. The patient should be followed closely by the physician. At our Hand Rehabilitation Center, weekly rounds are held where the patients are reviewed by the physician, progress is reported by the therapist and changes in the treatment plan are made. The patient's progress is measured objectively by keeping clear and accurate records of range of motion, strength, sensibility, etc.

Practically all patients are on a splinting program. Except for dynamic finger splints, most splints are custom-made by the occupational therapist at the Hand Rehab. Center. Custom fabrication is necessary to fit the patient's unique anatomic and dynamic needs. Splints need to be modified frequently and heat-molded thermoplastic splinting materials work ad-

mirably and can be adapted to the changing requirements as the patient progresses.

Functional activities that add interest and variety to the therapy program greatly aid in the patient's rehabilitation. It is important to relate the activities to those that the patients will do when they return to work. For example, people in construction trades, particularly carpentry, may be started on a gouging project such as making a wooden bowl. This will help improve dexterity, strength and endurance and add interest to his rehabilitation. The common modalities used in rehabilitation of patients can all be performed by the occupational therapists.

In short, the occupational therapist has an indispensable role as a team member in rehabilitating the patients by helping establish realistic goals, encouraging patient responsibility for their actions and rehabilitation, encouraging pride in accomplishment and instilling in the patients a genuine sense of concern for them as individuals. The Hand Center's work is not done until the patients have fully integrated the functional ability of their hands into all daily activities.

Hand Therapy—An Administrator's Viewpoint

By John Kerr, OTR, Director, OT Services, Loma Linda University Medical Center

As director of various occupational therapy services within a large acute care medical center it is imperative to me, that all services are revenue producing. The Hand Center at Loma Linda has been in existence for almost six years. When establishing the Center it was necessary to consider and obtain data regarding: (1) which physicians were going to refer patients; (2) source of third-party coverage of the patients treatment; (3) estimate of total number of treatments given per fiscal year; and (4) number of staff that could efficiently and economically provide the required treatments.

This data helped to provide guidelines for the establishment of reasonable charges which were based on our concept of treatment. Since the majority of potential patients to be treated were referred by our own hand surgeons (80%), we could estimate closely the number of patients that would be referred. With out hand sur-

geons, we review the types of patients they are seeing which enabled us to determine that 75% of the patients had work related injuries.

In California, workman's compensation insurance reimburses the cost of therapy, so this was positive for our program. However, workman comp. reimbursement for OT varies considerably from state to state. Our percentage of Medicare patients at the Hand Center is approximately 5-7% and reimbursement is good. Documentation is the key to verifying treatment provided to patients. In hand rehabilitation it is probably even more crucial to have specific evaluations, detailed progress notes and timely discharge summaries. In addition it is customary to write periodic letters to the insurance companies detailing program planning and progress. It is not unusual for insurance companies to send representatives to our physician/therapist rounds or to the clinic to observe

treatment with the therapist and to ask pertinent medical questions.

It was necessary to estimate the total number of treatments provided at the Hand Center to determine the staffing ratio and treatment approach. Our program plan was to combine group-type and individual treatments within a three hour block of time. Patients receive the individualized care they require, including essential splinting, while they are able to help one another in their exercise and activity programs. By establishing a patient/therapist ratio of ten to twelve treatments per day we were able to determine cost effective use of our staff. The employment of an OT aide facilitated group interaction and reduced personnel costs.

The Hand Center has steadily grown since it began. This has resulted in the planning and construction of a new facility designed to accommodate the 20-30 patients seen daily.

Pre-Operative Evaluations for Hand Surgery

By Virchel Wood, M.D., Chief, Hand Surgery Service, Loma Linda University Medical Center

There are two specific places in the pre-op evaluation where the hand therapist makes the greatest contribution to my practice. One is the assessment of patients for tendon transfers and the other is the assessment of patients for stroke and cerebral palsy reconstructive surgery.

Dr. Bunnell, the father of hand surgery, implicitly demanded that the patient's hand be supple, fully mobile and soft before any type of reconstructive surgery was attempted. The therapist is the one who knows when this dynamic state has been achieved. The therapist works with the patient every day while the hand surgeon sees him once a month or, at the most, once a week. In my practice I rely heavily on a therapist to tell me when the joints are fully supple and when the hand is completely free of edema. At this point

tendon transfers achieve the greatest success.

The second area in which I feel the therapist can provide a great service is that of evaluating stroke and cerebral palsy patients for surgery. There are five parameters that need assessment before surgery of any type is contemplated in a patient with a brain injury. 1) *Intact body perception.* We have seen several people who do not know that one side of their body is present. In those cases, sophisticated surgery is of no benefit. 2) *Patterned motion.* Reconstructive surgery does not benefit patients who have patterned motion. When the patient gets angry, the pattern motion will overpower any reconstruction. 3) *Position sense.* Can the patient place their extremity in a position that is helpful? If there is so much spasticity or rigidity that they

cannot put their hand to their nose, or in any place to be a helper, surgery will not help. 4) *Sensation.* In the stroke or cerebral palsy patient, sensation may be impaired in only certain parameters such as pressure sense which would inhibit the use of the hand with any sophisticated tendon transfers. 5) *Degree of spasticity.* Although spasticity is not an absolute contraindication; an extremity with a great deal of spasticity is difficult to perform satisfactory reconstructive surgery on. Many times the only way to even be sure that extensor tendons are functioning is to evaluate the muscles after a Xylocaine block has been given to the median or musculocutaneous nerves. Only then can the strength of the reconstructed muscles be properly evaluated.

(continued)

Hand Surgery

In my practice, if I find that the patient has three of the above five parameters persisting, surgery is probably contraindicated. Often the physician does not have time to do a sophisticated pre-op evaluation on this type of patient and therefore must rely on the occupational therapist's assessment.

This has been a brief review of two areas of particular importance in pre-op hand evaluations. I look for the therapist of tomorrow to take a much more active role in the area of pre-operative evaluation.

Physical Disabilities
Special Interest Section Newsletter; Vol. 5, No. 3, 1982

An Educator's Viewpoint on Hand Rehabilitation

By Edwinna Marshall, MA, OTR, Chairperson, OT School, Loma Linda University

"The domain of concern of occupational therapy consists of performance requirements within the context of age, occupational performance and the individual's environment" —Anne Mosey, **Occupational Therapy Configuration of a Profession,** *p. 74, 1981.*

Hand rehabilitation requires an occupational therapy program involving a close inter-relationship between the world of rehabilitation and work. The rehabilitation team consists of the hand injured/diseased patient, hand surgeon, OTR, COTA and office support staff who spend at least six hours a day in a work-oriented environment.

Individuals finding themselves face-to-face with hand trauma/disease enter the rehabilitation program through acute care intervention. It is the hand surgeon who initiates and sets the pace of the intensive therapy environment requiring performance within the context of self-care, work and leisure activities. The objective of the program is to return the patient to a satisfactory occupational role (meaningful life style) as soon as is possible.

The performance components of neuromuscular, cognitive and psychosocial functions are integrated with sensorimotor functions through treatment activities to develop self-care ability and to ready the person to re-enter the work force.

Rehabilitation takes on a new personality. The rapid transition from acute care to the world of work reduces health care costs as well as the damaging effects that long-term chronic rehabilitation have on temporal adaptation necessary for productive work.

Occupational therapy has a greater effect on the patients in a hand center assisting them in integration and interaction with family, friends and community (including the work environment). Disability is accepted as a functional disorder the patient can live and work with and not as a chronic disability that will interfere with adequate function in the mainstream of living.

Occupational therapy students claim that clinical experience in the hand center enhances their understanding of the performance requirements necessary for a balance of self-care, work and leisure activities within the context of occupational performance as it realistically relates to the patient's own environment.

"It's like seeing OT in a space capsule... the equipment/facilities are organized and efficiently used, the staff and patients are inter-related and are developing and accomplishing objectives that keep the patient in tune with home and work environments. The patient doesn't just hang around, he comes in, works and leaves. There isn't a lag between injury/disease onset and rehabilitation," so say the students. This is what rehabilitation should be in our modern age—a shuttle between acute health care and work.

Physical Disabilities
Special Interest Section Newsletter; Vol. 5, No. 2, 1982

Occupant Protection for Wheelchair Travelers

By Lawrence W. Schneider and Jolan Cossairt

In today's mobile society, independence and opportunity for severely disabled individuals is synonymous with availability and access to both public and private motor vehicle transportation. Increasing numbers of wheelchair-bound persons are traveling on today's roads and highways with their wheelchairs as the vehicle seat. Unfortunately, improved mobility of the handicapped has not been accompanied by equal concerns for the safety and protection of these persons in vehicle accidents. The typical wheelchair of today is little different in structure and design from that of 20 or 30 years ago and has simply not been designed for use as a motor vehicle seat, much less for occupant crash protection.

Effective crash protection for any person requires that the occupant be restrained in a controlled manner to provide "ridedown" of the vehicle deceleration. This prevents the second impact, human collision, with the vehicle interior surfaces, which is the common cause of serious and fatal injuries. The 3-point belt system provided in todays' automobiles are designed

(continued)

Wheelchair Travelers

to perform this function and wheelchair users should transfer to vehicle seats and use these systems whenever possible and practical. Effective occupant protection with proper placement of restraint belts should be provided for a person in a wheelchair structure. It is further complicated, however, by the fact that the wheelchair, weighing between 40 and 110 pounds, must be adequately secured or it will add significantly to forces on the occupant and generally reduce the effectiveness of vehicle anchored restraint systems. Furthermore, if the occupant restraint system consists solely of a wheelchair anchored-lap belt, ineffective wheelchair securement results in no occupant restraint at all. For the wheelchair-seated driver, inadequate wheelchair securement can result in loss of vehicle impacts and can lead to more serious vehicle impacts and occupant injuries.

Effective occupant protection systems for wheelchair-seated passengers and drivers must address both *wheelchair securement and occupant restraint.* Impact testing conducted over the past several years at the Highway Safety Research Institute (HSRI) of the University of Michigan (1,2) as well as by other groups including the California Department of Transportation (3) and Minicars (4) have revealed the inadequacies of many devices and systems in use today. In general, good crashworthiness design practices and principles have been ignored. With regard to wheelchair securement, wheelchairs are usually backed up to the vehicle side-wall. While this may be the most practical approach for entry and exit, it is probably the least safe direction to be facing during frontal impacts, the cause of most moderate and severe crashes. The wheelchair is difficult to secure for laterally directed forces. Standard belt restraint systems are almost totally ineffective and may even constitute a hazard. In this situation, the wheelchair arm becomes a side restraint likely to produce injury.

Use of the wheel-rim anchoring devices for wheelchair securement or attachment of tie-down straps to the wheelchair crossbars are also ineffective significant forces, such as with minibus or van transportation. Typical crash forces in these cases cannot be carried by the wheelchair cross-bars and wheel rims. But

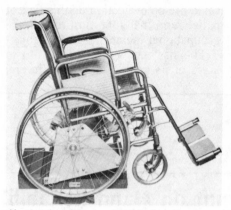

Newly developed wheelchair securement system.

if attachment is made to the stronger parts of the wheelchair, such as the junction of seat-back and seat-frame tubing on both sides, the force is lessened.

For vehicle drivers, there is the added requirement that both the wheelchair securement and occupant protection systems be automatic or switch activated. In the van, which is the primary vehicle available to wheelchair-seated drivers, the solution to automatic occupant restraint can be solved by vehicle anchored and "hung" belt systems. Such systems, to be effective, should include consideration for wheelchair modifications such as cantilevered chair arms to allow for proper belt fit over skeletal regions of the body. Inappropriate placement of belts over soft abdominal tissue can result in serious injury to internal body organs. It is also extremely important that these belt systems be constructed of appropriate webbing and stitching materials so that they comply with the Federal Motor Vehicle Safety Standards for seat belt performance.

A common device used to secure drivers consists of a screw motor-activated arm, which presses down on the wheelchair frame (on one side). Devices which rely on friction forces between the lock-down arm and the smooth wheelchair frame are completely inadequate for even minor declarations. They are essentially useless in forces of a 20 or 30 mph crash pulse generated by front-end collisions of van-type vehicles.

In the absence of Federal and State regulations dealing with this problem, it becomes the responsibility of transporta-

tion groups and users to educate themselves, to demand and expect better products and devices, and to implement improved practices. To some extent this is occurring. There have been developments in automatic wheelchair securement systems for drivers and passengers who routinely use the same vehicle. These new products generally require that some hardware be bolted or clamped to the wheelchair and provide suitable tie-down anchor points. A list of the companies involved in the manufacture and marketing of new wheelchair securement systems is available from the University of Michigan Rehabilitation Engineering Center. Prototype devices have been impact tested at HSRI. These systems generally represent a significant improvement in wheelchair securement systems for motor vehicle transportaiton.

There are many other considerations that enter into the problem of providing effective occupant protection for wheelchair travelers. Rear head restraints are needed for neck injury protection on rear end collisions. Vehicle interiors, especially driver controls, need to be designed with injury prevention in mind. Finally, wheelchair manufacturers may become responsible for developing a line of wheelchairs suited to the problems of motor vehicle transportation and occupant protection.

REFERENCES:

1. Schneider, L.W.: Dynamic Testing of Restraint Systems and Tie-Downs for Use with Vehicle Occupants Seated in Powered Wheelchairs. HSRI Report UM-HSRI-81-18. March 1981.

2. Schneider, L.W., and Tenniswood, D.N.: A Wheelchair Restraint System for Handicapped Drivers and Passengers. Proceedings of the International Conference on Rehabilitation Engineering, June 16-20, 1980, Toronto, Ontario, Canada.

3. Stewart, C.F., and Reinl, H.G.: Wheelchair Securement on Bus and Paratransit Vehicles. Interim Report No. 1, UMTA Contract CA-06-0098. California Department of Transportation, February 1980.

4. Khadikar, A.V., and Will, E.: Crash Protection Systems for Handicapped School and Transit Bus Occupants. Volume 1: Executive Summary. Interim Report. U.S. DOT Contract No. HS-7-01774. Springfield, VA, National Technical Information Services, 1980.

Lawrence W. Schneider, PhD is associate research scientist, at the Highway Safety Research Institute at University of Michigan, Ann Arbor, MI and Jolan Cossairt, MA, is editor/writer at the University of Michigan Rehabilitation Engineering Center, Ann Arbor, MI.

Disabled Drivers Program—An Occupational Therapy Approach

Occupational therapists working with disabled persons assist their patients to attain their highest levels of independence in ADL. Independent mobility is at the top of the list of important goals for rehabilitation. The best example of independent mobility is driving. Driving is a self-care activity which gives the patient the choice to go into the community, to work, play, and change the quality of their lives. Independence in driving is the ticket to this freedom.

In 1968, the occupational therapists at the University of Washington Hospital in Seattle began the "Disabled Driver's Program." We serve patients with neuromuscular disabilities, arthritis, spinal cord injuries, hemiplegia, post-polio and amputation. A car was donated to the Occupational Therapy Department by a former patient and hand controls were installed. The therapist, with the Department of Licensing and the local American Automobile Association, developed standards and tests to measure driving potential, designed training techniques, and criteria for licensing. As the program grew, the local car dealers provided a car for training purposes. The occupational therapists were instrumental in developing the philosophy that driver evaluation and training are important areas to be considered for all patients, despite the limitations caused by their physical disabilities. The primary concerns were the public safety and control of the vehicle.

The "Disabled Driver's Program" coordinator is actively involved in public education, specifically for vocational counselors, educators in school systems, private driving schools, automobile dealers, and medical equipment specialists. Through the University Learning Resources in the Magnunson Health Sciences Center, the project, "Healthy Living", has made a film of the driving program for television viewing by the community.

The "Disabled Drivers Program" is one of the services provided by the Department of Rehabilitation Medicine to persons in the Northwest Region-Washington, Oregon, Idaho, Montana, and Alaska. Referrals for driver evaluation and training come from inpatient and outpatient clinics, community hospitals and private physicians. The occupational therapist receives a physician referral identifying:

1. Medical-includes ROM, strength, spasms, medications, visual field.

2. Psychological-MMPI test interpretation. Patient's understanding of own limitations and overall adjustment.

3. Psychometric testing-cognitive, visual perception, problem solving and rapid decision making.

4. Rehabilitational-Functional Skills-Report by PT or OT or Discharge Summary.

The criteria used for referral are: (1) Medical stability, including seizure control for duration of no less than 6 months; (2) Sufficient perceptual-motor skills to make driving at least feasible; (3) Compliance with medication schedules and minimal or no use of ETOH and nonprescription drugs; (4) Absence of suicidal, homicidal, or other violent ideation or behavior; and (5) Compliance with medical program, especially safety factors, and compliance with vocational program.

All services through occupational therapy are individual with the charge based on an hourly rate. The coordinator of the "Disabled Drivers Program" works closely with the patient and "social services" to assure that funding will be available from insurance, Department of Vocational Rehabilitation or community agencies.

Staff Qualfications

An occupational therapist is the ideal health professional to thoroughly evaluate the potential driver. With background in evaluations including strength, ROM, coordination, visual perception, observation, self-care, and use of equipment, the therapist is skilled in using objective measures for comprehensive assessment of the patient.

The staff on this project have all received specific training in classroom and on-street driver's education.

Evaluation Process

The evaluation begins with an interview to gain background information, driving experience and licensing history. Measurements of active ROM, strength against resistance, proprioception/sensation, visual acuity, distance judgment, peripheral vision, color vision, reaction time and coordination. The AAA Psychophysical Test battery for general visual screening and brake reaction time is administered. A specially designed simulator has been developed by the University of Engineering program to measure steering, braking and acceleration. Incorporated in the simulator is a torque motor, adjustable to measure steering ability against a varying load of resistance at the rim of the wheel. This simulates manual, power or reduced effort/sensitized steering, thus allowing evaluation of functional steering. After completing an in-clinic evaluation and meeting minimum standards, the patient is seen for a parking lot, in-car assessment.

Specific vehicle use and operations tested include: transfer and body positioning in vehicle, wheelchair load/unload, dash control/ignition, seat harness, steering (steering devices), braking/acceleration (foot pedals vs. hand controls), emergency park brake and windows/door locks.

An on-street evaluation tests the patient's visual perception, distance judgment, balance making, appropriate knowledge of the rules of the road and driving attitude and judgment.

Driver's Training

All patients who will need vehicle modifications receive training in the University Hospital driver-training vehicles. Each patient is seen for 1-20 hours of instruction on a one-to-one basis with the same therapist who did the evaluation. Basic skills, maneuvers, residential, arterial and freeway driving, emergency vehicle control and preparation for licensing are all services provided during training. At the final stage of training the therapist takes the patient to the Department of Licensing for the written and driving tests. The patient uses the university vehicles for the test and has to pass a standard drive test given by the Department of Licensing examiner.

The "Disabled Drivers Program" serves an estimated 200 patients per year. The highest percentage of disability category is spinal cord injury, with 95% of those patients evaluated and trained becoming licensed drivers. The range of training hours is 5 to 7 hours for paraplegic, 5 to 15 hours for quadriplegic and 10 to 20 hours for high quadriplegics who require training in the van.

Vehicles and Equipment

We attempt to minimize the need and cost of equipment or vehicle modification and encourage the patient to achieve independence without equipment. Our vehicles have dual control brakes, hand controls, and regular foot controls. The vehicle most frequently used is a passenger car fully equipped for changing to specialized control to meet individual needs. Unique to this car are extended pedals for short clients, wide angle rearview mirror and gear shift crossover for left-handed operation. A van is equipped with a semi-automatic wheelchair lift, modified driver's seat, which elevates to wheelchair height, and a reduced diameter steering wheel with column extension, electric emergency brake and dash switch modifications.

New to the "Disabled Drivers Program" is a Ford van equipped with TARGET IN-

(continued)

Disabled Drivers Program

DUSTRIES modifications. With it we have been able to successfully evaluate C_5 quadriplegics and train them to drive independently.

Assisting the driving staff is the "Engineering Applications Program," which recommends modifications of the wheelchair for potential fit into the driver's station of a van, and the need and use of "Environmental Control Units" mounted on the wheelchair.

Vehicle Modifications and the Future

As therapists train drivers, they are able to identify what equipment is required for the car. In follow-up, the therapist is able to re-evaluate the client's vehicle after modification. Coordinating this re-evaluation with the client, vendor, and funding agency, an on-the-spot inspection can be made to ensure that the patient is as independent as possible and the necessary changes are done correctly.

With the advent of more sophisticated power wheelchair technology, it has become critical that the therapist complete comprehensive evaluations. We have to keep aware of the technological options such as power elevating head rests, power recline motor, and pact placement on wheelchairs. The wheelchair seat height can be lowered for increased visibility and the power leg rests operated separately from the recline back. This provides accessibility to the driver's station and wheelchair lockdown. The occupational therapists and the rehabilitation engineer complement the professional services for the patient.

Conclusion

The Department of Rehabilitation Medicine team members' philosophy is to assist the disabled individual to achieve the highest standard of independence. Driving becomes the turning point in the adjustment to their disability. They are freed from dependence on others for transportation, hence increasing their mobility and psychological well being. This freedom leads to improved self-esteem and self-control. Driving is an activity of daily living. Thus, it is the goal of the occupational therapist to evaluate, train, and assist the disabled driver in licensing equipment modifications.

Related Readings

1. Gurgold, G.D., Harden, D.H., Assessing Driving Potential of the Handicapped, *Am J Occup Ther*, January 1978.
2. Jacobs S., Reporting the Hanciapped Driver. *Arch Phys Med Rehab* 59:1978.
3. Less, M., Colverd, E.C., DeMauro, G.E., Young, J., *Teaching Driver Education to the Physically Disabled*, Library of Congress 78-62053, Human Resources Center, New York, 1978.
4. Evans, L., Langran, S.S., *Handbook for the Establishment of a Driving Program for the Physically Disabled*, Rancho Los Amigos Hospital, December 1975.

—Theresa Valois, OTR, is coordinator of the "Disabled Drivers Program" University of Washington Hospital, Seattle, WA 98195.

Physical Disabilities
Special Interest Section Newsletter; Vol. 5, No. 2, 1982

Driving for Physically Disabled Persons—A Program Description

Public transportation is not readily available in some parts of the country, particularly Los Angeles. Here transportation is usually inaccessible to individuals in wheelchairs. At Rancho Los Amigos Hospital, driver training is a part of the occupational therapy program because driving is considered a *critical part* of the activities of daily living. This article is a brief overview of the driver training program at Rancho Los Amigos Hospital.

In the driver training program, initiated in the late 1950s by an occupational therapist, patients learned to drive hand-controlled cars in the open fields on the hospital grounds. Occupational therapists now work together with trained driving instructors to teach physically disabled people to drive safely on surface streets and freeways.

In 1981 the program trained 150-200 patients, using two cars and a van equipped with basic commercial equipment. The majority of the patients have diagnoses of spinal injury, stroke or head trauma. Other diagnoses include lower extremity amputation, burns, arthritis, multiple sclerosis, Guillain-Barre and cardio-pulmonary problems. The population is primarily male and in the age range of 18-40 years. A small percentage of the population is 65 years and older and 80% have been licensed to drive before the onset of their disability. Many patients begin the program while they are inpatients and complete the training as outpatients.

The occupational therapist communicates with the physician about the patient's driving needs, resources, physical and cognitive abilities, and readiness for driving. The physician then orders driver training and the therapist refers the patient to the driver training program as early as possible to educate them and their families about the types of equipment available and the possibility of driving.

Once the referral is made, the patient's potential for driving is based on the combination of many factors including the individual's physical and cognitive functioning, equipment needs and resources, interest in driving and actual behind-the-wheel performance. Patients who have physical limitations but good cognition can usually be trained if they have proper equipment. Patients who have cognition deficits but good physical abilities require minimal equipment: however, they need an intensive evaluation to determine whether limited memory, judgment, attention span, visual perception or other problems will interfere with driving safety. Patients with both physical *and* cognitive limitations are complex because they re-quire equipment to compensate for physical problems but cognitive problems make safe driving inconsistent.

Patients who demonstrate the potential are trained to drive with the required equipment in different driving situations graded in complexity. Training begins in a protected environment and may progress to heavy freeway driving during rush hour traffic. If a patient can drive independently but cannot transfer or manage the wheelchair, he will need to be educated about the various vehicles and equipment that are available. The patient's financial resources are an important factor to be considered.

The average length of evaluation and training is 6 to 8 hours. Patients with brain injury may require 10 to 12 hours or longer. A small percentage of patients who are referred to the program do not demonstrate the ability to be safe drivers. These patients and families are counselled not to drive and alternative transportation is discussed. Patients may be re-evaluated at a later date if their physical or cognitive status changes and, if indicated, the Department of Motor Vehicles may be contacted about the decrease in their ability to drive.

The driver training staff includes an occupational therapists and two driving in-
(continued)

Driving for Physically Disabled Persons

structors. The occupational therapist is responsible for 1) reviewing the patient's physical and cognitive abilities; 2) determining the medical precautions and problems which will interfere with driving; 3) working with the driving instructors in behind-the-wheel evaluations to determine equipment needed, potential for driving and training method needed to assist the patient in reaching his or her potential; and 4) reinforcing medical safety

precautions with the patient while driving. The driving instructors teach the patients to drive safely and independently in multiple driving situations using vehicles with adapted equipment. This program works closely with the Department of Motor Vehicles, other local driver training programs and automobile clubs to keep current about changes and to work together to enhance driving services for the physically disabled.

A handbook entitled "Driving For The Physically Handicapped" is presently being revised and will be available soon from the Professional Staff Association of Rancho Los Amigos Hospital, Inc., 7413 Golondrinas, Downey, California 90242.

Prepared by: Charlotte Gowland, OTR, OT Supervisor on the Driver Training Program, Rancho Los Amigos Hospital, February 1982.

Physical Disabilities
Special Interest Section Newsletter; Vol. 5, No. 1, 1982

Project Threshold—An Approach to Using Assistive Devices

Heidi McHugh Pendleton, OTR and Nancy J. Somerville

Persons with physical disabilities may fail to achieve their maximum levels of independence often because of unsolved problems encountered in performing activities of daily living. Project Threshold is a client service delivery program that assists these individuals in overcoming such obstacles. Generally, these clients have severe physical disabilities, are no longer actively involved in rehabilitation programs and are living in community settings. Referral sources include the California State Department of Rehabilitation, and numerous other individuals or agencies. Project Threshold employs occupational therapists extensively, as well as other allied health professionals on a consultant basis. In addition, as part of the Rancho Los Amigos Hospital Rehabilitation Engineering Center, the project has ready access to engineering personnel and facilities.

The Project Threshold staff uses a comprehensive assessment and problem-solving approach to provide simple and cost effective solutions for problems related to independent living skills, home, work, or school environments. This is generally accomplished by using one or more of the following solutions: suggestions for adaptive behavior, recommendations for commercially available technology, and design and fabrication of custom equipment. The majority of solutions to problems presented by clients of the program, however, involve recommendations for commercially available assistive devices. Custom devices are considered only when all other

options have been exhausted.

During the past decade there has been a tremendous increase in the number of commercial products designed and developed specifically for use by persons with disabilities. Appropriate application of these devices can make an amazing impact on a person's independence with daily activities. However, considering the vast array of such devices, it is impractical, if not impossible, for consumers and allied health professionals to keep their knowledge in this area current and complete.

When searching for appropriate equipment, Project Threshold uses a variety of references and resources. These include books and periodicals (selected references are included in this newsletter), a comprehensive file of catalogues and brochures from equipment manufacturers, ABLEDATA (a computerized data base described in this newsletter), and ACCENT ON INFORMATION (another computerized information system for assistance with locating special products, devices, and how-to information available through Accent on Information, Inc., Box 700, Bloomington, IL 61701).

Once a functional evaluation of the client is completed by the Project Threshold staff, research is conducted for equipment items that seem suitable. The client is then provided with the opportunity to try out the equipment with the appropriate training. As occupational therapists have experienced, equipment trial is vital to definitive equipment prescription. In addition, this trial enhances

the clients' knowledge of techniques involved in using the equipment and optimizes successful integration of these devices into the clients daily life. Project Threshold has a Model Home stocked with a limited supply of major equipment items and hundreds of inexpensive assistive devices for the actual equipment trial. Although having this equipment readily available in the Model Home is a definite advantage, it is our experience that equipment manufacturers and distributors are often cooperative in loaning a specific device for short term trial or at least demonstrating the device at his or her facility.

In addition to the equipment trial, Project Threshold involves the client in as many of the problem solving aspects of the evaluation process as possible. As a result, many clients are able to extrapolate from this experience and apply newly learned skills to future situations, approach new obstacles in an organized, analytical manner and identify appropriate resources when equipment needs arise.

In summary, it has been the authors' experience that use of adaptive equipment to maximize independence hinges upon a comprehensive functional assessment as well as proper equipment selection. Successful integration of the recommended equipment into the client's lifestyle is further encouraged by the following: thorough research into products using a variety of resources, equipment trials prior to definite recommendation, and client involvement in the problem-solving process.

Physical Disabilities
Special Interest Section Newsletter; Vol. 5, No. 1, 1982

Case Example: Applications of Assistive Devices

By Kathryn L. Bowman, OTR

Tribbey Strehle balances a full-time job with the duties of a homemaker. Additionally, she was expecting her first baby and was continuing her active life despite her pregnancy. Typical of many young women today, Tribbey found her mixed roles fulfilling and challenging, if a bit hectic. But not typical was that Tribbey had arthrogryposis since birth, resulting in nonfunctional upper extremities, stiffness in her lower extremities, highly developed neck strength, and an ability to do many functional activities with her mouth. Why would such a successful lady need occupational therapy intervention and adaptive equipment? This was our thought at Project Threshold when we received her referral from the Department of Rehabilitation counselor for a functional evaluation and equipment recommendations.

During a home visit, we reviewed self care and home tasks. Tribbey is a very resourceful person who had developed her own methods of doing things. She had not been in contact with rehabilitation personnel as an adult, had never had much functional training, and was virtually unaware of adaptive equipment. Tribbey was quite self-sufficient in her home environment but needed assistance from her husband in several tasks.

She was ambulatory with good balance and could bend over safely to use her mouth for activities. She stated she was able to lift heavy loads with her teeth and demonstrated lifting and pouring a full half-gallon of milk. Her dexterity with her tongue was highly developed. For example, she strung tiny beads to make necklaces, which she sold at craft fairs and swapmeets, each bearing a tag, "Mouth-Made by Tribbey." She fed herself by mouth with no special equipment once set up, brushed her teeth and put on make-up with her hand supported at the sink, turning the faucet with her mouth. She used a pencil in her mouth frequently for such dextrous tasks as activating the nozzle on a deodorant spray can. She was unable to brush her hair, and needed assistance for dressing, bathing and toileting. Of major concern was the excessive wear on her front teeth due to manipulating and lifting objects. While her neck range was good and she had highly developed muscle strength, she did complain of some strain in this area. When eating, the position of her head at her plate was tiring and not conducive to social contact with others.

In the homemaking area, Tribbey was again quite functional. She did the majority of the cooking, needing help for only very

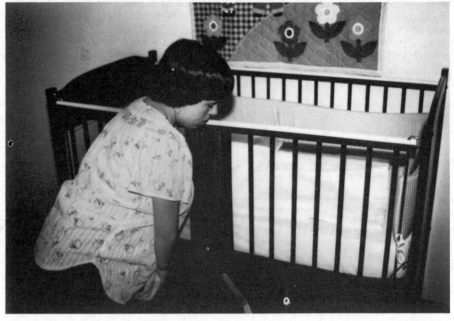

heavy items or reaching high places. She used a variety of utensils in her mouth to prepare food. She had standard kitchenwear and was often dangerously close to hot foods and flame while at the stove. Body mechanics and efficiency were not at their optimum when bending over to access standard countertops and cupboards.

Tribbey frequently used her desk at home for paying bills, cutting out store coupons (with scissors in her mouth, of course) and other common daily tasks. But telephoning was a burden since she picked up the receiver in her mouth, laid it on the desk top and then positioned her head near it as best she could. This was uncomfortable and did not allow her to write while on the telephone.

Resources for commercial equipment were explored to improve Tribbey's ability to be self-sufficient in her home. To improve posture and efficiency for feeding, the Universal Plate Positioner was recommended. This device, clamped to the table edge, positioned the plate several inches above standard table height by an adjustable mechanism and allowed for tilt at various angles. For assistance in handling her bathroom faucet, extended handles were recommended, which she could turn with her chin eliminating the need to use her teeth against the metal knobs. For hair grooming, a brush mounted on the bathroom wall allowed her to be independent. Bathing ability was improved markedly by the following: 1) a bench-style tub transfer seat allowing her to get into tub independently, 2) extended faucet handles, 3) a long-handled lightweight sponge to use in her mouth, 4) a suction

soap holder attached to the tub wall, 5) suction brushes mounted on the wall in three locations against which she could rub her body, 6) and a grab bar.

For homemaking, kitchen organization and accessibility were improved with use of slideout cupboards and turntables. A cutting board with stainless steel nails made using a knife in her mouth safer and easier. Nonskid matting and a pan holder for stove top also improved function. A telephone adapter that holds the receiver on a gooseneck extension positioned it at a convenient level for Tribbey. A simple lever is used to answer and disconnect.

Many of Tribbey's needs were met by commercial resources; however, custom equipment was also necessary. Custom equipment was devised for the following: 1) a set of mouth pieces was added to several standard kitchen utensils. These are "Y" shaped aluminum pieces coated with nontoxic plastic that use the back teeth for holding, bypassing Tribbey's front teeth, improving stability of the device in the mouth, and allowing for speech during use. In addition, those used for stove-top cooking were lengthened for safety. 2) An elevated platform styled with a table with a formica top was built to provide Tribbey with counter space conducive to better body mechanics. (She later used this table for many leisure activities as well.)

To prepare for her expected child, Tribbey and her husband had already done much problem-solving about ways in which she could handle the baby. Their ideas were valid but all in the preliminary

(continued)

Assistive Devices

stages with little resources to carry them out. Another area of concern was access to the crib and work areas for changing and bathing. Tribbey planned on nursing and needed a means of supporting the baby for this as well as just cuddling. Changing, bathing and feeding was not a problem once the child was positioned because Tribbey could manage disposable diapers, clothing with snaps or Velcro, spoons, wash cloths, sponges with handles and towels in her mouth.

A standard wooden crib was modified by making a hinge-style door opening with a lower lock Tribbey could release with her knee (Picture). Tribbey's ideas for a custom carrier were expanded upon and the design of a blanket with plastic insert for support, Velcro straps and a strong webbing handle was devised for carrying the baby. For nursing and holding the child, various commercial baby carriers were explored and the "Snuggli" was a feasible answer although Tribbey needed assistance to apply it. For holding bottles, lotions and powder, a commercially available plastic coated cuff-like handle with Velcro strap called the Quad-Quip Phone Holder was recommended.

A visit to Tribbey's place of employment where she worked as a keypunch operator was made. She was independent in most job activities, but again problems centered around excessive use of her front teeth, constant reaching with her neck and the frequent need to get up and down from her chair to access materials.

Exploration of commercial resources revealed no solution to Tribbeys' specific problems. Rehabilitation engineering was again involved. Custom mouthsticks were designed and fabricated. These mouthsticks incorporated the following terminal devices: 1) rubber tip for typing keypunch machine and sort cards, 2) pen/pencil attachment, 3) suction tip mouthstick operated by the breath control to enable her to

pick up cards without getting up and to access more storage areas. In addition, a mouthstick holder was made for easy accessibility from her desk. A vertical holder for computer cards to enable easy access with the suction mouthstick, a modification of the on/off switch on the keypunch machine from rear to front of desk for better body mechanics during operation, and a holder for rubberbands in which computer cards could be inserted and one rubberband slipped on with a mouthstick for grouping cards, were also fabricated.

Tribbey's efficiency and ease in performance on the job and at home were thus improved by an analysis of tasks and use of relatively simple adaptive equipment. We, in the field of rehabilitation, may become so familiar with common aids that we are unaware of those disabled persons who appear to be functioning quite independently but may have never seen a cutting board with nails perfectly suited to their needs. Occupational therapy's role with this type of client (one that has dealt with their disability for years) does not necessarily require providing the comprehensive, lengthy evaluations and treatment programs common to the acute rehabilitation setting. In Tribbey's case our involvement, while intense, was short and relatively inexpensive. The difference adaptive equipment made for her was in the quality of task performance.

Kathryn L. Bowman, OTR, is an occupational therapy consultant for Project Threshold.

SELECTED REFERENCES

1. *Accent on Living*, Cheever Publishing, Inc. PO Box 700, Bloomington, IL 61701. Published quarterly.
2. *Self-Help Manual for Patients with Arthritis*, Arthritis Health Professions Section of Arthritis Foundation, 3400 Peachtree Rd., NE, Atlanta, GA 30326, 1980.
3. Department of Education, Division of Rehabilitation Services and University of Nebraska College of Agriculture and Home Economics, School of Home Economics publish nine booklets related to homemaking activities for the physically disabled homemaker.
4. *The Green Pages RehabSourcebook*, Source-Book Publications, Inc., PO Box 1586, Winter Park, FL 32790, 1980. Published annually.
5. *Mealtime Manual for People with Disabilities and the Aging*. Institute of Rehabilitation Medicine, New York University Medical Center and Campbell Soup Company, 1978.
6. Lowman, E, Klinger, JL: *Aids to Independent Living Self Help for the Handicapped*. McGraw-Hill, 1969.
7. Laurie, G: *Housing and Home Services for the Disabled: Guidelines and Experiences in Independent Living*. Harper & Row, 1977.
8. Ford, J, Duckworth, B: *Physical Management for the Quadriplegic Patient*. F.A. Davis, 1974.
9. Gilbert, A E: *You Can Do It From a Wheelchair*. Arlington House, 1973.
10. Finnie, N: *Handling the Young Cerebral Palsied Child at Home*. New York, Dutton & Company, 1968.
11. Lifchez, R, Winslow, B: *Design for Independent Living: The Environment and Physically Disabled People*. New York, Whitney Library of Design, 1979.
12. High, E C: *A Resource Guide to Habilitative Techniques and Aids for Cerebral Palsied Persons of All Ages*. Job Development Laboratory, Division of Rehabilitation Medicine, The George Washington University, Washington, DC.
13. Cary, J R: *How to Create Interiors for the Disabled*. New York, Pantheon Books, 1978.
14. The Institute of Rehabilitation Medicine, New York University Medical Center: *A Manual for Training the Disabled Homemaker*. New York, 1955.
15. Accent on Living Buyer's Guide, Cheever Publishing, Inc., Bloomington, IL 61701, 1981.
16. Garee, B: *Ideas for Making Your Home Accessible*. Accent on Special Publications, Cheever Publishing, PO Box 700, Bloomington, IL 61701.
17. *The Sourcebook for the Disabled*: An Illustrated Guide to Easier More Independent Living for Physically Disabled People, Their Families and Friends. Edited by Glorya Hale, 1979, Paddington Press, Distributed in U.S. by Grosset and Dunlap, New York.
18. Washam, V: *One Handers Book: Basic Guide for Activities of Daily Living*. John Day Company, 1973.
19. *Do It Yourself Again*. Self Help Devices for the Stroke Patient, American Heart Association, New York, 1967.

Physical Disabilities
Special Interest Section Newsletter; Vol. 4, No. 4, 1981

Hands on: Pain Management—Occupational Therapy for the Spinal Pain Patient

By Jean Jackson, OTR, and Charlotte Klyan, OTR

J.K. is a woman who worked full time with her husband, entertained, kept house, and enjoyed recreational activities. As a generous and caring woman, J.K. often helped family members resolve their problems. She was accustomed to a high standard of living and valued being a high achiever in all of her roles—wife, mother, and career woman.

Four years ago, J.K. strained her right arm. To cope with the resultant pain, J.K. gradually decreased housekeeping activities, rested frequently, and often complained of pain. Her daughter responded by helping more with the housework. J.K. sought medical help and was given valium, codeine, and injections. She started to drink alcohol to relieve the pain.

By the time J.K. was admitted to RLAH she had not worked for nine months. Her

(continued)

Pain Management—Spinal Pain Patient

days were spent "wandering around" (in her own words). She felt depressed and her pain caused nausea, poor concentration, and exhaustion. She was on high doses of valium and codeine and was drinking alcohol regularly. In occupational therapy J.K. appeared depressed and quite fearful that her pain was imaginary.

As this case illustrates, many factors contribute to the experience of pain and pain affects many aspects of the patient's life. On the Spinal Pain Service at Rancho Los Amigos Hospital pain is viewed as a complex phenomenon. There is seldom a single simple cause for chronic pain.[1] In addition to biochemical causes of pain there are social and psychological sources of pain. Because of this multi-causal picture, medical and surgical procedures do not necessarily cure pain. Unfortunately, people who have not been cured by medical or surgical techniques are often seen as "crocks," "fakers," or people who are imagining their pain.

To treat chronic pain, a multidisciplinary team approach which uses behavioral methods in addition to medico-surgical techniques is often effective.[2] While the goal of traditional pain treatment is pain relief, the behavioral approach was a goal of increasing daily function and teaching people to be healthy even though they continue to have pain.

The Spinal Pain Service at RLAH provides a comprehensive approach to the treatment of disabling chronic back and neck pain. It is managed by a multidisciplinary team including orthopedic surgeons, a general practitioner, nursing, occupational therapy, physical therapy, and psychology. The program is divided into three phases. Patients begin with Evaluation Phase, which is a week of extensive evaluations by each team member. Based on initial evaluations, which are discussed at a team conference, patients are either accepted into the first phase or discharged.

Phase I

Phase I provides a program of continuing evaluation by the surgeons, therapeutic physical exercise, and education on back care. In physical therapy, patients participate in an anatomy class and in exercises designed specifically for the spine; leg strengthening, bicycling, and walking. The liaison nurse instructs patients about their medications, and the dietician provides information on proper nutrition. In occupational therapy patients attend relaxation, pacing, body mechanics classes, and work tolerance sessions. These activities are presented in a well-structured and full daily schedule to increase endurance. Those patients who will gain from a pain management program are progressed to Phase II.

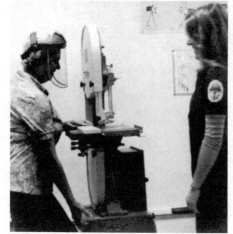
Jeanne Jackson instructs clients in proper body mechanics.

Phase II

Phase II is designed for those patients who are medically cleared, have demonstrated motivation to change their present disabled life-style and have goals consistent with rehabilitation. Phase II is based on a behavioral model of pain. Unlike Phase I, when treatment is based on finding and treating an underlying pathology, in Phase II pain is viewed as a complex system in which the patient's environment plays an important role in controlling pain. If patients receive reinforcement for "being sick," they learn attitudes and behaviors consistent with a sick role.[3] The overall goal of Phase II is to increase function and to decrease use of the medical system.

All Phase II treatment is designed to help all patients reach their personal functional goals. From those goals a quota system for improving physical tolerances is developed to increase each patient's function at a steady pace regardless of pain. Daily progress is charted on large bedside cards to provide positive reinforcement of well behaviors. The quota system is described further in the treatment section. In addition to Phase I classes, patients are taught body mechanics theory, and advanced anatomy by physical therapy; led in more advanced discussions of medications by the liaison nurse, and taught heavy lifting, pacing, recreational body mechanics, and assertive behavior, and provided prevocational guidance by the occupational therapist. Weekly group discussions are held with the clinical psychologist to identify the effects of stress and attitudes on pain and disability.

Occupational Therapy Evaluation

The occupational therapist evaluates all patients and their pain using the occupational behavior frame of reference. The patients describe their daily activities including self-care, household chores, work, and

leisure skills prior to the onset of pain and at the present time. Occupational therapy analyzes to what extent pain interferes with the patients' performance of these activities and evaluates their pacing and use of proper body mechanics. The interaction of family members with the patient's pain problem is assessed. Families can unknowingly reinforce the patient's pain by assuming responsibilities that were distasteful to the patient or by increasing attention given to the patient.

The patient's source of income, involvement in litigation, and court dates are discussed to assess the degree to which a patient is emotionally invested in hearings and demonstrating his or her disability.

A history and description of the pain is obtained. If there is a complaint of cervical problems, and upper extremity evaluation is performed. One objective is to assess the patient's own reaction to his or her pain problem to determine specific problems of pain. For example, a long history of pain can result in a learned disability role or a history of pain episodes closely related to stressful incidents may indicate a stress management problem.

The patient is questioned about his or her goals to determine whether he or she is being realistic and future-oriented. Throughout the evaluation pain behaviors are assessed. Pain behaviors include moaning, groaning, rubbing the back or neck, and verbal complaints. Pain behaviors indicate the patient's need to convey the intensity of the pain to others.

In general, the occupational therapy evaluation is concerned with extracting a picture of the patients' life situation and how pain interferes with their life roles. Occupational therapy also focuses on the inherent reinforcement in the patient's life situation which may contribute to a continued pain problem. This evaluation combined with those of other team members tries to present a complete picture of the patient and his or her pain.

Occupational Therapy Program

Most therapy is provided in group sessions to take advantage of group dynamics. The program includes instruction as previously outlined in relaxation, body mechanics, pacing and assertion coupled with work tolerance sessions and prevocational testing and guidance.

Back pain often induces a stress response in the body. This response increases pain by adding muscle tension and anxiety. Thus, a cycle develops which often escalates until the patient is unable to cope with pain. (Fig. 1) Relaxation is often an effective method for pain management because it breaks the cycle by reducing muscle tension and anxiety. In

(continued)

Pain Management—Spinal Pain Patient

this way pain is reduced to a manageable level.

Relaxation classes are held daily. In initially, Jacobsen methods are taught.[4] Patients learn to identify tense muscles, isolate problem areas, and relax those muscles. When this method is mastered, patients begin an advanced class where they learn to use imagery, autogenics, and deep breathing. Although classes begin in a quiet setting, patients are encouraged to use the techniques in more stressful situations.

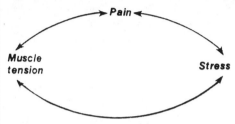

Fig. 1: Pain-Stress Cycle

All patients receive a lecture on the basic principles of body mechanics.[5] After the lecture patients attend daily classes to discuss and practice typical household chores and yard work.

In Phase I the goal is to be as active as possible during the hour while focusing on a task rather than on pain. Patients change positions as often as necessary. In Phase II patients are placed on quota programs to increase their sitting, standing, lifting, or carrying toleances to meet functional goals established at the beginning of Phase II. Daily quotas begin at comfortable time or weight levels and increase gradually.

In Phase II, the longer sessions enable occupational therapists to observe and further evaluate each patient's spontaneous use of body mechanics, pacing, pain behavior, and physical tolerances. It provides a time when patients can practice new skills to incorporate them into new habit structures. Patients can explore leisure activities and discover how they divert attention from pain. Many patients need this to reacquaint themselves with pleasurable tasks because chronic pain has disrupted their normal leisure activities.

To manage pain it is important to learn how to pace activities and avoid extremes. Some patients rush to finish tasks before their pain returns or increases, but this exacerbates their pain and causes fatigue. Others rest most of the day to avoid every increase in pain that accompanies activities. Principles of pacing are taught formally in lectures and informally during body mechanics and work tolerance sessions. Weekend schedules are used to help patients apply the principles of pacing during weekend passes. To be successful it is imperative that patients learn how to carry out the program at home. Hourly logs are used to evaluate all patients' ability to pace their weekend and apply principles and exercises from the progam.

Assertion classes are held twice a week for Phase II patients. Assertive behavior replaces pain behaviors and enables patients to implement their new healthy lifestyle. Much of the pain management program requires asserting oneself and taking charge of one's life. Topics covered in the twice weekly classes include (1) definitions of assertive, passive, and aggressive behavior, (2) relationship between pain, stress, and assertion, (3) assertive techniques, and (4) exercises to help patients identify their own behaviors. Occupational therapy uses role-playing, group discussion, and written exercises to teach the above.

Prevocational Assessment And Counseling

Within RLAH both prevocational and vocational counselors are available. The occupational therapist serves as a liaison with these services by screening patients and making referrals. Generally, patients fall into three categories: (1) those that return to former jobs, (2) those who must seek new employment, and (3) those for whom work is not a goal.

When a patient desires to return to his or her previous employment, the occupational therapist works with the patient in identifying specific job requirements and in problem-solving proper body mechanics and pacing. If necessary, job simulation is used to check body mechanics skills. Stressful situations are identified and the use of relaxation and assertive techniques is discussed. Job site evaluations and telephone discussions with employers are conducted if needed.

Some patients decide to seek new employment. An in-depth work history is taken to identify previous successful and unsuccessful work experiences. Specific skills and personal preferences for work conditions are discussed. The COPS interest test is given to explore job possibilities. The WRAT is used to assess academic level.

During daily work tolerance sessions the patient's response to a semi-structured work-like setting is assessed. Basic work skills such as (1) initiative, (2) planning and organization, (3) frustration tolerance, (4) relationship with supervisors and co-workers, (5) response to praise and criticism, emotional stability, and (6) leadership are assessed. The occupational therapist then either assists patients with a job search or refers them a vocational counselor for retraining, or to a prevocational counselor for development of basic work skills.

In some cases patients speak of vocational plans but emphasize negative factors that prohibit work. Those patients are confronted about the discrepancy between their stated goals and actual behavior. They are informed of available services to contact on their own.

Conclusion

Learning pain management requires learning a new life style, and patients need opportunities to practice their new skills and develop them into new habit structures. Occupational therapy provides the setting in which such practice can take place.

The complexity of pain can be effectively handled through the occupational behavior frame of reference because it addresses biological, psychological and social levels, all of which interrelate with chronic pain.

References

1. Melzack, R. Dennis, SG. Neurophysiological Foundations of Pain, in *The Psychology of Pain*, Sternback, RA, Editor. Raven Press. New York, 1-26, 1978.
2. McCaffery, M. *Nursing Management of the Patient with Pain*, JB Lippincott Co., Philadelphia, 1979.
3. Fordyce, W. *Behavioral Methods for Chronic Pain and Illness* CV Mosby Co., St. Louis. 1976.
4. Jacobsen, E. *You Must Relax*, McGraw-Hill Book Company, New York, 1978.
5. Watson, K. (Ed.), *Occupational Therapy in the Care of Spinal Pain Patients*, Professional Staff Association, Rancho Los Amigos Hospital, Downey, CA, 1980.

Jeanne Jackson, OTR, is a staff therapist at Rancho Los Amigos Hospital. Charlotte Kiyan, OTR, is a staff therapist at St. Joseph's Hospital in Orange, Calif., formerly supervisor at Rancho Los Amigos Hospital.

Rancho Los Amigos Spinal Pain Service was closed 7-29-81, as a result of budget reductions.

Physical Disabilities
Special Interest Section Newsletter; Vol. 4, No. 4, 1981

Chronic Pain Management: Occupational Therapy Role

By Carol Prenatt Sanborn, OTR

Chronic pain, more accurately described as long-lasting pain affecting a person both physically and emotionally, is estimated to affect more than 20 million Americans each year. Treatment of this disability totals somewhere between 35 and 50 billion dollars annually. Included in these high costs are lost wages, medical expenses and workman's compensation. This figure cannot begin to reflect secondary and tertiary losses to families, employers and insurance carriers who often absorb equally staggering losses over extended periods of time.

Working with chronic pain patients can be a very frustrating and often futile experience, particularly when treatment follows the traditional approaches using the medical model. Historically, the patient is seen as a passive figure in medical treatment. He or she goes to the doctor and seeks professional advice within a system where modern medicine is geared towards cure. Should the problem be diagnosed as one inoperable or untreatable by medication, patients are often referred to physical therapy. If this course is deemed unsuccessful, patients again may seek help by acupuncture, acupressure, hypnotism, mega-vitamin therapy, etc. Through this entire process, the patient often begins to view him or herself as rejected, having failed in procedures which focus on cures. The process fosters a feeling of failure by patients when they do not get well.

Common among most chronic pain patients is the role that a personal sense of control plays in the treatment approach. This is not to imply that control of pain can be purely voluntary and independent of any treatment, but merely points to a treatment approach used in theory and practice at the Pain Management Center at Daniel Freeman Hospital Medical Center.

Viewing the patient as the person most responsible for achieving and maintaining health rather than depending on doctors, drugs, and other allied health professionals has been found to be a successful approach to the remediation of chronic pain.

With this concept in mind, occupational therapy, using its modality of activity, is clearly established as an effective discipline in returning the chronic pain patient to the role of an *active* participant in his or her health care. At Daniel Freeman Hospital Medical Center, the occupational therapy progam offers the chronic pain patient a combination of activity and education to enhance his or her awareness of how to effectively cope with chronic pain

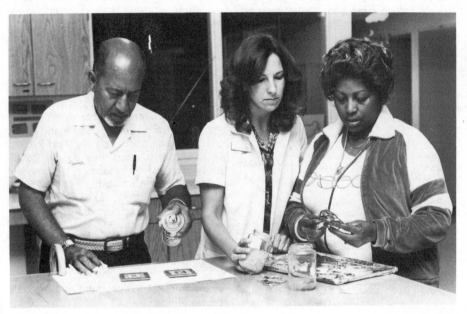

Jean Bergenstal, COTA, assists chronic pain patients in Work Tolerance Group while they try to increase standing tolerance during functional activity.

on a daily basis. This is provided through the holistic framework of viewing patients as bio-psycho-social beings.

The Work Tolerance Group is a group which emphasizes activity while seeking to increase a patient's sitting and standing tolerance in a simulated work environment. The work process is given attention, although this time is viewed as an opportunity to increase socialization skills and establish new leisure skills which both are often deficient areas in many chronic pain patients' lives. While engaged in functional, goal-oriented activity, patients make few complaints of pain or demonstrate little pain behavior. Patients begin to incorporate activity as a relaxation tool and a replacement for discontinued pain medication. Of prime importance is the patient's ability to remove himself from the once held passive role in treatment and given newly acquired coping tools that can be continued outside the hospital setting.

Educational material is also presented by the occupational therapist to enhance the patient's knowledge and increase his or her ability to return to a normal and meaningful life without a need for pain medication by effectively coping with pain on a daily basis so as not to interfere with activities of daily living performance. Assertion training, proper body mechanics instruction, goal setting, and pacing and scheduling techniques are some of the educational issues addressed by occupa-

tional therapy.

The occupational therapist is also available to explore vocational alternatives and return to work, although quite often this is an area which requires additional time from inpatient hospitalization before it becomes a completed reality.

All of the above would be most difficult to attempt without the supportive and consistent team approach used by the Pain Management Team. Team members include the team physician, a neurologist; a program co-ordinator, licensed clinical social worker, licensed clinical psychologist, physical therapist, nurses, certified occupational therapy assistant (COTA), physical therapy aide, and registered occupational therapist. Treatment consists of a five-week inpatient program which operates 5 1/2 days per week, allowing for therapeutic passes on the weekends to allow constant evaluation and adjustment for how these skills will correlate with a patient's home environment. The program has been in existence for approximately 3 years with patient and program success recently presented by invitation to the Third World Annual Conference on Pain in Edinburgh, Scotland.

(continued)

Carol Prenatt Sanborn, OTR, is a staff therapist at the Daniel Freeman Hospital Medical Center and is assigned to the Pain Management Team

Chronic Pain Management

Daniel Freeman Hospital Medical Center is located in Inglewood, California, and was recently named the outstanding rehabilitation facility in the United States by the National Association of Rehabilitation Facilities (NARF).

Bibliography: Pain Management

1. Benson, H., *The Relaxation Response.* Wm. Morrow and Company, New York, 1976.
2. Booraem, C., Assertion Training, Chapter in *Approaches to Assertion Training*, Flowers and Whitley, Editors. Brooks-Cole Publishing Co., Monterey, CA, 1978.
3. Bresler, D., *Learning to Control Pain*, Simon and Schuster, 1977.
4. Kiev, A., *A Strategy for Daily Living*, Free Press, McMillan Publishing Co., 1973.
5. Pellitier, K., *Mind as Healer, Mind as Slayer*, Dell Publishers, 1977.
6. Selye, H. *The Stress of Life*, McGraw-Hill Book Company, New York, 1978.

Physical Disabilities
Special Interest Section Newsletter; Vol. 4, No. 3, 1981

A Unique Outpatient Clinic for Burn Patients

By Kathy Torrell, OTR

Due to the long-term effects of burns, there is a need for prolonged rehabilitation follow-up after burn wounds have healed. Although physicians provide excellent medical follow-up care, many patients were found to regress in respect to joint range of motion and general functional status with an increase in scar formation. Occupational and physical therapy (OT/PT) identified a need for continuing rehabilitation as an adjunct to physician follow-up. In January of 1980, a monthly OT/PT outpatient clinic was established in collaboration with the physicians. The physician is an integral part of this clinic and must make a written referral. At present, there are six physicians participating in the clinic from this facility; in addition, referrals are also received from other facilities.

By having both occupational and physical therapy involved in this clinic, many parameters can be checked in a short period of time. The priorities of the clinic are range of motion, motor function, functional status (activities of daily living, mobility, and skin condition). The need for and/or effectiveness of special equipment, pressure garments and home programs is evaluated and revised. Since only a short period of time (15 minutes) is allotted for each patient, this is viewed as a screening clinic. If further therapy and/or medical treatment are needed, this is discussed with the patient and an appointment is arranged.

In addition to occupational and physical therapy, this clinic offers the opportunity to continue the team approach used in inpatient care. All staff members are invited to attend the clinic including physicians, nurses, social workers and students of all disciplines. Each discipline is notified of the patients scheduled for a given clinic at least one week in advance. A physician and social worker are present or on-call for each clinic.

Both therapists involved in the clinic are also responsible for acute burn rehabilitation, thus occupational and physical therapy services are consistent throughout the healing process. Patients are followed in this clinic up to one year post-burn.

An OT/PT burn outpatient clinic was developed with the objective of providing consistent follow-up care to help each patient obtain his maximum rehabilitation potential. The clinic is unique in that it was proposed, organized, and carried out by an occupational and physical therapist. It is hoped that the efforts of the clinic will maintain and/or increase the patients' physical and functional status, thus decreasing the need for some reconstructive surgery. Each patient is helped to obtain maximal rehabilitation potential, thus improving the quality of his or her life.

Kathy Torrell, OTR is staff occupational therapist at the Strong Memorial Hospital, University of Rochester Medical Center, Rochester, New York.

Physical Disabilities
Special Interest Section Newsletter; Vol. 4, No. 3, 1981

The Use of Hexcelite as a Splinting Material for the Acutely Burned Hand

By Peter J. Couchman, OTR

Of the more than 300 patients admitted each year to the Burn Center at Los Angeles County/USC Medical Center, one-third have burns of the hands. We have a yearly average of 100 patients that require handsplinting and use of our Hand Burn Protocol. More than 200 antideformity burn handsplints are required to meet the needs of those patients with hand burns.

While fabricating this quantity of splints each year, we became acutely aware of the problems that arise on the market today. For the past 10 years, we

(continued)

Use of Hexcelite

have been trying different splinting materials in an effort to find one that would be the most beneficial in the treatment of burned hand. Although studies have not been conducted, we think we are seeing a decrease in the length of time needed for healing the burned hand, a significant decrease in sepsis, and fewer hand problems, such as boutonniere deformity, have been observed since Hexcelite has been used for handsplints. We cannot state whether this is totally or in part due to the use of Hexcelite splints, or whether a greater awareness of the problem exists, with extra effort by the total burn team, to treat the hands carefully.

Problems Identified:

Some of the problems found during the use of other materials in our facility have led us to reassess the purpose of handsplints in the treatment of hand burns. The major purpose is to prevent hand deformity by keeping the extensor tendons as slack as possible; keeping the collateral ligaments at the metacarpalphalangeal joints taut; protecting the extensor mechanism over the proximal interphalangeal joints; and aiding in the reduction of edema of the hand. To accomplish this, we have been using fairly rigid thermoplastic splinting materials, with or without perforations. When these splints are applied to the burned hand, we have, in essence made an occlusive dressing that is not compatible with the use of topical agents in use today. It is commonly accepted that there must be an exchange of air while these topical agents are in use and, yet, we continued to use splinting materials that did not allow this free exchange of air.

Another problem with splints made of rigid materials is that they do not conform well as edema in the burned hands recede; the splints must be continually adjusted or completely remade. The length of time it takes to make the splints, conformability, ease of reshaping, setting time, and cost are some of the other problems.

With these problems in mind, we found that Hexcelite Orthopedic

Tape® met these specific needs just mentioned for our facility. Hexcelite is an open-weave cotton fabric coated with a high density resin. It was found to be strong, durable, remoldable, porous, impact and fatigue resistant, moisture resistant, fast setting and radioluscent. In addition, it has selective rigidity depending upon the numbers of layers used.

Hexcelite® Technique:

Hexcelite is heated tith hot water. Regular Hexcelite requires a temperature of 170° and "quick-dip and light" Hexcelite a temperature of 150°. Heating time for regular Hexcelite is 4 to 5 minutes for a roll, whereas quick dip and light Hexcelite take 30 seconds. Working time for regular Hexcelite is 3 to 6 minutes and for quick dip and light Hexcelite, it is 2 to 4 minutes. We have found that the best equipment for heating Hexcelite is a hydrocollator. Using tongs, the roll is held under water until the bubbles cease and then it is allowed to float for the remaining time required for the grade of Hexcellite used. The roll is then drained well or the excess water squeezed out with a towel.

When heated correctly, this material will drape very easily. We have found that using three layers of Hexcelite with the mesh pattern matched works the best; if more rigidity is needed, then a fourth layer is added. For additional strength, scraps can be added by aligning the pattern of the weave. When extra reinforcement is needed, well-heated pieces are laid on the cool splint and only the edges pressed down. If the entire surface is pressed, the open weave will close and the porosity is lost. The same applies in shaping the splint. Care must be taken not to slide the hand across the material or it will close the open weave.

Hexcelite is self-bonding and does not need any special adhesives or precleaning to attach one layer to another, or to add reinforcements or attachments. Hexcelite is easily shaped to make hooks, rolled, with or without

wire reinforcement, to make out-riggers and molded into the splint base. Adhesive-backed Velcro® can be directly bonded to Hexcelite, but a better bond is made if the Hexcelite and the Velcro adhesive are spot heated first before attaching. We do not use any straps to apply these splints to the burned hand. We have found that wrapping with Kling® bandage works best. Straps, when applied correctly, only led to increased edema between the straps and, in most cases, the pressure from the straps converted a second degree burn to full thickness burn.

Hexcelite splints are easily cleaned with soap and water or with 2 percent Staphene®, as is the case with burn splints. Splints can be gas sterilized but not autoclaved.

The only topical agent we have found not to be compatible with the use of Hexcelite has been Sulfamylon®. Sulfamylon, when used, becomes hard and cakes into the open weave of the splint material, thereby negating one of the primary advantages of allowing air to freely pass through the splint. When Sulfamylon is used, we revert back to using the solid types of thermoplastic splints such as Hexceplast. In some cases when Sulfamylon is used for 12 hours and Sylvadene® for the remaining 12 hours, two sets of splints will be used; one set is made of Hexcelite for use with Sylvadene and one set is made of Hexceplast for use with Sulfamylon.

We think that Hexcelite Orthopedic Tape is the best handsplinting material on the market today for our use in the acute treatment of the burned hand. However, we will continue to evaluate the use of Hexcelite handsplints in conjunction with our present hand protocol.

NOTE: Hexcelite Orthopedic Tape, Hexcel-Medical Products, 11711 Dublin Blvd., Dublin, CA 94566.

Peter Couchman, OTR is Occupational Therapy Supervisor I at the Los Angeles County/USC Medical Center—Burn Center, Los Angeles, California.

Physical Disabilities
Special Interest Section Newsletter; Vol. 4, No. 2, 1981

Psychosocial Aspects of Occupational Therapy in Burn Rehabilitation

By Cynthia Cooper, MFA, MA, OTR

Cynthia Cooper, MFA, MA, OTR is a staff occupational therapist on the Burn Program of the Plastic Reconstructive Service at Rancho Los Amigos Hospital.

Severe burn is one of the most catastrophic injuries that can occur due to its complicated functional, physical, and disfiguring sequelae. Unfortunately, there is a lack of literature which addresses the psychosocial implications of occupational therapy in burn rehabilitation. This article will begin to discuss some of these implications and the role of occupational therapy in facilitating psychosocial adjustment following burn injury. The content herein is based on the author's clinical experience in burn rehabilitation.

The Problem

During the acute phase of care, the emphasis is on the patients' physical status with measures taken to facilitate medical stability and the healing of open areas. In this phase of the treatment process, patients may or may not begin to deal with the large-scale implications of the injury. Among the psychosocial factors that most patients must deal with in a rehabilitation setting are changes in life role due to functional limitations, changes in body image and self-identity, continual and insidious progression of deformity, and family and community responses to disfigurement.

Bhalerao et al (1976) found the implications of physical disfigurement to include public non-acceptance and patients' feelings of inferiority. In an exploration of the social aspects of burn-related disfigurement, Andreasen and Norris (1972) noted the revulsion which strangers may express when facing a burn-disfigured person. They suggest that such revulsion stems from an unconscious dread of the physically deformed. Simon (1971) concurred and stated that most people are uncomfortable with others who are deformed. Even health professionals have been known to experience this discomfort. Patients develop their own ways of handling this problem. The author has worked with a severely facially disfigured male who initiates conversations by saying "Hi, ugly!" and jokingly referring to himself as "handsome."

The effect of disfigurement on body image and self-concept is described by Andreasen and Norris (1972) as an anxiety-evoking threat to one's self-identity. Woods (1975) described the way in which a distortion of body image is interpreted as

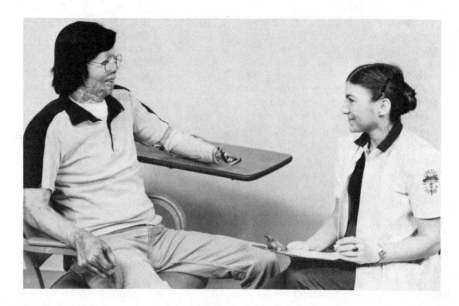

Cynthia Cooper is interviewing patient regarding his post-discharge activity level.

a distortion of self and thus evokes fear of rejection due to the bodily disfigurement. Body image and self-identity are interrelated elements which are both greatly affected by the responses of others. When a disfigured burn victim receives negative reactions from others, he may become convinced he does not look well and may even decide he does not feel well. Such feelings interfere with the experience of self-worth. These concerns must be acknowledged as valid components of the adjustment process, and all patients will eventually have to deal with them to some degree.

For instance, a badly burned woman who had undergone multiple facial reconstructive surgeries was surprised that a man she had dated pre-injury had remained her friend post-injury. The hands-on aspect of burn occupational therapy is an extremely important way to dispel such feelings of inferiority. Through touch the therapist suggests that the patient is still an approachable and valuable human being.

With severe burns, significant skin and joint changes can continue to occur for months following discharge from the acute care setting. These include changes in pigmentation, development of hypertrophic scar or keloid, and changes in soft tissue and joint structure leading to contracture formation. Any or all of the above changes may occur, resulting in increases in both deformity and disfigurement. Patients

may not be prepared for or even aware of the possibility of these changes occurring. Patients who have been informed may still express surprise at these ongoing changes. The therapist can help by repeatedly and realistically describing the possible changes to come. Having already undergone the pain and trauma of the original burn injury and its acute treatment, this insidious progression of deformity and disfigurement compounds patients' potential for psychological vulnerability.

OT's Role In Facilitating Psychosocial Adjustment

Occupational therapists deal with the psychosocial needs of burn patients on a daily basis as they implement programs to meet the physical and functional goals of treatment. The focus on function and the individual's life role together with the activities used in treatment provide a natural setting in which to address the psychosocial components of burn rehabilitation.

Helping patients acclimate to such a major insult as a severe burn injury requires sensitive acknowledgement of its impact throughout the treatment process, the use of the therapist's knowledge of and background in psychiatric occupational therapy, and an ongoing holistic overview in which physical and psychological considerations and their interrelationships are

(continued)

Psychosocial Aspects in Burn Rehabilitation

addressed. Furthermore, it is understood that the therapist must be aware of and not impose her own values on patients as she helps them to return to their maximum preinjury level of adjustment and style of life. *Occupational therapy can only facilitate the adjustment process.*

Patients must be ready and able to do the work required for their unique coping styles to be developed and for their adjustment potentials to be realized. Adjustment can be facilitated in the following ways: providing support; encouraging patient's awareness of and confrontation with the implications of the injury; and promoting the development of coping styles and self-directedness throughout the treatment process for eventual extension into the post-discharge setting.

Support: Certain aspects of the occupational therapy program reinforce the supportive role of the therapist. They include the intensity, frequent discomfort, long-term nature of burn rehabilitation, the number of hours spent in daily treatment, and the "hands-on" aspects of burn occupational therapy.

The therapist provides support in a variety of ways. The degree of support varies as patients' needs fluctuate and may peak with each new milestone in the treatment process. Facing an upcoming surgery or experiencing the first outing into the community are often times when patients need extra support. Requests for additional support do not necessarily indicate regression: a woman who had been passive and dependent pre-injury cried throughout her gradual development of assertiveness. Thus patients' emotional expressions overlap; the need for extra support does not negate the development of new coping skills. Throughout the provision of support, the therapist encourages patients to express their feelings and needs yet tries to monitor their needs so as not to encourage over-dependency.

Awareness/Confrontation: The therapist facilitates psychosocial adjustment by first eliciting awareness of the impact of the injury. This is achieved through building and reinforcing a climate which promotes exploration of problems that individual patients face in their unique adjustment process. Certain elements of the occupational therapy program tend to elicit such exploration. One of these is the frequent pain associated with ranging burn patients. Patients occasionally cry during occupational therapy. The pain of the moment may trigger the tears. Such a response, if handled sensitively by the therapist, often leads to a discussion of additional important issues such as fear of an upcoming weekend pass or concern about the effect of disfigurement on a spouse.

The activity-oriented, practical, and functional nature of occupational therapy with its focus on the life tasks of patients promotes confrontation with the implications of the burn injury. For instance, treatment such as retraining in self-grooming has prompted expressions of grief regarding facial disfigurement with ensuing discussions of altered self-image. Another case involves patient who sustained a flame injury. During the planning for a kitchen evaluation involving the use of the stove, a previously unidentified or unstated fear of fire came to the surface.

A final example relates to community outings. These are often stressful due to the responses of others to disfigurement and because they force the patient out of the protective environment of the hospital or home. The response of others in such places as the grocery store or restaurant can be an intense confrontation with the social implications of disfigurement. Such confrontation with the residual effects of the injury best occurs in a supportive environment before coping or optimal adjustment can take place.

Coping and Self-Directedness: The therapist promotes development of coping skills and self-directedness in part through clarifying patient expectations and advocating patient directed treatment. Burn patients and the public at large often have constructed a set of beliefs about the miracles of modern medicine in general and plastic surgery in particular. The influence of the advertising and entertainment media can be felt strongly here. For example, patients often assume that the accomplishments of plastic surgery far exceed its actual potential. This can result in significant discrepancies between the patient's and the team's expectations regarding post-operative cosmetic gains. The therapist often identifies this discrepancy early and helps reinforce more realistic expectations.

The same kind of discrepancy may also occur with expectations regarding post-operative functional gains. Patient involvement in treatment planning is especially helpful here. Patient participation through increased questioning and dialogue enables surgeons to address the problems that are the most significant to the individual, both functionally and emotionally. If patients are encouraged to verbalize their priorities regarding the order of their surgeries and to participate in planning their therapy programs, their expectations of post-operative gains may coincide more with the actual results. Additionally, patients often seem intimidated by doctors and therefore hesitant to ask many important questions. The therapist facilitates and supports patients in their efforts to ask questions and assert themselves. In this way the therapist is instrumental as an advocate of a patient-involved and patient-directed treatment process.

As with any patient population, burn patients are encouraged to be self-initiating in all aspects of daily living, including daily and vocational planning, socialization, and dealing with the public. The nature of the residuals of burn injury may require special assistance from the therapist. The therapist may help by discussing hypothetical situations with patients as well as actually providing psychological support through her physical presence and honest concern. She assists patients to make the transition from passive recipients to active participants with responsibility for their therapy programs and post-discharge plans. This instills feelings of self-worth and self-directedness and thus allows socially acceptable coping styles to emerge and develop while in a supportive environment.

Patients' pre-morbid coping styles vary greatly and may not be effective following injury. For instance, a woman who used her physical beauty as a method of meeting her needs may not be able to rely on her looks following a disfiguring facial burn. In another example, a burn amputee with limited mobility had to develop an alternative way of dealing with anger when she could not use her pre-morbid method of physical flight.

With major trauma such as burn injury, patients' coping repertoires may need to be redeveloped. The therapist facilitates the evolution of coping skills by carefully shaping the right challenge or frustration needed to elicit a new response. For example, the stress experienced on a patient's first public outing may, in fact, be the necessary turning point leading to the development of increased coping skills. Thus, the therapist intentionally but carefully chooses to interrupt the patient's "equilibrium" in order to facilitate improved coping skills and thus a higher level of function.

Furthermore, patients often perceive the treatment milieu as a nonthreatening forum for experimentation with self-expression. By encouraging patients to express themselves and giving them feedback, the therapist helps patients explore various communication and coping styles. Also related to this is the occasional patient's display of anger or patient's verbal abuse of the therapist. With some patients the opportunity for inappropriate expression such as swearing creates the imbalance needed to jar them and challenge their inventory of coping skills.

There are many methods for facilitating development and or improvement of coping skills, and each patient's uniqueness affects the evolution of these coping styles. At times, the therapist is most effective by recognizing the need for intervention by other team members. Therapists must also

(continued)

Psychosocial Aspects in Burn Rehabilitation

recognize that there will be times when they themselves need support and ongoing development of coping skills. The occupational therapist's role in facilitating psychosocial adjustment includes knowing her limits and being a liaison as needed so that other primary therapists can also be maximally effective. This ensures a good team approach and improves the overall quality of therapy.

Summary

Most patients eventually recognize the cosmetic and functional limitations of plastic surgery and rehabilitation. In so doing, they begin to deal with the prospect of permanent disfigurement and disability and with the social implications of the

effect of such disfigurement and disability on their friends and family. These implications can be overwhelming for both the patient and the therapist. Through the provision of support and facilitation of patient awareness, patient-directed treatments, and development of coping style, and with the positive effects of time, patients may be helped to return to activities which result in an altered yet meaningful life role.

References

1. Andreasen, NJC and Norris, AS: Long-term adjustment and adaptation mechanisms in severely burned adults. *Journal of Nervous and Mental Disease*, 154: 352-62, 1972.
2. Bhalerao, VR, Desai, VP, and Pai, DN: Study in females. *Journal of Postgraduate Medicine*, 22:3, 147-53, 1976.
3. Cooper, C: Activity level and its relationship to sex-

ual competence in adults who have sustained disfiguring burn injuries. Unpublished master's thesis, University of Southern California, 1981.
4. Simon, JI: Emotional aspects of physical disability. *AJOT*, 25:8, 408-410, 1971.
5. Woods, NF: *Human Sexuality in Health and Illness*. St. Louis, C.V. Mosby Co., 1975.

Pressure Garments

Did you know that two companies make pressure garments?

Jobst Institute, Inc.
P.O. Box 653
Toledo, OH 43694

Bio-Concepts, Inc.
7324 North 71st Street
Scottsdale, AZ 85253
(602) 948-6113

Physical Disabilities
Special Interest Section Newsletter; Vol. 4, No. 2, 1981

Use of the Thermoplastic Total Contact and the Foam Watusi Ring Neck Splints

By Elaine Sandel, OTR, and Christine Rath Khaleeli, RPT

The use of neck splints to prevent or correct neck flexion contractures, maintain or improve neck and jawline contours, and provide pressure to hypertrophic scars in the treatment of second and third-degree burns is well documented. There are a variety of materials and styles of neck splints from which an occupational therapist can choose.

During the last 4 years, 34 patients that were admitted to the New York Hospital burn center had burns on the neck that required the use of splints. A review of the effectiveness of the various types of splints led us to develop our present protocol for the use of the hard thermoplastic total contact neck splint and the foam "Watusi" ring neck splint.

The hard thermoplastic splint is made of either Polyform II® or Orthoplast®. Our reviews showed that when well conformed, the splint provided greater immobilization and produced less shear than other splints. Therefore, it is used post-autografting and over unhealed or newly healed skin because it is less likely to damage fragile tissue. This type of splint is also useful in preventing contractures and in maintaining or increasing neck range of motion and contour for patients with unilateral burns of the neck.

The foam "Watusi" rings splint was found to allow greater lateral and rotational mobility of the neck while maintaining neck extension (Figure 1). Since there

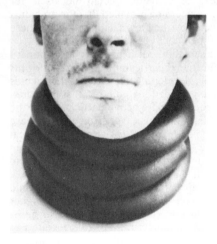

Figure 1.
The foam "Watusi" ring splint

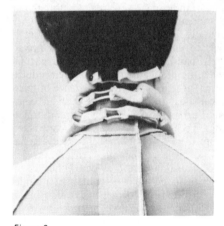

Figure 2.

Velcro and D-ring closure shown on foam "Watusi" ring splint made of adhesive backed Polycushion instead of the foam tubing.

is greater mobility, there is more shearing on the skin. The splint, therefore, is used only over well-healed skin which is less likely to break down. Its snug fit maintains constant pressure on the developing hypertrophic scar tissue and provides contour to the neck and jawline. It is lighter, softer and allows for mobility for performance of activities of daily living, thus, patient compliance is good. It is quick and easy to adjust as the patient's range of neck extension increases.

The foam rings can be made and adapted by untrained personnel including

the patient and his family. The materials are low in cost (approximately 70 cents per ring) and the construction time is short. The type of "Watusi" ring we use is made of a closed cell cylindrical foam padding, Orthoplast® strips, Velcro® straps and a D-ring. The foam tubing, which is commonly used to pad or build up handles of various implements, has an outside diameter of 1-3/8 inch and an inner hole with a diameter of 3/8 inch. A strip of Orthoplast approximately 18" long and 1/4" wide with a D-ring attached at one end and a 1/2" wide

(continued)

Use of Neck Splints

strap of Velcro hook and loop sewn together to make one continuous piece are prepared in advance. A piece of cylindrical foam padding is measured and cut to fit 2" past the patient's temporomandibular joint. Next, the Orthoplast strip is inserted through the inner hole of the cylindrical foam padding. The Orthoplast strip and Velcro strap are then adjusted so that when fastened, the ring will fit snugly on the patient's neck. The Velcro strap is riveted to the Orthoplast strip for closure with the D-ring. The procedure is repeated until the desired number of rings are made.

The basic procedure can be adapted as follows:

1. Larger diameter rings may be made by wrapping adhesive backed Polycushion® around the foam tubing. This adaptation is useful in adjusting for an increase in neck extension range when the gain is not sufficient to add another ring.

2. Smaller diameter rings may be made by wrapping adhesive backed Polycushion around the Orthoplast strip until the desired diameter is obtained. This method is helpful for use with children and adults with short necks.

3. The rings may be enclosed in a single length of Stockinette® or Tubigrip® for ease in donning and for skin care and comfort. The covering serves to absorb perspiration and to keep the collar clean.

In summary, two types of neck positioning splints are currently used at the New York Hospital. The hard thermoplastic total contact splint is used over well healed skin, and the foam "Watusi" ring splint is used over new grafts or over unhealed or newly healed skin. Thus, the skin condition is the major consideration in determining the type of neck splint to be used.

* All material for the "Watusi" foam ring splint is available from Be-OK Brookfield, IL.

Elaine Sandel, OTR is senior occupational therapist and Christine Rath Khaleeli, RPT is chief physical therapist; both are on the staff at the New York Hospital, New York City.

Physical Disabilities
Special Interest Section Newsletter; Vol. 4, No. 1, 1981

Project Teach: Technical Educational Aids for Children With Handicaps

In July 1978, the Bureau of Education for the Handicapped awarded a three-year demonstration grant to the Memphis City Schools, Division of Special Education. It was to demonstrate that severely physically handicapped children could participate more meaningfully in their educational program with the assistance of technical aids in the areas of seating, communication, mobility, feeding and toileting. Technical services were contracted from the University of Tennessee—Rehabilitation Engineering Center and appropriate aids were provided. Other objectives included the development of a model for the delivery of technical aids in an educational setting and the design of an instrument to aid in the prescription of technical aids.

Ten children were then selected to participate in the Project; each of whom exhibited some form of cerebral palsy and were non-verbal as a result of motor damage to the speech mechanism. Each child also demonstrated severe motor impairments that affected functions other than speech, i.e., trunk stability, head control, hand skills, or feeding.

The children attend Shrine School, a special education school for the physically handicapped, which is part of the Memphis City School System. Shrine School is located on the Sheffield School Complex, which consists of an elementary school, a junior and senior high school and a vocational technical center. This complex, conveniently, could be used for mainstreaming provided that the problems created by the physical limitations of these children could be minimized.

Each child participated in the standard educational curriculum appropriate for his or her developmental level. Technical aids were provided that allowed these children to become more active participants in the educational process. These aids were designed to permit easier access to educational materials to enhance communicative interaction and development, and to facilitate activities in daily living.

At the end of the first year each child had been evaluated to assess his or her technical needs. On an individual basis, training of prerequisite skills required to operate specific technical aids was initiated by the occupational therapist or speech pathologist. Preliminary communication aids, seating and mobility systems, and ADL (Activities of Daily Living) aids were then provided, based on the evaluation information. Initial inservice programs for teachers, teachers' aids, and parents were held. Dissemination activities were initiated.

Project TEACH, in its second year of operation, has shown that the use of technical aids, individually tailored to the needs of each child, can help them achieve the goals incorporated in the curriculum of the students' regular school program. For example, severely physically handicapped children are now able to participate in classroom activities because of customized seating and communication systems.

All ten children in Project TEACH have been provided with an alternative communication system. Each communication system has been individually prescribed based on the information gathered by the Technical Aid Evaluation developed by Project TEACH. Five children have wheelchair trays that have been custom-designed to accommodate the individualized communication boards. Two children have an optical strip-printer scanner developed by UT-REC specifically for a Project TEACH child. This item is now commercially available. One student has a commercially available Cannon Communicator with a custom-designed belt attachment. One child has been provided an Autocomm and another, with binaural amplification.

Without these technical devices, classroom participation and the related learning activities would be minimal. These communication devices have enabled the non-verbal children to communicate with their teachers, peers, and parents. Technical aids have increased sitting comfort and the time children can sit in their seats, i.e., wheelchairs. For both school and home, these seating systems have permitted safer transportation, provided proper work surfaces, and simplified other activities of daily living such as feeding. They have enabled three of the students to be par-

(continued)

Project Teach

tially mainstreamed, an especially positive experience for all involved.

The provision of technical aids through Project TEACH, in addition to the supplementary services of a Speech Pathologist and Occupational Therapist, has clearly demonstrated this approach as an essential supplement to the Individualized Educational Program of each of ten children involved in the Project.

Summary of Results to Date

Although the execution of Project TEACH did have limited scope (only ten children), after 2-1/2 years of involvement we feel confident in stating some of the following preliminary concepts.

1. *Seating Aids*

    Seating systems enable severely physically handicapped children to sit with greater stability in dynamic sitting posture in a classroom.

    As a result of the more stable posture, severely handicapped children are better able to use available hand skills.

2. *Communication Aids*

    With communication systems, children were able to increase expressive vocabulary.

    Children increased sentence length and complexity.

    Communication systems enabled the students to express abstracts concepts and feelings.

    Children were now able to respond to instructional tasks and participate in social interaction.

3. *Mobility*

    Technical aids enabled children to become more independent in following their daily school routine thus freeing teachers and aids for other activities.

    Mobility systems enabled children to independently initiate motion and so develop more initiative in general.

4. *ADL (Activities of Daily Living)*

    Feeding

    Feeding aids enable several children to feed themselves and so free teacher aids for other responsibilities.

    Toileting

    Adapted commode seats made toileting easier and safer for the children. It enabled several children to become toilet trained.

The following materials will be available for dissemination at the end of June 1981. For further information or copies of the below, contact:

Elaine Trefler, Rehabilitation
Engineering Center
1248 LaPaloma, Memphis, TN 38114
(901) 276-1752.
OR
Jeryl McCormick, Shrine School
4259 Forestview, Memphis, TN 38118
(901) 795-3930

— Project TEACH Brochure (available now)—Free
— Case Study Reports—Cost Unknown
— Project Model—Cost Unknown
— Technical Aids Evaluation Form—Cost Unknown
— 16mm film—15 minute film (available now)—Rental $20.00
— Slide sound—Rental Undetermined

Project TEACH
PRELIMINARY BIBLIOGRAPHY

Bigge, J., *Teaching Individuals with Physical and Multiple Disabilities*. Charles E. Merrill Publishing Company; Columbus, OH. This book has a chapter on technical aids as used in educational settings.

COMMUNICATION OUTLOOK — (an international information coordinator and resource newsletter) $10.00 ($12.00 overseas), Artificial Language Laboratory, Computer Science Dept., Michigan State University, East Lansing, MI 48824.

Elizabeth Codman High School, *A Resource Guide to Habilitative Techniques and Aids for Cerebral Palsied Persons of All Ages*. The Job Development Laboratory, George Washington University.

Equipment for the Disabled. National Fund for Research into Crippling Diseases, 2 Foredown Drive, Portslade, Brighton, Sussex BN42BB, England.

Goldberg, Paul, *Special Technology for Special Children*. University Park Press, Baltimore, MD. 1979. A publication which addresses technical needs of both cerebral palsy and hearing impaired children.

Handicapped Children—Strategies for Improving Services. Gary D. Breuer and James S. Kakalik. McGraw Hill, 1221 Avenue of Americas, New York, NY 10020, 1979.

Manual for Cerebral Palsy Equipment. Easter Seal Society for Crippled Children and Adults, Inc., 2023 So. Ogden Avenue, Chicago, IL 60612.

Nonoral Communication System Project. Beverly Vicker, Editor. Campus Store Publishers, The University of Iowa, 17 West College, Iowa City, Iowa 52242, 1964-1973. This publication has excellent program ideas.

Non-vocal Communication—Resource Book. Edited by Gregg Vanderheiden. Baltimore: University Park Press.

Non-Vocal Communication Techniques and Aids for the Severely Physically Handicapped. Edited by Gregg Vanderheiden & Kate Grilley. Baltimore: University Park Press. This and the preceding publication provide lists of basic inventors of assistive devices for communication.

Robinault, Isabel P., *Functional Aids for the Multiply Handicapped*. Hagerstown, Maryland: Medical Department, Harper & Row, 1973.

Technical Aids for Handicapped Children. Rehabilitation Centre for Children, Winnipeg, Canada. This is a resource book of both commercially available and custom made equipment.

Vanderheiden, G.C. and Luster, M.J. *Non-Vocal Communication Techniques and Aids as Aids to the Education of the Severely Physically Handicapped*. A State of the Art Review, Cerebral Palsy Communication Group, University of Wisconsin—Madison, Wisconsin 53706, 1975.

Physical Disabilities
Special Interest Section Newsletter; Vol. 4, No. 1, 1981

Specialized Seating: Assessment, Recommendations, and Resources

Many problems arise with a client's inability to maintain a sitting posture with the body in good alignment. The child who remains recumbent is unable to effectively investigate his surrounding, either visually or manually, and cannot develop self-care of manipulative skills. The inability of a child to sit securely, safely, and unattended places a burden on the family, making home management and mobility difficult, if not impossible. Many factors complicate the problem such as muscle imbalance, asymmetry, deformities and lack of sensation.

The greatest number of specialized seating problems are seen in the patient with nonambulatory cerebral palsy, muscular dystropy and spina bifida. The goal is to provide a sitting posture as close to normal as possible, and therefore as comfortable

(continued)

Specialized Seating

and functional as possible. Good body alignment in normal sitting is one in which the hips are flexed at 90 degrees and slightly abducted, the knees are flexed and the ankles are in neutral position. The trunk and head are maintained in erect posture and neutral alignment with 75 per cent of the body weight distributed over the ischial tuberosities and posterior thighs and 25 per cent on the supported feet.

Assessment And Positioning

The patient must be accurately and specifically evaluated in regards to joint range of motion, joint contractures and skeletal deformities. If the hips cannot be flexed to 90 degrees, positioning becomes very difficult and considerably narrows the options available. Contractures of the knee and ankle may influence distal weight bearing and hip position. It is essential to thoughtfully examine the spine—pelvis—hip complex, noting any deformities. Pelvic obliquity is often associated with scoliosis, a dislocated hip or leg length discrepancies; anterior pelvic tilt is seen with lumbar lordosis, severe hip flexion contracture and/or extensor tone; posterior pelvic tilt is associated with sacral sitting, kyphotic curves and/or flexor tone.

Specific muscle testing is usually not indicated except for the essential documentation of head and trunk control. In spinal cord injuries, the sensory level should be known and muscle weakness recorded. It is also important to note pain and skin problems.

The level of ADL function, especially in the areas of upper limb use, bowel and bladder continence, and mental retardation plays a significant role in selecting the correct seat.

The patient's predominate muscle tone and dominating reflex patterns directly affect positioning and, therefore, seating. The predominance of flexion, extension, hypertonicity or hypotonicity are significant. In the brain injured it is necessary to attempt to inhibit certain primitive reflexes when the patient is dominated by them and therefore not free to move normally. Some responses will aid in diminishing unwanted reflexes, patterns and tone. For example, if the patient demonstrates severe extensor tone, the goal would be to normalize extensor tone and therefore allow the flexors to work. This can be done by considering a seat—back angle or a roll seat, which promotes more than 90 degrees of hip flexion, posterior pelvic tilt, shoulder protraction, dorsiflexion of the feet and knee flexion. Because the hamstrings are two joint muscles, knee flexion will facilitate hip flexion.

In positioning, the pelvis is the keystone. It dictates foot and leg position, influences the position of the trunk and therefore the shoulder girdle, upper limbs, head and neck.

Lack of sitting tolerance in patients varies considerably. Lower tolerance is found in those cases with marked bony prominences, severe scoliosis, kyphosis or severe contractures of the lower limb.

A summary statement should be made including the presenting problems of the patient as described above, his present equipment and his position in his current chair. The prescription of seating needs should then be considered in the context of the family and home situation, schooling, recreation, mobility, comfort and function.

Recommendations

Considering the magnitude of some seating problems and the potential cost involved, it is ideal that the prescription be a consensus of the clinic team, including the family. There are alternatives to seating. The patient may be left in bed or on a bean bag. The patient may be braced, but, for the nonambulatory person, the orthosis may be uncomfortable, hot and difficult to put on and remove. Surgery may be considered, such as spinal fusion to align the spine over the pelvis, surgical release of contractures, or femoral head excision in cases of hip dislocation. Bracing and/or surgery may also be done in conjunction with seating.

If specialized seating is indicated, there are commercial and customized seating systems on the market, including the following:

COMMERCIAL SEATING SYSTEMS

Mulholland Growth Guidance Chair

This seating system is designed for the child with cerebral palsy and is based on principles of postural control. The adjustability of this chair and its component systems allow for precise body fit and positioning while allowing for growth and accommodating existing structural deformities. The patient cannot be positioned only in good alignment with proximal joint stabilization, but must be positioned in relation to his predominating muscle tone and dominating reflex patterns. The chair frame is composed of aluminum tubing with vinyl/nylon/naugahyde upholstery. The chair is completely adjustable with a large selection of options available.

Modular Plastic Insert (MED-MPI)

The Modular Plastic Insert Seating System is designed primarily for moderately involved children with cerebral palsy who have fair to good head and trunk control. This system interfaces with any wheeled base. It is composed of ABS plastic with back and seat interfaces available in several sizes. As the child grows, a new

back and/or seat may be inserted in the same system. It does not accommodate severe spinal curves, bony deformities or contractures. For the child without these problems, it offers seating stability and good alignment. Various support options and accessories are available.

Travel Chairs

Travel chairs are produced by many companies and are designed for use as strollers that provides support for positioning, comfort and cosmesis. They generally come in three sizes with various components available. The small size also functions as a car seat. The travel chair accommodates a child who is mild to moderately involved and who is unable to wheel his own chair. It does not accommodate children with severe spinal curves, bony deformities or contractures.

CUSTOMIZED SEATING SYSTEMS

ABS Plastic Insert Seats

The ABS seat was designed for neurologically handicapped patients with protective sensation who are confined to wheelchairs. It is a custom formed rigid seat that conforms to the full sitting surface of the patient, thus distributing weight evenly over the buttocks and posterior thighs. A pommel elevation between the distal thighs maintains hip abduction and keeps the patient from sliding forward in the seat. The precise fit provides pelvic stability for postural control, and alignment. Fabrication techniques require the use of a vacuum forming machine.

Desemo

The Desemo Body Support is a custom-molded foam module, precisely fitted to a patient. It can be designed for the seat alone or for total body positioning incorporating the pelvis, trunk and head in one integral light weight unit. The seat was designed to position the body in good alignment, to accommodate structural deformities and to be incorporated in various seating devices or to be self-standing. It is made by pouring epoxy resin into a thick rubber balloon filled with styrofoam beads. A vacuum is then applied with the patient positioned in the balloon. With this unique but simple dilatency technique, the foam beads mold to both the child and any base resulting in a double mold.

Foam-In-Place ((FIP) In Development)

The foam-in-place method uses a two component polyurethane soft foam which is mixed and stirred as a liquid. In this form, it is injected into a mold which has one stretchy side (top) made of latex sheeting. This stretchy surface is in direct contact with the patient during the foaming pro-

(continued)

Specialized Seating

cess. The remaining mold is made of wood and shaped to interface with the patient's wheeled base, usually a wheelchair. The foam molds to both surfaces, resulting in a double mold, and is thus adaptable to any base. The material used has been UpJohn-CPR Division, 1947 polyurethane foam. This material is a self-skinning closed-cell foam that appears to be a soft yet durable material for seating and spinal supports. Initial experience has indicated that customized foam components can be produced and interfaced into a wheelchair in less than two hours.—*Alice Bowker, MA, OTR, Orthotic Services, 1010 South Taylor St., Little Rock, AR 72204.*

Resources

MULHOLLAND GROWTH GUIDANCE CHAIR
   The Mulholland Corporation
   1563 Los Angeles Ave.
   Ventura, CA 93003
MPI
   Modular Plastic Seating System
   University of Tennessee
   Rehabilitation Engineering Center
   1248 La Paloma Street
   Memphis, TN 38114

ORTHOKINETIC TRAVEL CHAIR
   Ortho-Kinetics Inc.
   1610 Pearl Street
   P.O. Box 436
   Waukesha, WI 53187
ABS PLASTIC INSERT SEAT
   Little Rock Orthotics
   1010 South Taylor
   Little Rock, AR 72207
DESEMO SEAT
   Desemo Project
   P.O. Box 313
   University Station
   Birmingham, AL 35294
FIP
   Foam-In-Place
   University of Tennessee
   Rehabilitation Engineering Center
   1248 La Paloma Street
   Memphis, TN 38114

Bibliography
Seating For Children
With Cerebral Palsy

Bergen A.: Table and Chair Seat for Spastic Children. *Physical Therapy,* 51: 1305-1306, 1971.

Bobath B.: *Abnormal Postural Reflex Activity Caused by Brain Lesions.* London: Heinemann Medical.

Bobath, Berta: "The Very Early Treatment of Cerebral Palsy." *Dev. Med. and Child Neuro.,* 9, No. 4: August 1967.

Carrington, Ellen G.: A Seating Position for a Cerebral-Palsied Child. *The American Journal of Occupational Therapy,* 32, No. 3: 179-181, March 1978.

Christopher, R.P.: Recent Advances in Mechanical Aids in the Management of Children with Brain Damage. *Southern Medical Journal,* 67, 399-405.

Cristarella Mary C.: Comparison of Straddling and Sitting Apparatus for the Spastic Cerebral-Palsied Child. *The American Journal of Occupational Therapy,* 29, No. 5: 273-276, May/June 1975.

DiCarlo, Cheryl, BS and **Forbis Adelle,** BA: Chair for the Child with Hypertonic CNS Dysfunction. *Physical Therapy,* 57: 1151, October 1977.

Farber, S.: *Sensorimotor Evaluation and Treatment Procedures.* 2nd Edn. Indiana University: Purdue University at Indianapolis Medical Center, pp. 100.

Finnie, N.: *Handling the Young Cerebral-Palsied Child at Home.* New York, Dutton & Co. 1968.

Fulford, G.W. and **Brown, J.K.:** Position as a cause of Deformity in Children with Cerebral Palsy. *Develop. Med. and Child Neurol.,* 18, 1976.

Keegan, J. Jay, M.D.: Alterations of the Lumbar Curve Related to Posture and Seating. *Journal of Bone and Joint Surgery,* 35-A, No. 3: July 1953.

Montgomery, P. and **Gauger, J.:** Dynamic Trunk Stabilizer for Children with Cerebral Palsy. *Physical Therapy,* 58, No. 4: April 1978.

Robinault, I.: Functional Aids for the Multiply Handicapped. New York: Harper & Row. 1973

Slominski, A. and **Hamant C.:** In Willard, H.S., Spackman, C.S. (Eds.) *Occupational Therapy,* 4th Edn., Philadelphia: Lippincott.

Trefler Elaine, Hanks, Sam, Huggins, Paul, Chiarizzo, Sam, Hobson, Doug: A Modular Seating System for Cerebral Palsied Children. *Develop. Med. Child Neurol.* 20: 199-204, 1978.

Trefler, Elaine and Et Al: Seating for Cerebral Palsied Children. *Inter-Clinic Information Bulletin,* 17, No. 1: 1-8, Jan/Feb. 1978.

Physical Disabilities
Special Interest Section Newsletter; Vol. 4, No. 1, 1981

Equipment Information Dissemination—An Expanded Role for Occupational Therapists

Disabled individuals and rehabilitation professionals alike have long belabored the issue of inadequate dissemination of information regarding advances in rehabilitation technology. Numerous approaches to the problem have been tried both in the United States and abroad with varying degrees of success. The federal government, through its various agencies, has been evaluating the many approaches to information dissemination in the United States.

In 1978, the National Institute for Handicapped Research supported a program to establish three Rehabilitation Equipment Demonstration Units for the purpose of providing information, display, and trial use of rehabilitation equipment to consumers and health care providers. This attempt to get current information to the equipment user has since expanded with several methods of information dissemination being evaluated.

The University of Virginia Rehabilitation Engineering Center, a division of the Department of Orthopedics and Rehabilitation, is researching three approaches to information dissemination: 1) A demonstration/display unit, 2) An outreach program, and 3) An information system. Each of these programs employ occupational therapists in various roles. The programs are currently grant funded, but alternate sources of funding are being investigated.

The Demonstration Unit displays equipment on loan from the Veterans Administration, equipment manufacturers and distributors permitting a person to see, examine and try a variety of commercially available products. Engineering prototypes, designed or tested by the Rehabilitation Engineers, are frequently available for display. Videotapes of some equipment not in the unit are maintained and are available for viewing. Occupational therapists are on hand to help an individual assess his functional needs, and determine the most appropriate technique or equipment to meet them. Information

about the equipment and education or assistance in the equipment's use is routinely given. The Demonstration Unit employs a mechanical technician, and rehabilitation engineers are available to provide technical assistance. Consumer opinions regarding equipment features, use limitations, and recommendations are regularly given to the manufacturers to assist with design improvements. This approach evaluates use of an independent center staffed with rehabilitation professionals where people can see a variety of items from different manufacturers free from purchasing pressures.

The Community Outreach Team, an occupational therapist and a mechanical technician, serves the individual who requires equipment assessment at the home or work setting. Because of the rural nature of the area, and the lack of adequate transportation for the disabled, this program permits equipment to be taken directly to the home or to the work site for

(continued)

Equipment Information Dissemination

evaluation and trial. The Occupational Therapist assesses functional limitations, evaluates daily living skills, and through an understanding of adaptive equipment and techniques is able to assist the individuals to evaluate and understand their equipment needs. This research program also helps the consumer assess the needs for building adaptations, barrier removal, equipment modifications, or new equipment purchases. This approach assists the homebound individuals to determine the most appropriate purchases or modifications to meet their needs.

The Information System provides consumers with access to general information and literature searches on commercially available rehabilitation aids and equipment as well as other resource information. Information on product availability, standard features and options, use limitations, and prices are on file and a computerized retrieval system is being developed with the National Rehabilitation Information Center. The information consultant, an occupational therapist, works with equipment manufacturers, distributors and local resources in locating appropriate equipment, components and accessories to meet specific rehabilitation needs. The occupational therapists' awareness of disease and disability and concomitant capabilities and limitations enables a quick understanding of many problems. Again, the experience with adaptive equip-

ment and assessment of functional limitations helps make recommendations quick, informative, and appropriate. If a full understanding of the need requires observation within the home or at the work site, the Outreach Team is consulted. Referrals are made to the Rehabilitation Engineer, or other sources for custom modification and design if indicated. Referrals to physicians, therapists, agencies, etc. are recommended prior to equipment purchases when necessary.

Ongoing inservice education is conducted by the occupational therapists and is provided to professionals and consumers alike as a service of the Rehabilitation Equipment Demonstration Unit. A local file is maintained listing sources of equipment for purchase, rental, loan, repair, maintenance, and custom design and construction.

These programs offer the experienced occupational therapist an expanded role in rehabilitation. The unique training and background of the occupational therapist makes this professional an ideal equipment specialist. Throughout the years, in day to day practice, occupational therapists have been required to make judgments regarding equipment needs, and to design and modify equipment not readily available to them. The Rehabilitation Equipment Demonstration Unit has enabled the occupational therapist to further develop as a knowledgeable, experienced equip-

ment specialist who understands the problems, limitations, and capabilities of those with disabilities, and who can identify with their equipment needs. For further information on any of these programs contact: Rehabilitation Equipment Demonstration Unit, PO Box 3368, University Station, Charlottesville, VA 22903, (804) 977-1378. — *Carol Maier Clerico, OTR, Information Consultant, R.E.C., Charlottesville, VA.*

REFERENCES

Cheever, Raymond C., *Accent on Living Buyer's Guide*, Cheever Publishing Company, PO Box 700, Bloomington, IL 61701.

Mattingly, Stephen. *Rehabilitation Today*. Update Publications, Ltd. 33/34 Alfred Place, London. WCIE7DP, 1977.

Melichar, Joseph F., "Information System Adaptive Assistive Rehabilitation Equipment", Adaptive Systems Corporation, 1650 South Amphlett Blvd., Suite 317, San Mateo, CA 94402, 1975.

"Innovative Matching of Problems to Available Rehabilitation Technology", Research Utilization Laboratory, Texas Rehabilitation Commission, 1979-80.

(Development of a Model Rehabilitation Engineering Delivery System in California—A Beginning), Edward V. Roberts, Director State of California Health & Welfare Agency, Department of Rehabilitation, Sacramento, CA 95814.

(Suggested Approach for Establishing A Rehabilitation Engineering Information Service for the State of California), September 1978, Lo Christy, California.

Physical Disabilities
Special Interest Section Newsletter; Vol. 4, No. 1, 1981

Rehabilitation Engineering— Occupational Therapy's Friend or Foe?

Over the past fifty years, mankind has created incredible advances in all aspects of medical technology. Physical disabilities have presented physicians, engineers, and occupational therapists with innumerable opportunities to develop aids and equipment that provide people with disabilities the means to lead more independent lives.

The engineering specialist, who evolved to work specifically with the rehabilitiation client, is the Rehabilitation Engineer, who can be trained in any one of the engineering subspecialties (mechanical, electrical, etc.), but is basically an engineer who is challenged by solving people's problems.

The broad objective of rehabilitation engineering is to enhance the lives of the physically disabled through clinical involvement combining medicine and allied

health with engineering science and technology. The rehabilitation engineer is the person fulfilling the mission of the rehabilitation engineering plan begun in 1971 by the Rehabilitation Services Administration of the Department of Health, Education and Welfare (now the Department of Education's National Institute of Handicapped Research). He or she is to have identifiable competence in engineering with additional specialized training and experience in understanding disability and its many effects on human performance. In addition to the clinical role of applying and modifying rehabilitative devices or systems, the engineer also conceives, designs, tests, and evaluates innovative devices and systems for both the equipment industry and the consumer.

Most of the practicing rehabilitation engineers began their new role by being "grandfathered" into their profession with little or no clinical rehabilitative experience. Engineers at many centers throughout this country have had to receive on-the-job training from other professionals, including occupational therapists, to meet the basic clinical requirements of their job.

There are now fifteen federally sponsored centers conducting rehabilitation engineering research. Although the initial funding was to sponsor research, many of the centers are now in the process of creating networks involved in providing rehabilitation engineering service and variety of training programs. Also, a number of hospitals and rehabilitation facilities are

(continued)

Rehabilitation Engineering

looking for qualified engineers to help expand and increase the level of sophistication of their service programs. These programs are unable to fill the positions because engineers are also in demand in industry at higher salaries and only one graduate-level training program is in existence at the University of Virginia. Of interest to occupational therapists is the fact that the rehabilitation engineering training program is designed with a special educational tract for occupational therapists to become rehabilitation engineers. Twenty-five percent of the first class are occupational therapists who desired to further their professional base in physical disabilities with an engineering education. Several therapists nationally have entered into private practice as both partners and/or consultants to rehabilitation engineers. Opportunities are just beginning to abound for the occupational therapist and rehabilitation engineer to work together as equal members of the rehabilitation team.

Many occupational therapists have had difficulty with the rehabilitation engineer's role. None questions the role of the engineer; however, there is concern about the lack of formal training in rehabilitation and disability. At the same time, occupational therapists have spent many hours and have been quite successful in developing, customizing, and maintaining technical aids for their clients. However, they have also become overwhelmed at times with the time involved in meeting these technical demands, often at the expense of actual "hands-on" treatment with their clients. When rehabilitation engineers arrived on the rehabilitation scene to assume part of this responsibility, the occupational therapist met them with guarded optimism instead of open arms.

We physical disability occupational therapists must stand confident in our professional abilities and skills. Rehabilitation engineering has provided an opportunity for occupational therapists to pro-

ject their professional expertise into a new area. We must assist and influence rehabilitation engineering so that it can grow as a strong partner in the delivery of improved health care to the physically disabled. We must take every opportunity to become involved in rehabilitation engineering centers either as full time employees or as consultants so that the technical needs of our clients are met in the most practical and therapeutically sound manner. By dynamically bringing together the skills of the rehabilitation engineer and occupational therapist, our clients can only gain from a new level of technical service delivery.

—*Michael Boblitz, OTR, Medical Administrative Officer and Assistant Professor, Department of Orthopedics and Rehabilitation, University of Virginia Medical School, Charlottesville.*

Physical Disabilities
Special Interest Section Newsletter; Vol. 3, No. 4, 1980

Hands on: Cardiac Rehabilitation—Guidelines for Analysis and Testing of Activities of Daily Living With Cardiac Patients

By Linda Dempster Ogden, OTR, Cardiac Rehabilitation Specialist, Diamond Bar, CA

A key role of occupational therapy in the rehabilitation of cardiac patients in the late recovery period after myocardial infarction or cardiac surgery is evaluation for return to customary occupations involving moderate to heavy upper extremity work. These include homemaking tasks such as scrubbing, mopping floors, or carrying groceries, leisure activities such as gardening, home maintenance chores, and vocational activities.

Traditionally, the major evaluative tool used to determine readiness for return to these activities has been the maximal or submaximal treadmill or bicycle ergometer test. The patient undergoing either of these tests is presented with a graduated series of tasks involving lower extremity work. The intensity of the workload is gradually increased by controlling two variables, rate or speed and resistance to motion (provided by gravity when the incline is increased on the treadmill). The maximum workload achieved along with heart rate and blood pressure response, EKG findings, ischemia, and symptoms are used to predict the patient's potential tolerance of occupational tasks.

These tests, however, do not necessari-

ly predict responses to occupations requiring primarily upper extremity work for two reasons. First, heart rate and blood pressure responses to upper extremity work are generally higher than the responses to lower extremity work when the level of oxygen consumption, or MET

level, is held constant[1]. Second, with coronary artery disease patients, symptoms and arrhythmias may occur at lower workloads and at lower heart rates with upper extremity work, as opposed to lower extremity work[2]. In addition, functional

(continued)

Figure 1: Task Analysis and Scoring System for Monitored Task Evaluation

Number	Variable	Mild Influence	Moderate Influence	Strong Influence
1.	RATE	Slow (1	Moderate (2	Fast (5
2.	RESISTANCE	None or mild (1	Moderate (2	Maximal (3
3.	MUSCLE GROUPS USED	Small: fine motor tasks (1	Mixed fine and gross motor tasks (2	Large: gross motor tasks (3
4.	INVOLVEMENT OF TRUNK MUSCLES	Little (1	Moderate: mainly stabilization, balance (2	Strong involvement for bending or stabilization (3
5.	ARM POSITION	Waist height or below (1	Chest height (4	Overhead (6
6.	ISOMETRIC WORK: STRAINING	None or very little (1	Some isometric work, lifting, straining (4	Strong isometric: straining, breath-holding, Valsalva (6

145

Cardiac Rehabilitation—Guidelines for Analysis

tasks allow for much more individual variation in terms of working style and efficiency. It logically follows that prediction of cardiovascular tolerance of occupational tasks requiring mostly upper extremity work should involve testing the patient while he or she is actually performing these tasks or as close a simulation as possible of the upper extremity work involved in these tasks.

Monitored task evaluation, a technique described by the author in *AJOT* (May 1979), is similar to treadmill testing in that the patient is presented with a series of tasks graded to produce a gradual increase in cardiovascular workload and the patient is continually monitored for heart rate and blood pressure response, EKG, ischemia, and symptoms. The important difference is the fact that the tasks included in a monitored task evaluation are functional tasks requiring primarily upper extremity work and variations in body position. This means that in addition to the variables of rate and resistance, *at least* four additional variables are involved. These are muscle groups used (fine vs gross motion), position of the arms (waist level or below, chest level, overhead), involvement of trunk musculature (present when there is bending or trunk stabilization needed), and the presence of isometric muscle work producing straining or Valsalva (where there is a tendency to hold the breath, as with lifting, pushing, or struggling with tight jar lids). According to the literature, the variables that are most crucial because they can produce rapid elevations in heart rate and blood pressure are a very fast rate, arm position chest high or overhead, and the presence of isometric work[3-5]. It can be seen that organizing a monitored task evaluation so that tasks are graded from low to higher cardiac workload can become quite complicated.

On the basis of review of the literature and also on data gathered during four year's work with cardiac patients, the author proposes a method of task analysis and a scoring system to help the occupational therapist rank the functional tasks

Figure 2: Task Analysis and Scoring System Applied to Homemaking Tasks. Scores are Listed by Variable Number.

TASK VARIABLE #:	1	2	3	4	5	6	TOTAL SCORE
Wiping Counter	2	1	3	1	1	1	9
Sweeping, slow	1	1	3	2	1	1	9
Reaching into low cupboard	1	1	3	3	1	1	10
Chopping vegetables, standing	2	2	2	2	1	1	10
Reaching into high cupboard	1	1	3	1	6	1	13
Mopping, moderate pace	2	2	3	2	1	4	14
Scrubbing sink	5	2	2	2	1	4	16
Carrying grocery bags, heavy items	1	3	3	3	1	6	17
Washing windows	2	2	3	3	6	4	20

for the monitored task evaluation so that they are listed in an order from those that produce the least to those that produce the highest cardiac workload. The scoring system simply takes each of the six variables and assigns a score of 1 for a mild influence, a 2 for moderate influence, and a 3 for a strong influence. In addition, two extra points are added to strong influence of rate, moderate influence of arm position, and moderate influence of isometric work, and three points added to strong influence of arm position and strong influence of isometric work, because of the extreme nature of the effect on the heart of these variables. The completed task analysis and scoring chart can be seen in Figure 1. To use this system, the therapist chooses a group of tasks to be evaluated; for example, homemaking tasks in the kitchen. The tasks are listed, as in Figure 2, and each task is analyzed according to the chart. To do this, the therapist looks at each task and asks how strong is the influence of each of the six variables. The six scores are added to reach a total for that task. The tasks are then rank ordered from lowest to highest total score, and the patient is tested while performing the

tasks in this order, the lowest score being performed first. Figure 2 shows the scoring for each of the homemaking tasks listed.

It is hoped that this rough task analysis and scoring system will provide some preliminary guidelines for the testing of functional activities and perhaps serve as a basis for scientific inquiry. With continued research, occupational therapists may someday have a functional evaluation system for cardiac patients as carefully tested and scientifically validated as the treadmill test.

References:

1. Ogden LD; Activity guidelines for early subacute and high-risk cardiac patients. *AJOT* 33: 291-298, 1979
2. Wahren J, Bygdeman S: Onset of angina pectoris in relation to circulatory adaptation during arm and leg exercise. *Circulation* 44: 432-441, 1971
3. Astrand P-O, Rodahl K: *Textbook of Work Physiology.* New York: McGraw-Hill 1970, pp. 166-178
4. Astrand I, Guharay A, Wahren J: Circulatory responses to arm exercise with different arm positions. *J Applied Physiol* 25: 528-532, 1968
5. Kalbfleisch JH et al: Evaluation of the heart rate response to the Valsalva maneuver. *Am Heart J* 95: 707-712, 1978

Physical Disabilities
Special Interest Section Newsletter; Vol. 3, No. 4, 1980

Measurable Occupational Therapy Goals in the Treatment of Cardiac Patients

By Rebecca Kuntz, OTR

At Stormont-Vail Regional Medical Center in Topeka, Kansas, we have an active cardiac rehabilitation team and program. The majority of the patients on an inpatient basis have had myocardial-coronary revascularization surgery. They are seen individually and in educational classes. The occupational therapy class on activity uses the American Heart Association slide-tape presentation of "Move Into Action."

In an effort to minimize paperwork and uniformly treat all the cases, the occupational therapy department developed eight measurable goals for treatment. This was done in conjunction with the facility director of staff education who refined them into measurable goals. His assistance was invaluable as he was enough removed from the realm of treatment to be objective about the "measurability" of the goals.

The goals are printed on labels with adhesive backs and are inserted into the rehabilitation team notes. They are dated upon completion and, if necessary, any comments are written in an additional daily note.

The goals are as follows:

1. Patient is able to list 5 typical precautions pertaining to their particular recovery for activity of up to 6 weeks post-hospitalization.
2. Patient has increased activity level and work tolerance since the beginning of Stage III orders.
3. Patient is able to list those energy-saving techniques specific to their condition that can be applied to their lifestyle (given a list of 10 in the heart surgery book).
4. Patient is able to monitor and reduce (if necessary) an activity independently using the contraindications to activity such as increase pulse of 15 beats per minute over resting, shortness of breath, dizziness, nausea or fatigue.
5. Patient has decreased anxiety (if applicable) as reported by observations of team members, floor staff and physician.
6. Patient is able to express feelings that effect activity level and attitude towards activity to staff.
7. Patient is able to list appropriate number (at least 2) and kinds of leisure time activities for recovery period of three months.
8. Patient is able to develop a workable plan for a balance of work, leisure, play in lifestyle.

Physical Disabilities
Special Interest Section Newsletter; Vol. 3, No. 4, 1980

Cardiac Teaching

By Lori Smith, COTA

Research in the area of patient education reveals some startling information. Studies have shown that up to 75 percent of the information given to a patient is lost or only partially recalled. This creates a need for concise, reliable information that can be reinforced with a variety of methods.

The cardiac patient is no exception to the need for information regarding his or her condition. Circumstance has often placed the patient in the hospital unexpectedly. Even when a hospitalization is planned, as in the case of elective surgeries, adequate information continues to be lacking.

Occupational therapy has the capability to provide patient education in areas such as:

1. basic anatomy and physiology
2. home activities
3. graded exercise

Often the need for psychological support must be addressed before the education process can begin. We have found lectures with discussions and written handouts to be useful. Written information provides the patient and family with a reference after discharge.

Cardiac rehabilitation at Ford Hospital is a multidisciplinary team effort. Each member has a unique role in patient education and reinforcement of information. Education is started on an individual basis and progresses to class lectures. Lectures by team members cover basic anatomy and physiology, risk factors and intervention, warning signs, diet, stress and coping skills, home activities, energy conservation and graded exercise. At Ford, we have found that a team approach and the use of group dynamics effectively allows patient interaction and reinforces previously taught information.

The cardiac patient's need for education begins with hospitalization and continues two to three months post-discharge. Occupational therapy and other health care disciplines need to provide continued in-depth information as required by the patient. A variety of teaching methods with reinforcement will increase the likelihood of greater recall.

Lori Smith, COTA is a staff OT assistant on the Cardiac Rehabilitation Team at Henry Ford Hospital, Detroit, Michigan.

Emotional Reactions After a Heart Attack

The emotional reactions to having a heart attack can be divided into three phases: 1) initial response to symptoms, 2) hospitalization, and 3) period after discharge.

Initial Response to Symptoms: Even before symptoms appear, the patient may have a subjective fear of having a heart attack. The death of a close friend or family member, or the death of a national figure may cause the patient concern over the possibility of his or her own premature death. Chronic fear about heart disease, the aging process and family separations may also be part of the past history of a patient who has suffered a recent heart attack.

Nonspecific symptoms such as "nervousness," impotence, gastrointestinal upsets, fatigue, rapid heart beating and vague chest pains may occur prior to a heart attack. Rarely can a patient be found in whom heralding symptoms were not present. It is unusual for a heart attack to occur completely "without warning."

Though almost every middle-aged American is concerned about having a heart attack, the first response to severe chest pain is an attempt to explain why the pain cannot be serious. At this point, various emotional defenses appear. The person may "wish" the pain away or may blame the symptoms of food, "gas" or weather. These denial reactions cause delays in seeking medical attention. Since most deaths from heart attacks occur within the first two hours after the beginning of symptoms, this type of psychological avoidance can be fatal.

Ideally, one should go immediately to a hospital when chest pain is experienced. Most persons, however, will not take action until a few hours later, when their anxiety or nervous tension, not the pain, has built up to an intolerable level. A person is fortunate when a heart attack strikes in the presence of an "executive spouse" or another who will call the paramedics immediately without asking for permission.

Hospitalization: Most patients are very anxious upon arrival at the emergency department. The tension and fear usually lessen once the patient is attached to a cardiac monitor and is given intravenous and other medication. The patient quickly senses that his or her condition has priority and that care is constant. An unrecognized danger period, however, may occur after the diagnosis is established and before the patient is transferred to the Coronary Intensive Care Unit. At this time, if the patient is left alone, a feeling of intensely severe anxiety may result. If the patient is not attended by a nurse or physician, the least anxious family member or friend should remain present until the time of transfer.

At this phase of illness, the ability of a patient to deny the occurrence of an acute life-threatening illness may directly influence his or her survival. Anxiety, worry, fear, depression and anger all work against recovery. It follows that therapeutic measures should support the patient's capacity to deny the presence of a grave illness, as long as the treatment plan is not obstructed. Repeated reassurance and a positive approach toward recovery also are important.

The patient should be allowed to ask questions that clarify what is happening. Optimism must be bolstered and denial supported without compromising truth. The patient should be aware of his illness and the physical limitations imposed at various stages. This understanding will help avoid disappointment and will help deal with depression. When feasible, linkages to the world should be maintained such as a radio, TV, newspapers, publications and the sensible use of the telephone.

The Period After Discharge: The "homecoming depression" is nearly universal in patients recovering from a heart attack. Patients should be advised that hospital bed rest and limited activity decrease physical strength and that it takes some time to regain one's strength after a heart attack. A graduated program of increasing physical activity helps. Patients want to know what they can do and what they can't do. They fear harming themselves through excessive physical or emotional stress. For example, concern about sexual performances may occur. Again, reassurance by the physician and a gradual return to previous sexual activities lessens the nervous tension.

Much has been written concerning the risk factors, including emotional stresses that may be important in the production of coronary artery disease and heart attacks.

James J. Lynch, in his book, *The Broken Heart, Medical Consequences of Loneliness*, published by Basic Books, Inc., New York, agrees that human relationships are important.

This is a book of life, death, love, companionship, sex health, and loneliness! The author's stand is that human relationships do matter. They are vital not only to our mental, but also to our physical well-being. Social isolation, the lack of human companionship, the death or absence of parents in early childhood, sudden loss of love and chronic loneliness contribute significantly to premature death.

Special attention was given the Framingham studies, which began in 1948, to help answer the question of what caused fatal heart attacks? Those studies of Framingham, Massachusetts, a peaceful town of 28,000 just 30 miles from Boston, indicated the risk of coronary heart disease to be: 1) elevated blood pressure, 2) cigarette smoking, 3) elevated serum cholesterol, 4) electrocardiogram—evidence of left ventricular hypertrophy and 5) glucose intolerance. The study indicated stress and heart disease were unrelated! But Framingham offered few stressful situations. The people were religious, church-going, nondivorcing, dependable and socially well integrated. The people were accustomed to and well versed in the group approach to their problems. Emotional stress, which is brought on by social disintegration and family disruptions, was obviously minimal there.

Considering the city of Las Vegas with a high divorce rate, and an extremely mobile population, these risk factors would have varied. In fact, present statistics indicate that social and psychological factors may not only influence the course of heart disease, but they may also be the most important of all risk factors.

Lynch furthers his point by giving the studies of children who experience early disruption of parental contact. These children, upon maturation, contribute in increased numbers to the rank of those who encounter interpersonal difficulties. Raising the question: Does the heart disease begin in the lonely and broken hearts of children?

The animal studies presented by the author indicated that social deprivation adversely influenced the health of the animals. Furthermore, a series of experiments were reviewed which demonstrated that the early social experiences of various animals routinely used in medical research, significantly influenced their ability to resist experimentally induced diseases. Resistance to diseases as varied as heart disease, cancer, malaria, and tuberculosis, was altered by early social experiences.

The author recognizes the social paradox. Very few people want to be lonely. What then can be done to help alleviate the spread of loneliness induced disease in our society? The author indicates that medicine must move beyond science to deal with this problem. The scientific objectivity may very well be the cause of the loneliness.

(continued)

Physical Disabilities
Special Interest Section Newsletter; Vol. 3, No. 4, 1980

Permanent Pace Makers

The occupational therapist is part of the multidisciplinary team treating patients. In such a role, it is important to understand all situations a patient faces, whether they be our discipline's primary responsibility or not. Understanding a patient's pacemaker is one of those facets of cardiology that effects discussion of activity and OT's treatment of the patient.

The following information is reprinted from "The Beat Goes On," a newsletter for the Stormont-Vail Regional Medical Center Cardiac Monitoring Program.

Pacemakers are used for a variety of cardiac conduction defects, ranging from complete atrioventricular block, partial or incomplete bilateral bundle branch block, to sinoatrial arrest and block.

Heart attack victims with persistent bradyrhythmia usually need permanent pacemakers. So do patients with complete heart block and slow ventricular rates from congenital or degenerative heart disease, or from cardiac surgery.

Pacemakers help patients whose "block" causes serious hemodynamic problems or those who suffer recurrent Stokes-Adams attacks. Pacemakers can also be used to treat Wolff-Parkinson White syndrome. Patients with sick sinus syndrome can't be treated with digitalis or some antiarrhythmia drugs without aggravating their bradycardia.

The determination that a given patient should have a permanent pacemaker is usually made by a cardiologist in consultation with the primary physician, the patient, and the family.

Regardless of the indications for permanent pacing, the unit used will have three basic components:

— A pulse generator to provide the electrical potential required to trigger cardiac contractions at a rate or interval determined by pacer setting

— The lead, an insulated wire from the pulse generator to the heart

— An electrode (or electrodes) embedded either in myocardium or positioned against the endocardium of the right ventricle. The electrode is usually bipolar, in which two conductive elements transmit the impulse to the heart and the cardiac signal to the pulse generator. The electrode may be unipolar in which a single conductive element is used with the body acting as a ground.

Pacemakers themselves are classified according to their pacing mode.

— *Fixed rate* (asynchronous) pacemaker, is the oldest type but is rarely used today. It is designed to fire at a fixed rate and it is not affected by the heart's intrinsic rhythm. In the patient who retains some spontaneous rhythm, competition between the pacer and the intrinsic rhythm could result in life-threatening ventricular tachycardia.

— The *demand* (inhibited, synchronous, sensing or noncompetitive) pacemaker is designed to fire when the patient's heart rate falls below a preset point. Such pacemakers permit the patient's own heartbeat to override the pacemaker at any time.

— *AV synchronous* pacemakers require two electrodes. A sensing electrode in the atrium detects spontaneous atrial depolarization. Then a stimulating electrode in the ventricle discharges within a fraction of a second later. If the atrial rate exceeds 130 beats, the pacemaker will automatically transmit only every second impulse to the ventricle. If the rate falls below 60, the pacemaker will initiate fixed pacing at a rate of 60. This pacemaker is difficult to implant. A thoracotomy is usually necessary for accurate and stable electrode attachment.

The Omnicor series produced by Cordis Corporation can be adjusted faster or slower by a control device that is held against the skin over the pacemaker.

Mercury-zinc batteries, lasting 2-3 years, power most pacemakers. Lithium batteries will power a pacemaker for 9 years. The longest-lasting power source, radioactive plutonium, has been driving pacemakers since 1970. Nuclear pacemakers are rarely used. Their cost is upwards of $5,000. They come under the federal Nuclear Regulatory Commission's control.

Pacemaker implantation has become a well-established procedure during the past decade. Local anesthesia is recommended for the procedure. Under fluoroscopy, a pacing catheter is advanced through a cutdown made in the right cephalic vein, until the tip is lodged in the trabecular cordis lining the apex of the right ventricle. The catheter and pacemaker are tested. If no problem arises, the surgeon will then create a pocket in the right infraclavicular region large enough to encompass the pacing unit encased in a Dacron pouch. (Connective tissue grows into Dacron fibers, anchoring the unit into the chest wall.) The distal end of the pacing electrode is attached to the implanted pacing unit. If pacing proves satisfactory, the incision is closed and the wound dressed. For the next 24 hours, the patient remains in bed while his or her EKG, vital signs and general condition is carefully monitored.

Before discharge, a complete EKG study and chest X-ray series are invariably done to provide a baseline for future evaluations. Copies of these studies, plus a full description of the implanted device, including manufacturer, model and serial number, type, and rate setting, site and type of lead, site of pulse generator are normally forwarded to the referring physician. The patient should have this information on his or her person at all times. Most manufacturers prefer that every installation of their pacemakers be registered with them, which enables them quickly to contact patients in the event of pacemaker recall.

Acceleration, slowdown, irregular pacing and failure to capture the heart rate, are the principal problems. Any slowing or acceleration of a pacemaker requires prompt attention. Electrode failure is most likely to occur within three months of placement. Electrode breakage usually cannot be predicted. Electric component

(continued)

Permanent Pace Makers

failure tends to be both erratic and unpredictable.

Although lithium batteries last much longer than the older mercury batteries, their exhaustion occurs slowly, requiring careful long-term monitoring to detect changes that may signal failure.

Complications such as infections and rejection of the pulse generator by the body are more common after the first battery change.

Nurses should assume a responsible role in patient and patient-family education. Teaching must be geared to the patient's intellectual capability.

As a rule, advise patients not to wet the incision site until after it has healed and the sutures are removed. Then they can even swim. The patient should be shown how to take his or her pulse and when to report discrepancies. Some types of electrical apparatuses such as microwave ovens will inhibit a demand pacemaker. Patients should be advised not to go near operating microwave ovens.

The patient must be advised to state he or she has a pacemaker before receiving any medical treatment. Diathermy as well as other high frequency apparatus will inhibit the demand pacemaker.

Though pacemaker circuitry is designed to withstand a direct current shock, it is advised that if a patient is defibrillated, for example, he or she be monitored closely to detect any disturbances.

Other hazards are met at airports where pacemakers may ring the alarms of metal detectors. The patient is well advised to warn the authorities in advance. Patients will be seated away from the galley of the plane where microwave ovens are operating. The patient and a responsible family member should learn about checking the pulse for a full minute. If their pulse rate drops below the pacemaker's fixed rate, they should notify their physician. If you see that there is difficulty in pulse taking, this patient should be recommended to a pacemaker clinic. With pacer monitors, patients can have their pacemakers checked while in the comfort of their homes.

The patient must be made aware that the earliest signs of pacemaker problems are dizziness, shortness of breath, prolonged hiccoughs, and a very fast or very slow heart rate.

Contrary to what many patients believe, a pacemaker won't cure all their heart problems. So remind them to stick to their diets, take their medications as ordered, and get checkups.

Above all, encourage your pacemaker patient to enjoy life.

Bibliography

Bilitch, Micheal, et al; *When Your Patient Has a Pacemaker*, Patient Care; June 1978; pp. 76-97.

Proctor, Diane; *Temporary Cardiac Pacing*, Nursing Clinics of North America, Vol. 13; No. 3, September, 1978; pp. 409-422.

Furman, Seymour; *Recent Developments in Cardiac Pacing*, Heart & Lung; Sept/Oct 1978; pp. 813-826.

O'Brien, Garry; *The Nursing Care of Patients with Cardiac Pacemakers*, Nursing Times; January 1979; pp. 147-152.

Sweetwood, Hannelore; *Patients with Pacemakers*, Nursing 77; March; pp. 44-51.

Physical Disabilities
Special Interest Section Newsletter; Vol. 3, No. 3, 1980

Hands on: Stroke—Importance of Physiological Screening to Occupational Therapy Assessment

By Jane Baumgarten, OTR

Introduction

Each year 1.7 persons out of every 1,000 in the United States suffer a *cerebral vascular accident*. Frequently, patients who have suffered a stroke are unable to derive maximum benefits from activity and exercise programs that are an important part of their overall rehabilitation. From clinical observation, these patients fatigue easily and require frequent rest periods. There are several possible causes for this and any single patient may suffer one or any combination of these causes.

The deconditioning effect of bedrest following the acute phase, as well as a previous sedentary lifestyle must be considered. Prolonged bedrest usually has a harmful effect on the ability of the circulatory system to respond to increased physical exertion. Negative effects of deconditioning may be detected through clinical observation as well as through several physiological measures including decreased blood and plasma volume, which increases the chance for clot formation; orthostatic hypotension

(continued)

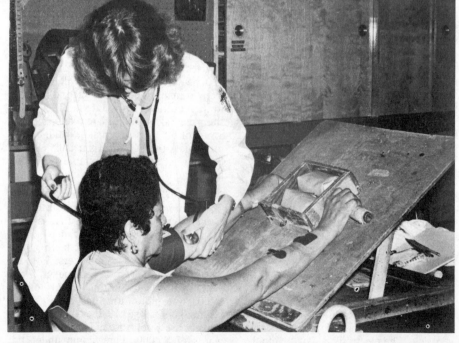

Jane Baumgarten, OTR, monitoring blood pressure of patient during treatment session.

and resultant venous pooling, and an abnormal increase in heart rate in response to activity, which decreases physical work capacity.

Physiologic Factors to Consider

An increased metabolic cost for activities due to the loss of coordinated motor response in the hemiplegic extremities may also be a factor. Metabolic cost for wheelchair propulsion and ambulation has been investigated in the stroke population, and reported to be 64 percent higher per unit of work than in the normal population.[1] Studies have not been done on other activities of daily living, although documentation exists indicating that patients with ischemic disease are more likely to show abnormalities during ADL at a lower heart rate than with an exercise test.

Another important factor for consideration, is the high incidence of co-existent cardiac abnormalities in rhythm. Some common changes in cardiac rhythm associated with central nervous system deficits include atrial fibrillation, paroxysmal atrial tachycardia and premature ventricular contractions. In 1968, Iseri evaluated 195 patients with nontraumatic hemiplegia who were admitted for rehabilitation. Seventy percent of these patients were found to have demonstrable heart disease, and 30 percent had significant heart disease that caused limitations to their lifestyle before their stroke. Therefore, we can expect that approximately one out of every three patients will have significant heart disease capable of interfering with the rehabilitation process. This study reveals the importance of physiological screening and assessment for all stroke patients.[2] Physiological screening aids the therapist in identifying those patients in danger of compromising their cardiovascular system. It also enables the therapist to provide the most vigorous and yet safe rehabilitation program possible, while allowing for the most effective use of rehabilitation time. Physiological assessment is valuable not only as a means of initial screening, but as an ongoing process, especially when significantly increased demands are placed on patients as they progress through their program.

Physiological Screening

Physiological screening begins with a review of the patients' medical history. At this time, the therapist is alerted to the patients' current cardiovascular status, as well as to any past medical history that might interfere with successful participation in a rigorous stroke rehabilitation program. In general, we see two patient populations with potentially inhibiting cardiac problems. One group with a documented history of heart disease, and one group with less specific vascular histories such as hypertension, arteriosclerotic disease and/or diabetes, which, because of its systemic nature, may affect cardiac function. All of these medical problems are common in the stroke population. In addition to the patient's history, attention should be focused on the list of medications that the patient is currently taking. Frequently, the reason for administering certain medications is not evident in the summary of the medical history. A basic understanding of cardiac-related medications will give the therapist additional insight into the patient's cardiac status. The information obtained from the medical chart determines the course of action to be taken by the therapist.

There are specific cardiac conditions that indicate the need for activity ECG monitoring either immediately or within one week. The conditions that indicate need for immediate ECG monitoring are: a history of myocardial infarction or cardiac arrest within 6 weeks of date of initial contact, a history of atrial flutter or fibrillation, a history of ventricular tachycardia or fibrillation, or a history of a second or third degree heart block. ECG monitoring should be completed within one week or before instituting a full therapy program when the medical history reveals myocardial infarction, cardiac arrest or congestive heart failure within the past 6 months, idiopathic or alcoholic cardiomyopathy, organic heart disease or a history of angina. If a patient does not fall within either of these categories, the therapist may proceed with the measurement of the blood pressure, and arrhythmias, with close observation of physical signs and/or symptoms. Physiological response to changes in body position and to sustained UE activity are assessed to determine the effects of inceased cardiovascular demand.

The occupational therapist monitors the patient in a supine position, sitting upright and after activities such as combing hair, or upper extremity exercise. It is important to wait at least two minutes before monitoring each of these activities to allow the cardiovascular system to adapt to change in position or in physical demand. Initially, one would expect a transient decrease in blood pressure when the patient moves from supine to sitting. Normally, blood pressure will return to the baseline measurement within seconds. Frequently, however, stroke patients' blood pressures will not adapt secondary to orthostatic hypotension. This hypoadaptive response frequently indicates deconditioning.

Record blood pressure and heart rate initially at rest, and note whether arrhythmias are present. Take pulse for ten seconds to determine baseline rate, but, if arrhythmias are noted, take pulse for one to two minutes to establish rhythm, and to determine the number of times arrhythmias occur within a full minute. When checking the patient with an arrhythmic pulse, the therapist should distinguish between an essentially regular pulse with occasional missed beats, and consistent irregularity that may indicate atrial fibrillation, which is common in the stroke population.

Since blood pressure is a vital part of the physiological screening, proper technique in measuring is important to ensure accuracy. Blood pressure should be taken on the uninvolved upper extremity when measuring patients with unilateral involvement. The normal size cuff is usually adequate to transmit pressure to the artery and surrounding tissue for accurate measurement; however, a larger thigh cuff may be used when taking blood pressure on extremely obese patients to avoid falsely high readings. The cuff should be applied approximately one inch above the crease in the elbow to leave adequate room for palpation of the pulse and for stethoscope placement, and the artery should be at heart level, regardless of the position of the patient. Blood pressure should always be taken within 15 seconds of stopping the activity to obtain the most accurate picture of the response during the activity.[3]

During the routine physiological screening, the therapist should also observe the patient for any of the physical signs and/or symptoms such as dizziness, diapheresis, shortness of breath, excessive fatigue or chest pain and these should be recorded. Clinically significant observations from the physiological screening that indicate the need for activity ECG monitoring and physician consultation include:

1. Decrease in systolic blood pressure with increased activity.

2. Diastolic blood pressure greater than 110mm Hg.

3. A combination of decreased systolic and increased diastolic blood pressure with increased activity.

4. Decreased heart rate with increased activity.

5. More than 5 missed beats per minute during or post activity.

6. More than 10 missed beats per minute at rest.

Therapy Program Modifications

For patients who are medically cleared for continuing rehabilitation programs,[4] therapy program modifications must be made to ensure the safest course of treatment possible. Examples of some common modifications include:

1. Use of elastic hose for patients demonstrating orthostatic hypotension and resultant venous pooling when challenged to assume upright postures.

2. Focus of initial treatment on general conditioning activities rather than resistive strengthening activities.

3. Use of warm-up and warm-down exercises to avoid sudden increases or decreases

(continued)

Stroke—Physiological Screening

in cardiovascular demand and to avoid sudden changes in blood pressure.
tion: the effects of valsalva's maneuver and need to avoid strenuous exercise after meals.

5. Continue physiological monitoring throughout the treatment process to allow for safe change as the rehabilitation program progresses.

Conclusion

The high incidence of cardiac disease and abnormalities documented in the stroke population should be taken into consideration by any therapist treating stroke patients. Screening includes a review of the medical history, accurate monitoring of heart rate, blood pressure and arrythmias, and careful observation and recording of signs and

symptom associated with any cardiac abnormalities. Routine physiological screening and ongoing monitoring is easily accomplished by any therapist and should be an integral part of the initial occupational therapy assessment. The only equipment necessary is a blood pressure cuff and a watch or clock with a sweep second hand. Close attention to potential problems initially will help to ensure safe rehabilitation and possibly aid in the prevention of further morbidity and even mortality in this patient population.

References:

1. Fisher SV, Gullickson G, Energy Cost of Ambulation in Health and Disability: A Literature Review. *Arch Phys Med Rehabil* 59: 124-133, 1978
2. Iseri LT, Cardiovascular Problems and Functional Evaluation in Rehablitation of Hemiplegic Patients. *J Chron Dis* 21: 423-434, 1968
3. Lancour J. How to Avoid Pitfalls in Measuring Blood Pressure. *Am J Nurs* 76:773-775, 1976
4. Winchester P, Verbal Communication, Research Physical Therapist, Rancho Los Amigos Hospital.

Jane Baumgarten is an OT II at Rancho Los Amigos Hospital in Downey, California. Her clinical experience has been primarily with the adult who is neurologically disabled and a special interest in the cardiac problems of patients following central nervous system impairment. Recently, Jane was a featured speaker at a two-day conference and discussed the importance of assessment of physiological factors to OT evaluation and treatment planning.

Physical Disabilities
Special Interest Section Newsletter; Vol. 3, No. 3, 1980

Stroke Rehabilitation—Setting Realistic Occupational Therapy Goals

By Dorothy J. Wilson, OTR, FAOTA, Guest Editor

Introduction:

Many clinicians have tried to identify the specific factors that can be used to predict the functional outcome of stroke rehabilitation. Approaches to this problem include predicting on the basis of neurologic symptoms that are prevailing after the stroke, either singly or in clusters or setting targets of improvement during the rehabilitation process. However, many therapists feel that the most accurate goals can be determined by analyzing the overall effect of multiple neurologic and functional deficits. This paper names the factors identified during initial OT evaluation that most influences upper extremity (UE) function at three different levels.

Use As A Minimal Stabilizing Assist

The goal of use of the impaired upper extremity as a minimal stabilizing assist during bilateral activities is defined as use of the arm and hand to stabilize objects being manipulated or acted on by the uninvolved extremity (e.g., stabilizing paper while attempting to write). This function can be accomplished by the weight of the arm alone and does not require voluntary use of motor control.

Before setting this goal, the therapist must analyze the results of the initial assessment of the patient's cognition and judgment, motor control, muscle tone, pain, sensation and the patient's ability to

interpret the sensation for purposeful use.

One requirement for achieving this level of function is cognition sufficient to enable the patient to follow specific motor instructions and generalize use of the arm from a few specific therapeutic activities to all comparable functional activities. The patient must exhibit the judgment to realize how much the arm can be realistically used and when the extremity is potentially unsafe to use during bilateral tasks.

Although there is no requirement for voluntary active motion, the muscle tone in the impaired extremity must be normal for use as defined, or, at the least, minimally hypertonic.

Range of motion at the shoulder joint must be sufficient to allow comfortable placement of the arm on a table top and if pain is present, it must be alleviated to the point that it does not interfere with the patient's participation in a use training program. This pain requirement applies to any goal that is set for use of the arm and hand in functional tasks.

Purposeful UE function requires at the very least protective sensation ... the ability to discriminate between hot and cold, sharp and dull, etc. In addition, normal stabilization activity requires proprioception at the shoulder and elbow joints. Peripheral sensation in itself may be critical to safe use of the arm and hand, but it is not very functional unless the patient can

integrate the sensation and interpret the input for use in purposeful activity. Integration deficits of unilateral neglect, denial and severe apraxia, which is arbitrarily defined for this paper as deficits in initiating, planning or sequencing motor acts, will interfere with even this minimal level of functional use of the arm and hand.

Use As A Minimal Active Assist

Minimal active assist of the UE is defined as use of weak shoulder and elbow voluntary motion to assist in accomplishing single sequence activities or a single part of an activity such as placing the arm in a wheelchair sling or actively placing the arm away from the body during dressing and hygiene tasks.

Requirements for establishing this goal are the same as discussed above in the areas of cognition and judgment. In fact, the basic levels of cognition and judgment described apply to all the goals that are established for the UE.

Motor control and muscle tone requirements differ only in that the patient must exhibit some voluntary motion. This motion may be limited to synergistic motion in one direction such as a flexion synergy or weak selective control (F+ or below). Again, absence of excessive or counterproductive tone is necessary in order not to block the weak or beginning motor control. *(continued)*

Stroke Rehabilitation

Range of motion should be at a functional level in all joints in order to prevent pain when placing the arm and hand in the many positions required for use. Although there have been no conclusive studies to define the range of motion necessary for performance of activities of daily living, some suggested minimum ranges have been used by therapists as guidelines. These ranges are a minimum of 100 degrees of shoulder elevation in either the flexion or abduction plane, at least 45 to 90 degrees of elbow flexion, 30 degrees of pronation supination and wrist extension. The hand must be flexible, even if there is no active motion, in order to prevent pain from an accidental pull on the fingers during performance of functional activities.

Sensation of the impaired upper extremity should be present throughout with only minimal impairment acceptable in propioception and tactile discrimination. Body image or body scheme must be basically intact. Some degree of apraxia may be present such as minimal impairment of motor planning and sequencing, but the patient must be able to initiate motor activity if he or she is to succeed in achieving this goal.

Maximum Active Assist

This goal is defined as use of the impaired upper extremity in all activities that require active pushing, pulling, stabilizing and grasp and release. The additional factors to be considered are the quality and strength of UE motor control and the presence of intact peripheral sensation and higher levels of sensory integrative function.

Although the patient's previous life style and remaining social support systems cannot be deemed requirements for UE function, the impact of these factors are of increasing importance in predicting outcome as more is expected of the patient. For this reason, these factors will be discussed in conjunction with requirements for achieving the higher goals.

The motor control requirements are contained in the preceding definition of this goal. They must have, in addition to stabilization capability, voluntary elbow flexion, gross grasp and either active finger and thumb extension or at a minimum, ability to relax the hand following gross grasp. The elbow motion should be able to take resistance in order to provide a stabilizing force downward or an active pull upward. Spasticity, which is assessed to be greater than minimal, would definitely interfere with activities associated with this goal. Active grasp and relaxation of that grasp must be present but severely increased muscle tone will not allow functional release during performance of bilateral tasks.

At this level, use depends on intact peripheral sensation. It cannot be said that intact sensation guarantees use but it is a generally accepted fact that absent sensation precludes a patient reaching an upper extremity use goal at this level. In spite of intact peripheral sensation, deficits in planning and sequencing motor acts and inability to accurately perceive and interpret visual input interfere in this level of function, not only of the impaired arm, but bilaterally. In addition, deficits in body image, depth perception and failure to accurately perceive the position of the body in space provide functional obstacles that are difficult to overcome.

The patient's previous life role greatly influences residual behavior. When use of the impaired upper extremity as a maximum active assist is established as a goal, the patient is expected to be independent in performance of self-care skills as well as participate in numerous home and community skills such as assisting with meal preparation. The patient is expected to use available motor control and sensation and be encouraged to participate in a variety of activities by this family. The family should be willing to allow the patient opportunities to participate, at his level, in activities such as cleaning, laundry and cooking. Family support can be enhanced by education to the value of the patient's participation to eventual recovery. This requires understanding and patience from able-bodies family members who could probably perform the activities faster and more efficiently without the patient.

Incorporation In All Bilateral Activities

This final goal is defined as incorporation of the impaired arm and hand in all bilateral tasks associated with activities of daily living. This is the highest goal we can realistically establish unless there is total spontaneous recovery of normal arm and hand functions. This level represents ability to assist with most activities but therapists should remember that the extremity is still not normal.

Motor control at this level must be selective in the shoulder, elbow, forearm, and wrist, but still may exhibit vestiges of synergistic patterns and abnormal muscle tone, particularly in the hand. Strength should be at least F+ and counterproductive tone should be absent throughout except perhaps minimal increase in thumb and finger flexors. Speed and timing of motion are important to consider at this level as most of the higher level activities require more versatility than demanded by the previous goals. Ability to perform alternating motions smoothly and in the proper sequence and rhythm are essential.

At this point the patient must have intact integration of sensation. Praxis, body image, visual perception, depth perception, etc., all must be intact. Even mild motor planning deficits can interfere with the timing of motion necessary to complete these tasks.

The importance of the patient's previous life style and expected life role assumes major importance in connection with this goal. The patient is more efficient in using his or her arm and hand and can complete most tasks independently rather than assisting someone else. The therapist can actually help the patient decide priorities in use of energy and assist in re-establishing role through prevocational or pre-educational exploration, inventory of interests, and patient-family education and training.

Conclusion

Occupational therapists can set realistic functional goals for use of an impaired upper extremity as a result of stroke by careful initial assessment and by analyzing factors that influence upper extremity use. The importance of accurate prediction of outcome of treatment cannot be overstressed in our current era of emphasis of quality assurance and cost containment in all arenas of health care.

BIBLIOGRAPHY

Bard G, Hirschberg GG: Recovery of Voluntary Motion in Upper Extemity Following Hemiplegia. *Arch Phys Med Rehabil* 46:567-572, 1965

Bobath B: Adult Hemiplegia: Evaluation and Treatment. London, William Heinemann Medical Books, Ltd., 1970

Cailliet R: The Shoulder in Hemiplegia. Philadelphia, F.A. Davis Co., 1980

Feigerson JS, Polkon L, Meikle R, Ferguson W: Burke Stroke Fine-Oriented Profile (Bustop): An Overview of Patient Function. *Arch Phys Med Rehabil* 60:508, 1979

Gordon EE, Drenth V, Jarvis L, Johnson J, Wright V: Neurophysiologic syndromes in Stroke as Predictors of Outcome. *Arch Phys Med Rehabil* 59:399-403, 1978

Johnstone M: *Restoration of Motor Function in the Stroke Patient.* New York, Churchill Livingstone, 1978

Kaplan PE, Meredith J, Taft G: Stroke and Brachial Plexus Injury: A Difficult Problem. *Arch Phys Med Rehabil* 58:415, 1977

Kitowski VJ: Rehabilitation of Patients with Cardiac Disease and Associated Cerebral Vascular Accident. *So Med J,* 72:303, 1979

Lehman JF, Delateur BJ, Gowler RS: Stroke Rehabilitation: Outcome and Prediction. *Arch Phys Med Rehabil* 56:383-389, 1975

Licht S: *Stroke and its Rehabilitation,* Baltimore, Waverly Press, Inc., 1975

Ottenbacher K: Cerebral Vascular Accidents: Some Characteristics of Occupational Therapy Evaluation Forms. *AJOT* 34:268-271, 1980

Savinelli R, Timm M, Montgomery J, Wilson D: Therapy Evaluation and Management of Patients With Hemiplegia. *Clin. Orthop* 131:15-29, 1978

Stern PH, McDowell F, Miller JM, Robinson M: Factors Influencing Stroke Rehabilitation. *Stroke* 2:213-218, 1971

Wilson DJ: Training For Daily Living: Occupational Therapy in Rehabilitation of Patients With CVA. *QAB* 4(11), 1978

Physical Disabilities
Special Interest Section Newsletter; Vol. 3, No. 3, 1980

A One-Step Modification to the Bobath Sling

**By Diana Williams, OTR,
Geisinger Medical Center,
Danville, PA**

It is common knowledge that the Bobath sling can be successfully used by patients with long-term uper extremity proximal weakness. The sling provides just enough support to prevent shoulder subluxation while allowing freedom of elbow and hand motion. The problem with its use, however, is the difficulty in independent donning and doffing. A "D"-ring attached to the strap over the involved shoulder with a Velcro attachment is a modification that permits independence and ease in donning the sling. It is worn under the clothing to permit support without exposure.

Reference:

Bobath, Berta: *Adult Hemiplegic Evaluation and Treatment* 2nd Edition, William Heinemann Medical Books Limited, London, p. 106-107.

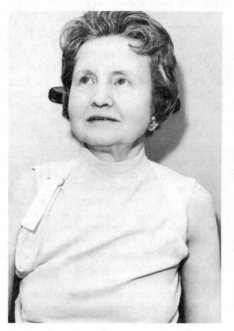 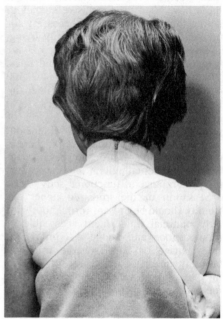

Physical Disabilities
Special Interest Section Newsletter; Vol. 3, No. 2, 1980

Accountability—No Choice

By Ruth Ann Watkins, MBA, OTR, FAOTA

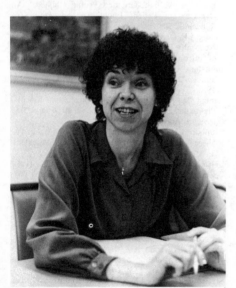

Guest Editor: Ruth Ann Watkins, MBA, OTR, FAOTA, is the associate administrator of Allied Health Services at the Rehabilitation Institute of Chicago. She received her BS *in occupational therapy from the University of Illinois, and her MBA from the University of Chicago. During her career she has been active on National and State AOTA Committees. She was the first chairperson for the AOTA Physical Disability Specialty Section, served on the AOTA Physical Disability Specialty Section Steering Committee, was on the AOTA Task Force for developing AOTA Standards of Treatment for patients with arthritis.*

Accountability is more than a buzz word in the health care field; it is a concept that is here to stay.

Changes brought about by state and federal regulations and advances being made in medicine and research present challenges to the occupational therapist that are greater than ever. Assurance of quality of care is being demanded by the public and monitored by local, state and federal licensing and/or accrediting agencies.

As an occupational therapist you are accountable to your consumers—patients/ clients, employer, sources who refer patients/ clients to you and the general public.

The concept of accountability not only addresses the quality of services you provide but the economic value of those services. Do the benefits of your services exceed the costs of providing them? Are you confident enough to predict specific outcomes that will occur as a result of your services? Do the Federal Drug Administration regulations for medical device manufacturers apply to you? If you manufacture any medical device (such as an orthosis) for however small a clientele, they might. Does your local PSRO have an occupational therapist on the board?

These are samples of the many questions you, as a practicing occupational therapist, must ask yourself. Accountability is here to stay; you can not ignore it hoping that AOTA and your employer will wrestle with it and leave you uninvolved. You must become involved.

This newsletter presents a bibliography and approaches to the accountability issues that are being taken.

Accountability and Productivity

By Louise R. Thibodaux, MA, OTR

Sound fiscal management consists of organizing and monitoring the available resources within a department so that service is rendered at a reasonable cost. Recent attempts to control the rate of inflation within the hospital industry have pointed out the need for fiscal accountability among all levels of occupational therapy staff. Even though the practice of occupational therapy has not yet been transformed by the rampant technological change which characterizes other medically related professions, the effect of these changes on the day to day operation of most departments cannot be denied. If nothing else, occupational therapists have been forced to think of themselves as "product-oriented," providing as their product specific and identifiable services geared toward predictable patient/client outcomes. This new emphasis on product and outcome calls for new methods of documenting and measuring services to guarantee that all departmental resources are used to the best advantage.

In the realm of fiscal management, the departmental budget is the major tool. Not only does the budget insure adequate financial support for the program, it also identifies the resources available to the department. These resources include manpower hours, capital equipment, supplies, space and overhead. The department will within any given year "use up" these resources (usually identified in terms of direct and indirect costs) in order to produce a given number of products or outcomes (generally identified as projected revenue). This is not exactly the view of budgeting to which most occupational therapists are exposed in school. However, the resource-based understanding of budgetary process points out that the budget must be flexible and that continuous monitoring is necessary to insure that the most efficient service can be provided at a reasonable cost.

Management decisions based on flexible budgeting approach should work to the benefit of the total institution. One occupational therapy department recently staggered its work hours to provide 10-hour coverage. The staff reports for work in three shifts between 7 am and 9 am and provides coverage through the evening meal. Although each staff member works only an 8-hour day, 2 extra hours are available for productive interaction with the patient and his family. It has been possible to provide more time for individualized ADL instruction and to involve the family in the care of the patient during their evening visits without additional drain on departmental resources. The change in work hours has been monitored by the number of treatment units generated within a month. If this should somehow result in a decrease in the number of patient/therapist interactions corrective action should be taken promptly so that an adequate balance between outputs and resources is restored. The process of monitoring changes in productivity within a department has been simplified by computer technology (although it can be implemented manually to some degree). Information on the number of units of service may be gathered by therapist, by program, by department or by a given unit of time. In 1977 Congress mandated to DHEW the task of identifying productivity measures for all revenue-producing departments in hospitals (PL 95-142). The AOTA Commission on Practice has developed, in response, *Uniform Terminology for the Reporting of Occupational Therapy Services.* The report of this Task Force is available from the AOTA Distribution Center. Further study was devoted to the development of a method which might assign weighted values to the work-output of occupational therapists. This information is as yet experimental and has been passed on to DHEW to be published by them.

The relationship of productivity to cost is one which must be emphasized. If the staff of a department is able to increase the number of units of service provided while at the same time achieving full utilization of budgeted departmental resources, the total cost of providing treatment will be reduced. As the share of the cost is distributed equitably among all users, the resources costs incurred by an individual patient or client should decrease. Thus the concept of flexible, resource-based fiscal management is basic to the concept of accountability to total institution by organizing and monitoring the available resources so that the patient/client may obtain maximum benefit at a reasonable cost.

References

1. American Occupational Therapy Association, Inc., "Uniform Terminology for Reporting Occupational Therapy Services", January 1979.

2. Baum, M. Carolyn "Management and Documentation of Occupational Therapy Services" in *Willard and Spackman's Occupational Therapy,* 5th edition, Philadelphia, J.B. Lippincott and Co., 1978 pp. 675-685.

3. "Cost Finding and Rate Setting for Hospitals," Chicago, American Hospital Association, 1968.

4. Sibson, Robert E. *Increasing Employee Producitivity,* New York, American Management Associations, 1976.

5. Soper, George "Uniform Reporting System", *The Pyramid,* American Physical Therapy Association Section on Administration, vol. 8 no. 3 August 1978.

Health Accounting—A New Method of Quality Assurance for Occupational Therapy

By Julie Shaperman, MA, OTR

As part of the AOTA's quality review educational program, the Division of Professional Development is presenting a series of seminars on Health Accounting Principles and Techniques. The primary goal of the series is to train core faculty, and the thrust of the seminars is to develop the skills of the faculty trainee.

Health Accounting is a method of public accountability which meets AOTA's *new* quality review standard, the *new* JCAH Audit Standard, and the PSRO's *new* approach to quality review. The methodology is a natural evolution and a necessary addition to the retrospective chart audit AOTA has been teaching. Health Accounting focuses on outcomes; it does not rely on charts, and it can include a health benefit analysis.

(continued)

Health Accounting

The first series of seminars was taught by Patricia C. Ostrow, MA, OTR, at Daniel Freeman Hospital in Los Angeles, and included an actual quality review in occupational therapy. A member of each AOTA Specialty Section was invited to observe the process. The Health Accounting process includes 5 stages: Priority Setting, Initial Outcome Assessment, Definitive Assessment, Improvement Action and Outcome Reassessment. It cannot be learned by "reading an article," but requires supervised practice to become an effective tool. It appears that Health Accounting will be useful to occupational therapy in many ways: (1) to improve documentation of the results of our services and to define cost-benefit relationships; (2) to improve services to patients by focusing on one high priority problem at a time. These problems must be important, solvable and cost effective; they are selected jointly by occupational therapists, patients, associate health care providers and others who influence outcomes; (3) to learn how to proceed through a series of steps, systematically, to resolve the problem; and (4) to measure outcomes. Health Accounting is especially well suited to occupational therapy. The method is useful not only for quality review required by outside agencies, it is very promising for improving the quality of practice. Occupational therapist should not miss the opportunity to learn Health Accounting if a seminar is offered in their area.

Physical Disabilities

Special Interest Section Newsletter; Vol. 3, No. 2, 1980

A Method of Ensuring Accountability

By Eila Cagle, OTR

The occupational therapy department of a general hospital and rehabilitation unit developed a functional graph in 1970, to be used with the Problem-Oriented Medical Record to establish a more efficient and complete system of recording. To date, the occupational therapy department continues to evaluate the use of the functional graph which is used with all patients seen in the 38-bed rehabilitation unit. Initially, the occupational therapy department agreed to use the functional graph in conjunction with the problem-oriented medical record to:

1) Provide an efficient and thorough means of communication with all members of the rehabilitation team.

2) To establish a realistic treatment program with coordinated short and long-term goals and plans.

3) To provide a loop system of follow through for established goals and plans. The idea for such a functional graph resulted from reading Erdman, Wm. J., M.D., Scranton & Fogel's Article "Evaluation of Functional Levels of Patients During and Following Rehabilitation" *Archives of Physical Medicine and Rehabilitation,* January 1970, Volume 51, No. 1, pp 1-21. In this paper the authors found that patients improved in level of function in all of the variables identified for the purpose of evaluating the effectiveness of the rehabilitation program, with the greater improvement in the physical area than in the psychosocial area.

The functional graph is a tool that documents deficits of patients and instantly discloses to team members progress made in fulfilling objectives in treatment plans. Coordination of disciplines and interdisciplinary communication, both of which are critical to meeting treatment goals, can be accomplished by use of the functional graph.

(See illustrations.)

The functional graph, one for each rehabilitation discipline, can meet the specifications of such a tool for the physical medicine and rehabilitation department, or for any rehabilitation discipline, separately. Functional graphs for nursing, physical therapy and occupational therapy staff members lead efficiently to effective results in one hospital and rehab unit.

Retrospective audits of the performance of the rehabilitation staff members are facilitated by the functional graph. What treatment was performed and reviewable by the supervisor, department manager, administration, and outside auditors.

The functional graph can be a performance standard for the rehabilitation staff member. A tool for the following is available:

A) Self-review by the individual therapist, continuously, as treatment progresses.

B) Supervisory review, continuously, as treatment progresses.

The functional graph is a flow sheet comprised of twenty categories or problem areas. Progress notes are recorded on the reverse side of the flow sheet, and the updating of the flow sheet periodically constitutes the follow-up phase of the record-keeping process. At the time the functional graph was implemented, a grid or definition sheet defining every level of achievement for each of the 20 categories was developed at the same time. The definitions were coordinated with terms used in the various physical medicine and rehabilitation departments. The occupational therapist's information for the functional graph is obtained through a thorough patient evaluation. Subsequent to evaluation results, each week the PM and R professions assume an integrated and an easily audited role in solving the patients' problems. It also serves as an educational function for each rehab team member, to constantly review the problem list and enter observations under the appropriate heading.

With standardization among therapists in the development of the data base (identified on the functional graph) correct formulation and management of the solutions of all of the patient's problem is better assured.

The implication of the problem-oriented medical record used with the functional graph is mainly that the therapist is taught to find solutions to specific problems.

Documentation with the functional graph has the capacity to be systematic, well organized, and clearly delineated, so that the therapist may logically pursue each problem. With each subsequent evaluation, there is a continuing audit of all the patients problems.

Contributing Authors

1. Eila Cagle, OTR, Manager of Occupational Therapy, Wyandotte General Hospital, Wyandotte, MI.
2. Patricia Ostrow, MA, OTR, Director, Quality Review Program, American Occupational Therapy Association, Rockville, MD.
3. Julie Shaperman, MA, OTR, University of California, Child Amputee Prosthetics Project, Los Angeles, CA.
4. Louise Thibodaux, MA, OTR, Director, Occupational Therapy, Lake Shore Hospital, Birmingham, AL.

(continued)

Ensuring Accountability

FUNCTIONAL PROGRESS CHART

	DATE	SCORE	QUARTILE
INITIAL			
PROGRESS			
PROGRESS			
DISCHARGE			

UNIT NO._____
AGE _____
ROOM _____
PHYSICIAN

NAME _____
DIAG _____
ADM. DATE_____
SEX

Therapist:

CATEGORY	0	1	1.5	2	3	4	5	COMMENTS
1. Bathing	0	LESS THAN 25%	MAXIMUM 25%	MODERATE 50%	MINIMUM 75%	GUARDING ASSISTANCE	INDEPENDENCE	
2. Dressing	0	LESS THAN 25%	MAXIMUM 25%	MODERATE 50%	MINIMUM 75%	GUARDING ASSISTANCE	INDEPENDENCE	
3. Feeding	0	SEVERE	POOR	FAIR	FAIR +	GUARDING	INDEPENDENCE	
4. Grooming	0	LESS THAN 25%	MAXIMUM 25%	MODERATE 50%	MINIMUM 75%	GUARDING	INDEPENDENCE	
5. Homemaking Skills	0	LESS THAN 25%	MAXIMUM 25%	MODERATE 50%	MINIMUM 75%	GUARDING	INDEPENDENCE	
6. Transfers	0	MECHANICAL LIFT	MAXIMUM 25%	MODERATE 50%	MINIMUM 75%	GUARDING	INDEPENDENCE	
7. Bed Mobility	0	TRACE	POOR	FAIR	FAIR +	GOOD	INDEPENDENCE	
8. Sitting Balance	0	TRACE	POOR	FAIR	FAIR +	GOOD	INDEPENDENCE	
9. Fine Motor Skills	0		TRACE	POOR	FAIR	GOOD	NORMAL	
10. Wheelchair Use	0	TRACE	POOR	FAIR	FAIR +	GOOD	INDEPENDENCE	
11. Strength - Right Upper Extremity	0	REFLEX	TRACE	POOR	FAIR	GOOD	NORMAL	
12. Strength - Left Upper Extremity	0	REFLEX	TRACE	POOR	FAIR	GOOD	NORMAL·	
13. Range of Motion Right	0	LIMITATION	FULL PASSIVE	ACTIVE 25%	ACTIVE 50%	ACTIVE 75%	NORMAL	
14. Range of Motion Left	0	LIMITATION	FULL PASSIVE	ACTIVE 25%	ACTIVE 50%	ACTIVE 75%	NORMAL	
15. Upper Extremity Use	0	SEVERE BOTH UPPER	UNAWARE	WEIGHTED ASSIST	GROSS ASSIST	FUNCTIONAL	NORMAL	
16. Sensory Loss	0	NO SENSORY 2 LIMBS	LOSS IN 1 LIMB	DULLED 4 LIMBS	DULLED 2 LIMBS	DULLED 1 LIMB	NORMAL	
17. Cognitive/Perceptual	0	SEVERELY IMPAIRED	MODERATELY IMPAIRED	MILDLY IMPAIRED	GUARDED	SLIGHTLY IMPAIRED	NORMAL	
18. Attitude	0	SLIGHTLY REALISTIC	MILDLY REALISTIC	FAIRLY REALISTIC	MODERATELY REALISTIC	QUITE REALISTIC	REALISTIC	
19. Pain	0	SEVERE UNABLE	SEVERE LIMITS	SEVERE WITH	MODERATE	MINIMAL	NONE	
20. Endurance	0	SEVERE	POOR	FAIR	FAIR +	GOOD	NORMAL	

Copyright 1980
Wyandotte General Hospital

TP-148

DEFINITIONS

SUPERVISED ACTIVITY TO INDEPENDENCE — PATIENT REQUIRES GUARDING ASSISTANCE FOR SAFETY

MINIMAL DEPENDENCE — PATIENT WILL REQUIRE MINIMAL ASSISTANCE (25%) WITH MOST ACTIVITIES OF DAILY LIVING

MODERATE DEPENDENCE — PATIENT WILL REQUIRE MODERATE ASSISTANCE (50%) WITH MOST ACTIVITIES OF DAILY LIVING

SEVERE DEPENDENCE — PATIENT WILL REQUIRE MAXIMAL ASSISTANCE (25%) WITH MOST ACTIVITIES OF DAILY LIVING

Initial:

	DATE	SCORE	QUARTILE
Evaluation			
Evaluation			
Evaluation			
Evaluation			

1st Quartile: 0-30 — severe dependence
2nd Quartile: 31-50 — moderate dependence
3rd Quartile: 51-80 — minimal dependence
4th Quartile: 81-100 — supervised activity to independence

DATE	PROBLEM			

Physical Disabilities
Special Interest Section Newsletter; Vol. 3, No. 1, 1980

Hands on: Arthritis and On-Site Job Intervention

Work: From the Old English WYRCAN: to bring to pass: Effect miracles.

By Catherine Budic

Introduction and Overview

There are psychological, social, financial, and physical benefits to be derived from gainful employment. Work is an active concept; it is occupation; it is purposeful. Statistics indicate that, of the 31 million people who have arthritis, more than 7.5 million report a decrease in their capacity to perform—to work, to go to school, keep house or participate in recreational activities. The costs in lost work productivity were more than 5 billion dollars in 1978.

The main goal for people with arthritis is to remain productive at work without exacerbating their symptoms. To this end, on-site job intervention may be a valuable adjunct to health care for the patient, employer and the therapist.

There are several indications for job intervention by the occupational therapist in the treatment of arthritis: 1) The physician or patient expresses a concern that current job activities are capable of causing an increase in symptoms; 2) There are questions regarding the extent of disability; and 3) The potential for the patient to return to partial or complete gainful employment needs to be established.

The Department of Health, Education and Welfare has defined morbidity, impairment and disability to provide a common language for all parties concerned. There is also a booklet entitled: *Disability Evaluation under Social Security: A Handbook for Physicians*, in which is stated—very simply, very directly:

"The determination of whether a man is disabled under the social security statute requires two separate judgments. *One* is an assessment of a man's remaining capacity to perform physical or mental activities. The *second* is an assessment of the physical or mental capacity demands of a group of jobs which falls within a man's vocational spectrum. When remaining capacity to perform is less than the demands of the job, he is disabled."

The person with arthritis presents a particular problem in that the amount of disability is not constant. The occupational therapist has a difficult decision to make regarding which phase of the disease to deal with in the process of job intervention. Arthritis is a disease with exacerbations and remissions. The problems of a paralytic, an amputee, or a brain-damaged patient are established. The patient with arthritis has a disease which may follow a malignant course in one person, periodic flare-ups in another, or a slow, relentless progress toward severe crippling in a third. Long-range planning is difficult; vocational counseling is involved and frustrating. Physicians tend to place job intervention low on the list of priorities because the situation may not yet be critical. Patients prefer to handle the situation themselves out of fear of losing their jobs if it appears they need special consideration.

Factors Affecting Employment

The assessment of the patient's capacity to perform is part of a comprehensive evaluation for functional rehabilitation. The functional capacity is determined by the effect of the local joint/muscle changes on the person's ability to carry out activities of daily living. The occupational therapist must evaluate the patient's total function and the physical therapist must evaluate the patient's joint/muscle function before formulating a realistic program.

Features of arthritis that can be occupational hazards are:

1. Morning stiffness;
2. Ease of fatigue and decreased activity tolerance;
3. Recurrent pain and active inflammation in multiple joints over extended periods;
4. Joint deformity, instability and limitation, with muscle wasting and weakness.

To plan a realistic approach, it is important to know something about the patients' personality and social background and to evaluate their close family relationships, their intellectual capacity, and the extent to which they have accepted their disease. The familys' knowledge of and attitude toward the patient's problems and their ability to give realistic support when they return to work are of great importance in the results

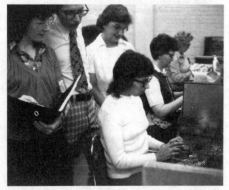

Kitty Budic, OTR (left), with an area supervisor and the industrial health nurse, completing an on-site job evaluation at Master Lock Company, Milwaukee.

of intervention.

When job intervention is indicated, the emphasis changes from medical management to psychophysiological management. Arthritis is a disease which affects every aspect of the person's life patterns. There is frequently little relationship between the person's capacity to perform and the extent of the impairment.

Occupational readiness is then assessed by considering the following:

> *Psychosocial Aspects*
> —Motivation
> —Education of patient and family
> —Cooperation; attitude
>
> *Physical Aspects*
> —Max. physical status
> —Functional ability to manage:
>   self-care ambulation
>   transport
>   functional requirements of job
>   activity tolerance
>
> *Occupational Aspects*
> —Job opportunity
> —Suitability
> —Availability

The individual factors affecting employability cannot be dealt with without having an awareness of the needs of management, the laws governing hiring and employing the handicapped, unions, and the state of the economy.

Management has two primary concerns: safety and dollars. The therapist must be aware of the costs of workers compensation, of hiring a new individual to replace the skilled, long-time employee, of insurance dollars paid and risks incurred with a chronically ill person. Gains must be offset against losses, and management skillfully made aware of their responsibilities to the handicapped and disabled.

Recent legislation and rulings have facilitated the return of arthritis patients to work in a time when a sense of community and public relations have honed management's awareness of the needs of the disabled. *The Rehabilitatin Act of 1973,* originating in the Department of Health, Education and Welfare, states "reasonable accommodations" must be made to the handicaps of applicants and employees. *The Workers Compensation Act of Wisconsin* states "one of the primary purposes . . . is restoration of an injured employee to gainful employment."

Hand-in-hand with management's attitude of the helpful benefactor is the state of the economy—business, local and national. When jobs are scarce and money is tight, employers don't hire; they expect max-

(continued)

Arthritis and On-Site Job Intervention

imum production, and the public relations programs are decreased.

The unions play a role in the particular job environment of the industrial worker. The therapist must have some knowledge of their effectiveness and power if changes are being considered for a patient's job. Changes made to the environment or tasks must be appropriate for all workers, not just the handicapped employee. It behooves the therapist to have a working knowledge of time—energy conservation techniques and be able to convince all concerned of the dollars that are saved when an employee operates efficiently and still retains quality.

If a therapist believes an on-site job evaluation would be beneficial to the patient, he or she should explain the purpose and value of such a procedure and obtain the patient's written permission to contact his or her employer. Management, usually the director of personnel, is contacted by the therapist to determine how to proceed with-

in the work environment. Key contact people would usually be someone familiar with a variety of jobs throughout the setting, the safety director, and the job supervisor. The therapist proceeds with the evaluation only after management has cleared his or her admittance and has arranged for a knowledgeable person to accompany him or her.

The therapist observes the job and the patient's current environment and then visits other work positions which may be more appropriate. A letter of recommendation is sent to the physician, the industrial health nurse, and the personnel director.

Conclusion

Work is therapeutic, and there are psychological, social, financial, and physical benefits to be derived from gainful employment. Recent legislation and rulings define the responsibilities of the employer to make jobs available to the injured or handicapped. The occupational therapist has the

expertise to evaluate a patient's functional problems and assets, to analyze the work environment, and to work with the patient, the management, and the physician to facilitate the employee's return to a modified job or an alternate assignment. On-site intervention is a valuable and integral part of this process and facilitates management's understanding of the person with arthritis.

Catherine Budic is chief occupational therapist at Columbia Hospital, Milwaukee, WI.. Her program has incorporated on-site job intervention for the past three years. Her clinical experience of eleven years has been primarily in physical disabilities, seven in management capacity. Recently, she was appointed to the Wisconsin Arthritis Foundation's Industrial Subcommittee for Public Education and Information. Cathrine lives with her husband and three sons in Mequon, WI.

Physical Disabilities
Special Interest Section Newsletter; Vol. 3, No. 1, 1980

Community Arthritis Education

A person with arthritis can live in a world of pain, disability, fear, and quackery with family or friends who do not understand the problems posed by this disease. Just read a newspaper, review advertisements or count copper bracelets, get a feel for the magnitude of forces influencing a person with arthritis. The less a person knows about the disease, the more influential these elements can be.

To improve the patient's total life, the issues of family education about arthritis and quackery need to be addressed, as well as pain relief, joint protection and functional adaptation.

There are an estimated 110,000 people with arthritis in Santa Clara Valley, California. Given the needs of such a large population, it became apparent that a program other than traditional therapy referral was needed.

To meet this need, the Occupational Therapy Department helped initiate a community arthritis education course for people with arthritis and their families. The course involves six 2-hour sessions over a 1-month period. The course is taught by an OT, PT, and nurse team.

To help determine the need for such a program a survey was conducted with a sample arthritis population in Santa Clara Valley. In summary, the survey disclosed that general knowledge was low and that people who used modalities or did exercises knew more about their disease.

The goals for the course were: a) the person with arthritis would be able to do exercises and use modalities at home; b) the participants would increase their knowledge of joint protection and energy conservation measures and they would be able to practice these measures at home between classes; c) participants would increase their knowledge of the disease process; d) both patient and family would learn about theories of adaption to chronic disease or crisis; and, e) participants would be more aware of resources available in the community.

Over the 2-1/2 years the course has been in operation, we have found that the following features of class structure work particularly well. First, the family is strongly encouraged to attend. Second, all instructors are periodically updated on the content of classes taught by others to encourage uniformity and to allow for effective staff backup. Third, although the class discussions often cover popular material, the classes themselves focus on basic material. Patients are encouraged to join the local arthritis club for continued support and to learn about topics of current interest. Fourth, we try to schedule occasional "reunion" groups to reinforce the material and answer questions. When the class members have been retested it has been documented that the material taught has been fairly well retained, and that people with arthritis are continuing with some but not all of the measures taught. Fifth, allied health professionals

have been able to attend the classes to increase their knowledge of arthritis, and treatment measures. The length and duration of the sessions seems to be well tolerated.

Program logistics: To keep the cost of the program low, available resources were used as much as possible. The Hospital provided space (the therapy department after closing time), a small fund of money for reimbursement of teaching time, and a commitment toward developing a community program. The rheumatologists at our facility support the classes through referrals and review of class materials. A former class member teaches about community resources, and schedules people who have been referred to the class. Eventually, exploration of funding sources uncovered a local foundation, which provided funds for non-expendable materials, e.g., slide projector, paraffin unit, etc.

Through these classes we have been able to reach many more people than would be possible within the hospital setting and they appear to benefit from the group experience. We found we could provide a needed service at a reasonable cost to the consumer. Prior to this experience we would have said this kind of program would be possible only with a grant or other funding, not as an outgrowth of an existing program at a communit hospital.—*Suzanne Guthrie, OTR, O'Connor Hospital, San Jose, CA.*

Physical Disabilities
Special Interest Section Newsletter; Vol. 2, No. 4, 1979

Hands on: Prosthetics

Effective Function! That is the goal of the occupational therapy program at the Child Amputee Prosthetics Project (CAPP) at UCLA.[1] Joanna Patton, OTR, and Susan Clarke, OTR, are working with a team of other health professionals to establish a basic model for habilitation of limb-deficient children. An important goal of the CAPP program is the education of professional personnel to carry out the techniques developed at CAPP. For occupational therapy, this includes teaching others to provide direct services to clients and to intervene as the client's advocate, teacher and supporter in the community.

Two Principles of the CAPP Treatment Model

1. Clients should be helped to achieve goals consistent with the normal growth and development process. Since most limb-deficient children develop at the same rate and sequence as normal children, occupational therapists present tasks consistent with developmental norms and individual interests to teach children to operate prostheses and to apply skills to daily activities.

For example, children are taught to operate the terminal device when they are interested in holding objects with it. If the child has a prosthesis during his early life, he will usually incorporate it into activities at each developmental stage.

2. Clients should be encouraged to use artificial limbs only if they enhance function and are accepted by the amputees. It is surprising to many people that prostheses do not always provide amputees with the most effective way to function. Most of the time, a prosthesis offers an alternate way of functioning, and the amputee needs to develop skills and habit patterns with the prosthesis that are sufficiently advanced so that he can make an informed decision about the role of a prosthesis in his life.

Specific Functions of the Occupational Therapist

1. *Patient Services:* The occupational therapists monitor the child's development and help parents to see their child's progress in relation to the achievements of other normal children. Therapists evaluate the amputee's needs for a prosthesis. They orient the family and the amputee to available components, and to the implications of choosing between the available alternatives. Therapists then contribute information to the prescription conference so that components selected will meet functional needs.

After a prosthesis has been made, the occupational therapists participate in the evaluation of the limb, especially to see if it functions as intended by the prescription and

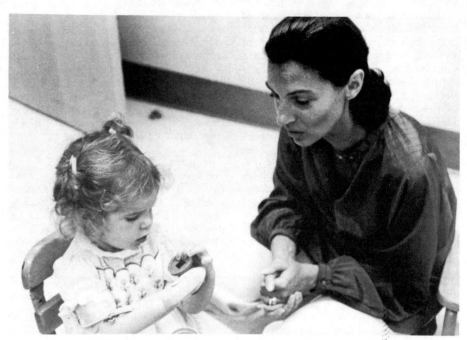

Joanna Patton, OTR, has been a clinical occupational therapist at the Child Amputee Prosthetics Project at UCLA for seven years. Her responsibilities include direct patient care, teaching and writing.

the overall treatment plan. Therapy sessions then are planned to help the client develop practical prosthesis wearing patterns, to orient the client and family to methods of caring for the prosthesis and recognizing the need for repairs. Instruction in operation of the controls and active use of the prosthesis are accomplished by presenting purposeful activities which encourage the amputee to work out practical solutions by "creative problem solving". This means that the therapist gives cues and suggestions on ways to perform the task, but methods are chosen by the amputee himself.

One of the most important services of the occupational therapist is helping the client and his family develop confidence in dealing with the public so that the amputee will not be excluded from opportunities to participate in community programs and to reach occupational goals.

2. *Teaching Programs:* Lectures, demonstrations and practice sessions are provided to occupational therapists in treatment centers in California and other western states. Much of the teaching is conducted for therapists in the public schools, where the local therapists can facilitate the child's ability to function in a classroom with nonhandicapped students. Also, Occupational Therapy for the Limb Deficient Child, a comprehensive three-day workshop is presented annually. In addition, teaching includes a unit on prosthetics at each of the local occupational therapy schools annually.

Some teaching programs are conducted jointly with other team members. Programs are planned for nurses, physicians, physical therapists, teachers and counselors. Also, occupational therapists attend three other child amputee clinics in California serving as consultants on overall management of patients. Teaching is also provided through writing articles and contributing sections to publications, such as the new edition of the book, "The Limb Deficient Child," which will be ready for publication in the near future.

Public education involves giving information to newspaper and magazine reporters for feature stories, and explaining about habilitation of amputees to philanthropic groups. Although sometimes time consuming, this has proved to be a valuable part of the teaching program.

The CAPP Research Program

In addition to the program for patient services and teaching described above, there is a research program at CAPP to design, develop and test new components for limb deficient children.[2] Carl Sumida, CPO, designs all of the new components and develops prototypes for testing. Julie Shaperman, MA, OTR, FAOTA, organizes and oversees the clinical testing program. A number of new components developed at CAPP have already become available as production items. Most recently, the CAPP

(continued)

Prosthetics

Terminal Device, Size No. 1, completed the design, development and testing program; it is now in production. The Size No. 2 CAPP Terminal Device is now in development and should be ready for testing in approximately one year. An active clinical testing program of two other components is being completed. These are the CAPP Two-Way Shoulder Joint and the CAPP Multi-Position Post.

The CAPP Terminal Device, Size No. 1, offers an alternative type of grasping device to children from infancy through 8 to 10 years of age. The terminal device has a wide frictional resilient covering which is somewhat compressible, like human soft tissue, to hold objects securely without requiring excessively strong pinch force or precise positioning. These features are well suited to the developmental abilities of young children. Also, the shape of the terminal device has a flowing line to blend with the forearm as a continuous unit. The voluntary operating mechanism uses a braided dacron control line which can be routed either for center pull or outside pull. The CAPP Terminal Device was tested extensively by children in 20 centers.

The CAPP Two-Way Shoulder Joint was designed to give patients a very narrow, cosmetic shoulder contour. It can be used with either a two-way humeral module (for flexion-extension and abduction motions) or with a one-way humeral module (for flexion-extension only). The friction control mechanisms are designed for reliability and fine adjustment. The joint was made as a complete, covered unit to give the prosthesis a finished look and to assure the patient a narrow shoulder contour. It can be assembled to endoskeletal or conventional laminated prostheses. Testing to date has included children from 2 through 19 years of age in 4 clinics. The shoulder joint has been applied with a variety of other components, mechanical and electrical. Although testing of the CAPP Two-Way Shoulder Joint is nearly completed, some prototypes with the one-way humeral module are still available for testing from CAPP.

The CAPP Multi-Position Post was designed to provide selective sizes of grasp for partial hand amputees. The post has a manual push-button mechanism which allows the amputee to place the opposing piece at varying distances from the palm of the hand. The testing program to date has included 35 amputees (children and adults) in 9 clinics besides CAPP. The design and development staff has been surprised to find such a large number of clinics and patients requesting this component in so short a time after a single announcement of availability. Early results of testing indicate that the concept of the device is valid; most patients found the CAPP Multi-Position Post acceptable and functionally beneficial, although some features need revision. The large and

enthusiastic demand for the CAPP Multi-Position Post makes it important to proceed with these revisions so the post can become widely available. (See photo)

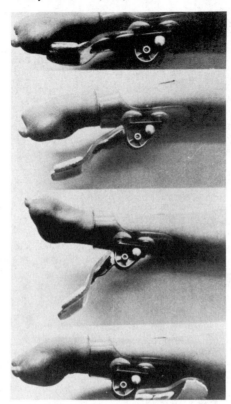

[1] Supported by Training Grant No. 204, Maternal and Child Health Services, Department of Health, Education and Welfare.

[2] Funded by Grant No. MC-R-060004, Bureau of Maternal and Child Health-Research, Community Health Services, Department of Health, Education and Welfare.

Bibliography: Upper Limb Prosthetics

Journals

Bulletin of Prosthetics Research: Publication of Rehabilitative Engineering Research and Development Service, Department of Medicine and Surgery, Veterans Administration, Office of Technology Transfer, Veterans Administration, 252 Seventh Ave., New York, NY 10001. Published twice yearly. Contains in-depth reports of current research on externally powered components for adult amputees. See issues for 1970 (Spring and Fall), 1971 (Fall), 1972 (Spring and Fall), 1973 (Spring), 1975 (Fall), 1976 (Fall) and 1977 (Spring).

Inter-Clinic Information Bulletin: Publication of Assn. of Children's Prosthetic and Orthotic Clinics. prepared by Department of Prosthetics and Orthotics, New York University, Post-Graduate Medical School, 317 East 34th St., New York, NY 10016. Published bimonthly. Contains clinically oriented articles, many by occupational therapists, on treatment of limb deficient children and other orthopedically handicapped children. Some references by topic are:
Training Techniques—1970 (June), 1975 (Sept.-Oct.), 1976 (Nov.-Dec.)
Sports for Amputees — 1970 (April, Nov.-Dec./ Bowling), 1971 (Jan./Badminton), 1973 (Oct./ Skiing), 1975 (June/Hockey), 1977 (May-June/Camping)
Musical Instruments—1974 (July), 1972 (March, December)
Bathing and Hygiene—1970 (Feb.), 1975 (July-Aug.), 1976 (May-June)
Components—1972 (April/Munster socket), 1973 (March/Partial Hand, June/ACAC Electric Hook), 1974 (Jan./Simulated Prosthesis, March/Myoelectrics,

Sept./Hands), 1977 (Jan.-Feb./Three-State Myoelectrics, Shoulder Joint), 1978 (May-June/Thumb Device, Universal TD)
Psychosocial Development—1973 (May), 1975 (July-Aug.), 1976 (May-June), 1978 (Jan.-Feb.)
Cases with extensive limb deficiencies—1972 (Nov.), 1975 (July-Aug.), 1976 (May-June, July-Aug., Sept.-Oct.), 1977 (Nov.-Dec.)

Prosthetics and Orthotics International: Publication of the International Society for Prosthetics and Orthotics, National Centre for Training and Education in Prosthetics and Orthotics, University of Strathclyde, 73 Rottonrow, Glasgow G4, ONG, Scotland. Published three times yearly: April, August, December. Contains articles on new developments in prosthetics and orthotics from many countries. See 1978 (April/Italy, August/Japan and Partial Hands—USA).

Professional Journals

American Journal of Occupational Therapy, 1971 (June), 1974 (July), 1975 (Aug.), 1977 (May, Sept.), 1979 (May).
Archives of Physical Medicine and Rehabilitation, 1974 (Feb.), 1978 (March)
Canadian Journal of Occupational Therapy, 1977 (March)
Orthotics and Prosthetics, 1972 (Sept./External Power Applications), 1974 (March/Bilaterals), 1975 (March/Children), 1976 (March/Partial Hand)

Books

Bender, LF: *Prostheses and Rehabilitation After Arm Amputation,* Springfield, IL: Charles C. Thomas, 1974
Blakeslee, B (Ed.): *The Limb Deficient Child,* Berkeley, CA: University of California Press, 1963. In revision, Second Edition will be published by Charles C Thomas, Springfield, IL.
Friedmann, LW: *The Psychological Rehabilitation of the Amputee,* Springfield, IL: Charles C Thomas, 1978.
Klopsteg, PE and Wilson PH: *Human Limbs and Their Substitutes,* New York, NY: Harper Company, 1968.
Leavy, JD: *It Can Be Done,* PO Box 515, Lake Almanor Peninsula, CA 96137
Roskies, E: *Abnormality and Normality, the Mothering of Thalidomide Children,* Ithica and London: Cornell University Press, 1972
Swinyard, CA (Ed.): *Limb Development and Deformity,* Springfield, IL: Charles C Thomas, 1969
Talbot, Darlene: *The Child with a Limb Deficiency: A Guide for Parents,* Los Angeles, CA: Child Amputee Prosthetics Project, 1979

Films

A Day in the Life of Bonnie Consolo, 1974, 16 min, 16mm sound, color. Available from Arthur Barr Productions, Inc., PO Box 5667, Pasadena, CA 91107. (Shows a woman, born without arms as she goes through a typical day)
2,3 Fasten Your Ski, 1972, 20 min, 16mm sound, color. Available from Denver Childrens' Hospital, Handicapped Sports Program, 1056 E. 19th Ave., Denver, CO 80218. (Ski program for amputees)
The CAPP Terminal Device, 1978, 12 min, 16mm sound, color. Available from UCLA Media Center Library, Royce Hall 8, 405 Hilgard Ave., Los Angeles, CA 90024. (New child's terminal device)
Shari, 1978, 15 min, 11mm sound, color. Available from UCLA Media Center Library, Royce Hall 8, 405 Hilgard Ave., Los Angeles, CA 90024. (Triple amputee, age 16, uses feet and prosthesis for daily activities)
Wendy, 1973, 30 min, 16mm sound, color. Available from Area Child Amputee Center, 235 Wealthy Street, SE, Grand Rapids, MI 49503. (Bilateral upper limb amputee, age 12, demonstrates extreme agility in daily activities)
Musical Instruments for the Limb Deficient Child, 1972, 8 min, 16mm sound, color. Available from UCLA Media Center Library, Royce Hall 8, 405 Hilgard Ave., Los Angeles, CA 90024. (Upper limb amputees play various instruments)
The Infant to School Age Child, 1964, 15 min, 16mm, black & white, sound. Available from UCLA Media Center Library, Royce Hall 8, 405 Hilgard Ave., Los Angeles, CA 90024. (Unilateral below-elbow amputees fitting and training procedures for children)

Myoelectrics Today

By Elaine Trefler, OTR, assistant professor, College of Community and Allied Health Professions, University of Tennessee.

Much has been written on myoelectric controls for artificial limb components. In 1960, the first practical myoelectrically controlled components were fitted in Russia, a system developed by Kobrinsky. Since then, several systems have become commercially available in the United States. Also, the Rehabilitation Institute in Montreal and the University of New Brunswick in Fredericton, Canada, have developed systems and made them available on a limited basis.

There is no dispute that the technology is available. Both the two-state and the three-state systems controlling electric hands, elbows and wrist rotators are being worn by amputees throughout the world. A two-state control is an on-off system. This means that one muscle site controls one function. In order to operate a prosthetic component, such as a hand, with a two-state system, the amputee would need two muscle sites—one to open the hand and one to close it. On the other hand, a three-state system has three levels; off, first and second. To operate a prosthetic component, such as a hand with a three-state system, the amputee needs only one control site; off, slight contraction to close the hand, and a strong contraction to open the hand.

As occupational therapists, our major concern is to determine when to recommend a system, and what type of system is most appropriate for our patients. Myoelectrically controlled prostheses are at least twice as expensive as standard artificial arms. They require more patient care in order to maintain constant performance. They also necessitate the use of heavier, more costly, and often more maintenance-prone components.

Then, why bother fitting myoelectrically controlled limbs? There are a number of important advantages of these systems which should be considered. With a forequarter and other high level amputees, the loss of muscle strength and excursion precludes the use of a standard prosthesis in a really functional manner. With myoelectrically controlled components, the amputee can functionally operate both an electric hand and elbow if indicated. Minimal body motions are required if the patient has learned to control the muscle sites under the electrodes. See Case No. 1 below.

In the case of the unilateral amputee who either dislikes or cannot tolerate a harness, a suction socket or "Munster" type of socket combined with myoelectric controls will allow for both suspension and component operation without any harness. See Case No. 2 below. The Otto Bock Z-6 Hand, the size

worn by pre-teen and teenaged children, has approximately 18-20 pounds of pinch force while a mechanical hook's pinch force is less than half of that.

Perhaps even more important than technical and financial factors are the human factors in selecting myoelectric controls. The amputee must really want a myoelectric system. That is, he must have a higher level of "gadget tolerance," and he must be able to establish good control over the number of muscle sites required to operate the prosthetic components. Since occupational therapists work with patients to select and develop skill in controlling muscle sites, and then teach patients to use prostheses in daily activities, therapists are in an especially good position to observe and influence these factors.

As with any prescription for a prosthesis, there are many important considerations in the selection of myoelectrically controlled components. The more committed the patient and the team to the use of myoelectric controls, the higher the success rate.

Case No. 1: Rocky, age 19 years. Diagnosis: Malignant histiocytoma resulting in forequarter amputation in August 1975. Fitting: Endoskeletal (Otto Bock) forequarter prosthesis with University of New Brunswick three-state myoelectric controls for an OCCC Electric Elbow and Otto Bock Hand. Control sites are the middle trapezius for operation of the hand, and remnant fibers of the latissimus dorsi for operation of the

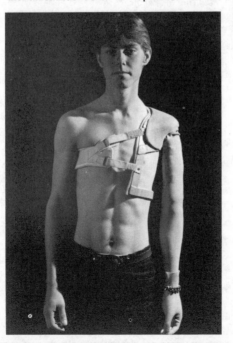

elbow. Since the middle trapezius was the control site with the best contraction, it was used to operate the hand—the most frequently used component. The operation of the hand with the three-state system uses the strong contraction to open the hand, as this allows quick release of objects without the worry of selecting a mid-range control. The prosthesis was fitted in February 1977. See pictures this page. Functional Result: Rocky works full time on the maintenance crew of a golf course. He wears a shoulder cap when doing heavy chores and tractor work, but he wears his prosthesis at all other times.

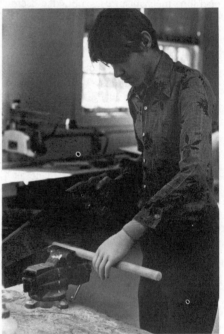

Case No. 2: Nancy, age 14 years. Diagnosis: Left below-elbow amputee due to a benign tumor at age 3 years. Fitting: Modified "Munster" type of below-elbow prostheses with Otto Bock Hand (two-state system). Control sites are on the radial and ulnar parts of the stump to avoid interference from elbow flexors. Previously, nancy had worn a prosthesis with a hook terminal device. Functional Result: Nancy wears her arm all waking hours and incorporates it in a dynamic bimanual approach to hand skills. She likes the appearance of her myoelectric hand, but even more, she enjoys not having to wear any harness.

Both of these individuals were carefully chosen to receive myoelectric components because of their functional needs as well as

(continued)

Myoelectrics Today

their concern for aesthetics. Neither has had any serious mechanical problems with the prosthesis in more than three years of wear. Occupational therapists who understand the advantages and requirements of myoelectric prostheses can offer a valuable service to amputees.

BIBLIOGRAPHY

Scott, R.N. "Myoelectric control of prostheses," *Archives of Physical Medicine and Rehabilitation*, 47:3, 174-181, 1966.

Childress, D.S., et al. "Myoelectric immediate postsurgical procedure: a concept for fitting the upper extremity amputee," *Artificial Limbs*, 13:2, 55-60, 1969.

Kay, H., et al. "The Munster-type below-elbow socket, a fabrication technique," *Artificial Limbs*, 9:2, 4-25, 1965.

O'Shea, B. "Research in prosthetics in New Brunswick," *Canadian Journal of Occ. Therapy*, 35:3, 92-97, 1968.

Physical Disabilities
Special Interest Section Newsletter; Vol. 2, No. 4, 1979

The Upper Limb–Deficient Child: A Brief Review of Treatment Strategies and Modifications as the Child Grows

By Felice Celikyol, OTR, director of Occupational Therapy, Kessler Institute for Rehabilitation, West Orange NJ 07052

The importance of providing activities which coincide with the child's developmental level rather than chronological age is well known to therapists treating children. The occupational therapist working with the limb-deficient child must be able to identify readiness levels and match these to the necessary mechanical requirements needed for operating the prosthesis. Therapists need to be attentive to parental attitudes toward the child and the prosthesis. When possible and appropriate, the parents should be allowed to participate in the problem-solving and decision-making process concerning the prosthesis and therapy strategies for their child.

Treatment strategies and goals for the unilateral upper limb child amputee are discussed here, since these are the children most frequently seen in clinics by occupational therapists.

Sensorimotor Period (to age 1 1/2 years)
The primary goal is acceptance of the prosthesis. Parental attitudes and expectations will determine the child's acceptance or rejection of the prosthesis at this stage. Therapists should educate parents as to types of prostheses available which are suitable to their child's level of amputation, using samples, photographs and films if available. Also, parents should be introduced to parents of other children having similar limb deficiencies to allow them to share experiences, discuss common problems and offer mutual support.

For the child, the prime goal in the sensorimotor period is assimilation of the prosthesis into the body scheme as an extension of his own limb. Early fitting and full time wearing is recommended to ensure acceptance. The age of choice for the initial fitting, by most clinics, is 6 months of age, or when sitting balance has been attained, since visually *controlled* reaching occurs normally at approximately 5 months of age. (Some

clinics advocate fitting as early as 3 months of age.)

Therapy Strategies: Parents are the prime trainers at this stage, with frequent clinic visits initially, followed by visits at approximately three-month intervals. During these beginning sessions, it may be necessary to review instructions given at previous visits not only because parents are unfamiliar with prosthetic components, but because initial anxiety may cloud their attention to details. Parents should become thoroughly familiar with the prosthesis, its care, as well as skin care. The child will probably be first fitted with a prosthesis having no cable attachment to the terminal device. The parents will be expected to pre-position all joints, including operation of the terminal device at this early stage, and to place objects into it. Gradually, the child should be encouraged to place objects in the hook while it is held open for him. Bilateral gross motor activities are appropriate at this time, as in grasping large balls or blocks, for encouraging natural, spontaneous use.

Pre-School Period (1 1/2 to 4 years)
Instilling motivation for prosthesis *use* is the prime goal, since cable attachment is provided now. For most children, the focus is still on terminal device use only. Treatment sessions should be scheduled at the child's "peak" time and not when he is tired and apt to reject training. The parents are still very much involved in the training process, e.g., the therapist actively moves the prosthesis in position for terminal device opening and instructs the parents to use this technique until the child understands this concept. An object can be placed in the terminal device for the child while he is encouraged to release it at a pre-determined area, such as dropping a block into a container. Bilateral gross motor activities are still appropriate and static holding—such as

is required for holding handle bars of push scooter, tricycles and swings—can be encouraged to instill spontaneous use. Remember that the child must appreciate the value and purpose of the prosthesis in order to use it spontaneously. Eventually, terminal device selective opening can be taught using toys and objects of varied sizes and shapes. The child can be taught to don and remove the prosthesis, or at the very least, to assist.

The therapist should consider having group treatment sessions of 2 or 3 children. This approach can be most rewarding for parents who can then share experiences with other parents.

Early School Age Period (4 to 10 years)
Therapy Strategies: This is the time to emphasize more skilled use. Terminal device pre-positioning can be taught, and the child with an above-elbow deficiency can learn elbow control. Emphasis should be on activities which are commensurate with the child's level of development, including such desk skills and self-care skills as tying laces and cutting food. If the parents report that the child is reluctant to participate in sports activities in school, the child should be given the opportunity to experiment with the activity in the clinic to eliminate fear of failure. Parents may also wish to discuss musical instruments appropriate to the child's capabilities.

In addition to periodic individual treatment sessions (usually at 3-to 6-month intervals), group sessions can be very helpful to the *child* at this stage. Exposure to children with similar deficiencies may make the child place greater value on independence (if this is a problem) in order to "keep up" with his peers.

School Visits: During early school years, the child is strongly influenced by his teachers. Therefore, contact with the

(continued)

The Upper Limb-Deficient Child

teacher, even before the child enters school, can be a great help to the child. The teacher should understand the use of prosthetic components, have realistic expectations for the child's function in the classroom, and, if necessary, help lessen the child's apprehension. The therapist may also want to visit the school, particularly if parents have accepted minimal responsibility for encouraging prosthesis use, because the teacher can then become a primary source of encouragement for the child.

Adolescence

Cosmesis often becomes of paramount importance to the adolescent, and a functional prosthesis may be rejected in favor of a cosmetic limb. This occurs frequently with the unilateral amputee who can function well as a one-handed invidiual. One answer in this situation is to prescribe a functional prosthesis with special features that emphasize cosmesis, such as a functional hand or an endoskeletal prosthesis. Therapy strategies for the adolescent are to increase skill and

speed, especially in self-care skills such as homemaking and grooming.

As the child grows, he is expected to take on more responsibilities, and he should be permitted to make the choice of what type of prosthesis he prefers and if, in fact, he wants one at all. It is the therapist's responsibility, with the clinic team, to expose the parents and child to the appropriate prostheses and to teach them its value, but the parents, and later on, the child, should make the final choice.

Physical Disabilities
Special Interest Section Newsletter; Vol. 2, No. 3, 1979

Hands on: Spinal Man

By Penny Machmer

The treatment of patients in groups is not a new technique in rehabilitation. Occupational therapists in psychiatric settings have used groups very successfully and much has been written concerning group treatment for other disabilities such as amputees, multiple sclerosis, CVAs, sensorimotor integration and developmental disabilities.

In the rehabilitation of spinal cord injuries, patient groups are frequently used in the counseling aspect of their program, but there is very little in the literature describing or indicating that groups, or classes as I will call them, are used extensively in the physical rehabilitation of the paraplegic or quadriplegic.

I will attempt to explain here how the Occupational Therapy Department, together with other disciplines at Craig Hospital, use classes/groups successfully in treating spinal cord injuries.

I believe a large part of our success can be attributed to the milieu in which we function. It is one in which the patients are not considered to be "sick" individuals. Once stabilization and other medical problems are under control, patients are up in their wheelchairs, dressed in their own clothes, and expected, as their sitting tolerance and endurance increase, to be up and involved in therapy the entire day.

Generally, the patients do not have rigid schedules for therapy. Patients are usually treated by both occupational therapy and physical therapy in one large "gym." Each patient is given the responsibility, once his or her program is underway, of getting to therapy, asking for assistance for a set-up when independent strengthening is possible and attending assigned classes.

Those of us who work in spinal cord injury rehabilitation many times play a larger role as educators than we do as therapists, in the

traditional sense. We teach our patients why they must continually be concerned with their skin. We help to educate them about bowel and bladder management, and work with the team in helping them to make decisions. We introduce them to various orthoses, show them how to use adaptive equipment, some of which may be extremely specialized, and ultimately encourage them to decide whether they are comfortable in using the adaptive equipment.

The patients, in all aspects of spinal cord injury, become the "experts." Patients are encouraged to learn about their injuries with the changes that result, how to function within their disabilities, to teach others to provide the care they cannot, to learn how to prevent unnecessary complications, and how to modify the plan of care if the need arises.

How are we able to carry out this immense job of education in the short three to four months that each paraplegic or quadriplegic spends at our facility?

We have found that by using groups or "classes," patients provide support for each other and learn from each other in ways that would otherwise not be possible. Group therapy tends to be more dynamic than individual therapy and also allows patients to assert their independence and self-identity. We believe in using groups not only for patient education, counseling, and socialization, but also for exercise and learning and practicing techniques taught during individual therapy sessions.

The major group that the Occupational Therapy Department is responsible for meets for 45 minutes, four times a week, with a special class or outing on Fridays. It is labeled "Chair Class," differentiating it from a class the physical therapists hold daily, which is called "Mat Class."

This class changes occasionally in that its

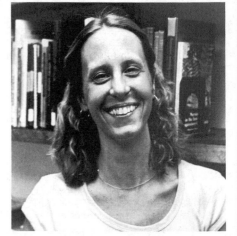

Penny Machmer *has been working at Craig Hospital for four years, two of which were in a supervisory capacity. Her experience before Craig consisted of pediatric and homebound adult rehabilitation. She is a graduate of Colorado State University.*

Craig Hospital is the Rocky Mountain Regional Spinal Cord Injury Center. It is an 80-bed rehabilitation hospital located in Englewood, CO.

organization and format are restructured and improved upon but the objectives of the class remain fairly consistent. I will list them first, not necessarily in any order of importance, and then further explain how the groups are run.

OBJECTIVES:

1. Strengthen available musculature, with concentration on neck, shoulder girdle, and upper extremities.
2. Improve balance in the wheelchair for both improved mobility and use in other functional activities, in and out of the wheelchair.
3. Acquaint patient with the wheelchair, its removable parts, maintenance of the chair, and/or to become capable in instructing others in all of the above (to include electric wheelchair).

(continued)

Spinal Man

4. Increase body mobility in the wheelchair, and to be able to instruct others in repositioning them in the chair.
5. Increase endurance and wheelchair mobility through wheeling increasing distances over smooth and rough terrain.
6. Teach patients to instruct others in safely managing the wheelchair over rough terrain, over curbs, ramps, and stairs.
7. Teach skin precautions (i.e., clothing, heat, cold) and various methods of shifting weight in the chair.
8. Instruction and practice in dressing skills, hygiene, and homemaking.
9. Socialization and group interaction.
10. Teach methods of relaxation; discuss and teach methods to increase vital capacity.
11. Acquaint patients with community resources, organizations for the disabled, public transportation, and how they may locate or obtain assistance once back in their own community.
12. Through outings into the community acquaint patients with architectural barriers, allow them experiences in relating to the public from a wheelchair and opportunities to practice skills learned in the hospital.

Because higher-level wheelchair skills for the paraplegics are taught by the physical therapists, the majority of those patients in our classes are quadriplegics. Paraplegics may start out in the occupational therapy class for beginning strengthening and endurance, as well as some of the more advanced homemaking skills, but normally they will not continue in the class.

The Chair Classes are divided into two groups which run concurrently. The classes are co-led by therapists who plan the week around a specific theme or set of objectives. Each patient is put in the group most appropriate for him or her, depending on the level of injury and needs at that point in the program. Sometimes the classes are beginning and advanced in nature (i.e., exercise, ADL skills) allowing a patient to progress from one class to another, depending on his or her level of injury.

A somewhat newer format allows for patients of all levels to be in one group that may be discussing vocational possibilities, how to hire an attendant, skin precautions in hot weather, or to be responsible for planning and setting up that week's outing.

On Fridays, when our classes are not scheduled for an outing into the community, the classes are somewhat less structured and include more "socialization." Nonetheless, they are geared toward patients using skills they have learned or in encouraging them to experiment with new ones. These activities may include:
1. Volleyball, using a large lightweight beach ball.
2. Table games or recreation room activities, encouraging use of hand braces and mouthsticks (i.e., checkers, ping-pong, monopoly, pool.)
3. Group cooking experiences (i.e., pizzas, ice cream sodas, or cookie decorating.)
4. Relays of various kinds.
5. Games such as charades and in-hospital scavenger hunts.

The "outings," as we call them, consist of 6 to 12 patients from the OT Chair Classes who are chosen by their therapists as appropriate for a particular experience, such as a movie, lunch at a restaurant, visiting an art or history museum, having a barbeque in the park, or taking a shopping trip to a nearby mall.

We are fortunate to have a bus and van available to us that can accommodate wheelchairs. Family members are frequently encouraged to accompany the patient. There is usually a staff/patient ratio of 1:2 depending on the number of higher-level quadriplegics and the nature of the outing. We encourage the patients to practice skills they have learned at the hospital, as well as wheeling themselves for increasing their endurance. Classes the following week may include discussions about the outing, problems with architectural barriers, and their feelings about interacting with the public from a wheelchair.

Besides the Chair Classes, other groups may be organized during a therapy day. A smaller group of patients on one floor may all need work on specific skills such as dressing or using hand braces for ADL, communication or simple homemaking skills. The group may consist of only three to four patients, but they will be set up together or gathered into a room where they can easily communicate and/or observe each other. Patients seem to communicate well in these smaller groups and learn well from each other. One therapist can frequently run this group, freeing up other therapists for needed one-to-one therapy with other patients.

Needless to say, Occupational Therapy is only one department that uses patient groups effectively for therapy and/or patient education. Physical Therapy, Nursing, Family Services, and Recreation Therapy all accomplish many of their goals through various types of classes and counseling groups.

In conclusion, I feel it is important to recognize that groups do not replace the necessary individual therapist-to-patient relationship, but we find groups to be extremely effective in treating and educating patients with spinal cord injuries. They are successful not only in the psychological benefit they provide (for patients and staff alike), but are also beneficial in increasing the amount of teaching and learning that can be accomplished in a set time period, with more effective use of staff time and improving the quality of patient care in our institution. — *Penny Machmer, OTR, Englewood, CO*

Physical Disabilities
Special Interest Section Newsletter; Vol. 2, No. 3, 1979

Spina Bifida: Areas of Concern

Spina bifida is the second most common birth defect. Eleven thousand affected U.S. children are born each year. The most serious form is spina bifida with myelomeningocele in which portions of the spinal cord, as well as its meningeal coverings and spinal fluid, protrude in a sac from the baby's back. Hydrocephalus is present in about 75 percent of these children, mental retardation in 25 percent. Because of modern shunting procedures which control the hydrocephalus, these children are surviving.

The goal of occupational therapy is to help the child with spina bifida achieve the maximum degree of independence, physically, socially, and later, economically. This independence is governed by the level and extent of the neurological deficit that determines the motor level, the sensory level, cortical function, and continence.

MOTOR LEVEL. Myelomeningocele can occur at any level of the spinal cord but is rare above the 10th thoracic. At T_{10} the child is a complete paraplegic with no sensation below the waist. The ultimate goal is complete independence in a wheelchair. At L_2 the child has hip flexors, and sensation interiorly down to the knees. The ultimate goal is complete independence in a

(continued)

Spina Bifida

wheelchair, but they may need to be extensively braced to perform limited ambulation. At L_4 the key motion present is knee extension. Sensation is present except in the buttocks area and the back of the legs. The goal is ambulation with AFOs. At S_1 key motions present are knee flexion, foot eversion and plantar flexion. These children are able to ambulate without orthoses. Sensation is still absent in the buttocks area and the back of the legs.

SENSORY LEVEL. Because of sensory deficits these children have a high risk of tissue trauma. Both parent and child will require education in skin care.

CONTINENCE. Since the nerves to the bowel and bladder are at the S_{3-5} level, incontinence is a major problem at all levels of impairment. Crede, intermittent catheterization, or other programs must be initiated.

DEVELOPMENT. It is of primary concern that children be assisted in meeting developmental milestones at appropriate age levels regardless of their ambulation status as adults. Attempts must be made to normalize the environment by providing orthoses and assistive devices to mobilize the child. Equipment such as scooter boards, trunk supports, caster carts, A-Frames, and parapodiums are used.

CORTICAL FUNCTIONS. In addition to hydrocephalus, a significant number of these children demonstrate perceptual problems and poor manipulative ability. The relationship of visual perception and ocular motor function to body movement, particularly hand movement, is documented. The lack of opportunity to manipulate objects in infancy, together with immobility, may contribute to the visual-spatial problems seen in some of these children. This may apply especially to those who have prolonged and repeated hospital admissions.

CONCLUSION. To the occupational therapist, striving for independence for the multiply handicapped, spina bifida presents many challenges, some of which are addressed above.—*Alice Bowker, MA, OTR, Little Rock, AR*

Physical Disabilities
Special Interest Section Newsletter; Vol. 2, No. 3, 1979

Tendon Transfers for Quadriplegics: Implications for Therapy

INTRODUCTION

The loss of grasp and pinch affects the functional abilities of quadriplegics. Traditionally, occupational therapists have used tenodesis splints, adapted equipment, and special techniques to improve levels of independence. However, these in themselves have limitations. A variety of surgical possibilities to improve hand function is available to quadriplegics at different levels.[1-3] One surgical option is the tendon transfers for a "strong C_6 quad" performed at the University of Minnesota Hospitals by Dr. James House, orthopedic surgeon[4]. The transfer of selected wrist and forearm tendons can restore active grasp, lateral pinch, and sometimes finger and thumb extension to C_6 quadriplegics. Criteria for selecting patients, a brief description of the surgery, and implications for therapy will be discussed.

SELECTION

Candidates for successful tendon transfer surgery must be carefully selected. First, the patient must have an adequate number of intact muscles, including the brachioradialis (BR), the extensor carpi radialis longus (ECRL), the extensor carpi radialis brevis (ECRB), and the pronator teres (PT). An intact flexor carpi radialis (FCR) is beneficial. Generally, patients must be at least one year post-injury to allow maximal physical return and adequate strengthening of these muscles. The use of tenodesis splints is encouraged at this center, both to strengthen key muscles and to develop tenodesis grasp. This action in grasping and releasing objects helps to develop a coordinated pattern that is consistent with desired hand function

post-surgery. Wrist and hand PROM must be maintained and spasticity absent. Patients should have protective sensation of thumb, index, and middle fingers. The one-year wait post-injury also allows patients time for psychological adjustment to their disability. Patients demonstrate the necessary motivation by their level of ADL independence and their vocational/avocational interests. Good candidates for surgery meet these criteria.

Since the tendon transfer surgery is optional, patients must understand the surgery, the hazards of the convalescent stage, and the expected outcome. A variety of media is used to educate prospective patients. During the patient's initial rehabilitation, the therapists informally discuss and explain the surgical possibilities. The patient and family view an educational film describing tendon transfers and showing a patient doing hand activities pre- and post-surgery. After the film, the therapist clarifies information and answers questions. Visiting with patients who have undergone tendon transfer surgeries is a most valuable experience for prospective patients.

SURGERY

Tendon transfer surgery[4] is done in two stages. In the *Extensor Phase*, the tendons of the extensor digitorum communis, the extensor pollicis longus, and the rerouted abductor pollicis longus are tenodesed to the distal radius to provide passive finger and thumb extension at the wrist flexes. Second, free tendon grafts routed through the lumbrical canals of the index and middle fingers help prevent metacarpal phalangeal (MCP) hy-

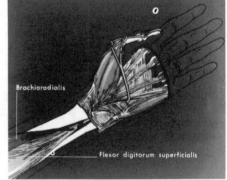

Figure 1

perextension and enhance interphalangeal extension as the wrist flexes. In the *Flexor Phase*, the ECRL is transferred to the flexor digitorum profundus to provide finger flexion. Its transfer removes a strong radial deviating force and is synergistic with finger flexion. The ECRB is maintained for wrist extension. The FCR, if present, is preserved to provide action wrist flexion. To develop a lateral pinch, the PT is transferred to the flexor pollicis longus, and the BR is transferred to form an adduction-opponensplasty (Figure 1). An alternative is a carpometacarpal (CMC) fusion of the thumb to provide thumb stability in the lateral pinch position. This is done when only two muscles are available for transfer in the flexor phase, or when the BR is used to provide active finger and thumb extension.

POST OP

The immediate post-surgery stage (approx-

(continued)

Tendon Transfers

imately 3-5 weeks) can be a frustrating and potentially hazardous time for patients. While the forearm is temporarily immobilized, patients often experience an increased dependence in ADLs and transfers, and have difficulty in weight shifting. Alternative wheelchair cushions that may assist in preventing skin breakdown may be explored and prescribed. A temporary wheelchair armrest extension, raising the height of the arm rest and assisting patients in performing pushups from their forearms has been constructed. If adequate shifting is impossible, patients must make plans for temporary assistance.

When the cast is removed, patients wear their half cast forearm shell for protection and receive therapy sessions twice a day for about one week. After the extensor phase of surgery, if the first CMC joint has been fused, a thumb post opponens splint is constructed to prevent movement in the joint and allow further healing. This splint positions the thumb in apposition and slight extension and allows full wrist extension. If the hand shows evidence of clawing, a temporary splint preventing MCP hyperextension (in 30 degree flexion) is constructed or combined with the thumb post opponens splint.

THERAPY

Occupational therapists and physical therapists, the orthopedic surgeon, and the physiatrist are involved in the program. The goals of therapy include improving ROM, strength, endurance, coordination, and the level of ADL independence.

AROM is the primary modality used to increase ROM, strength, and endurance during the first month. During the first week of therapy, the whirlpool is used to cleanse the wound, promote healing, and assist in AROM. While *GENTLE* PROM may be done, if it is too aggressive, the anastomized tendons may detach at this early stage. Biofeedback is used to assist the patient in learning the new function of the transferred muscles and to monitor progress. After the flexor stage of surgery, light hand activities are used to reinforce coordinated patterns for grasp and lateral pinch. More resistive activities, such as writing or shaving are begun after adequate healing.

A reassessment of ADL techniques and equipment is beneficial. Many pieces of adapted equipment are no longer necessary and more one-handed activities are possible. Patients often discard tenodesis splints, universal cuffs, and writing devices. Sometimes new equipment may enable patients to perform new tasks. To avoid undue stretch on the flexors, patients may need to learn new transfer techniques. Patients are encouraged to transfer with fingers flexed or relaxed over the surface edges instead of in full finger/wrist extension.

CONCLUSION

All patients, post-surgery, have obtained grip (2.7-9.1 kg) and lateral pinch (1.8-6.8 kg) readings where there was no recordable strength before surgery. Most patients have chosen to have surgery on their other arm to increase bilateral hand function. All patients have increased their speed in doing functional activities, decreased the amount of equipment necessary, and are pleased with their surgery results.

We wish to thank Dr. James House, Edna Maneval, and Jean Magney for their assistance.—*Virgil Mathiowetz, OTR and Mary Brambilla, OTR, Minneapolis, MN*

References

[1] Zancolli, E: Surgery for the Quadriplegic Hand with Active, Strong Wrist Extension Preserved—A Study of 97 Cases. *Clin Orthop* 112: 101, 1975.

[2] Moberg, E: Surgical Treatment for Absent Single-Hand Grip and Elbow Extension in Quadriplegia. *J Bone Joint Surg* 57A: 196, 1975.

[3] Freehafer, A.A., VonHaam, E., and Allen, V: Tendon Transfers to Improve Grasp After Injuries to the Cervical Spinal Cord. *J Bone Joint Surg* 56A: 951, 1974.

[4] House, J.H., Gwathmey, F.W., and Lundsgaard, D.K: Restoration of Strong Grasp and Lateral Pinch in Tetraplegia Due to Cervical Spinal Cord Injury. *J Hand Surg* 1: 2, 1976.

Physical Disabilities
Special Interest Section Newsletter; Vol. 2, No. 3, 1979

NYU Engineering Program: Clinical Evaluation of Electronic Assistive Devices

Since October 1974, the Institute of Rehabilitation Medicine, New York University Medical Center, has been conducting a formal clinical evaluation of electronic assistive devices. During the first three years, the investigation was limited to those devices that were operable by persons with spinal cord injury at or above the level of C-5. Scope of the project is currently inclusive of the total severely physically disabled population with continued emphasis on the high level quadriplegic. The multidisciplinary evaluation team includes a physiatrist, occupational therapists, electrical engineers and technicians, a psychologist, and a rehabilitation nurse.

The objective of the study is to determine the usefulness of specific devices within the rehabilitation of specific diagnostic populations. This is pursued via clinical evaluation of each device. All devices of a particular category are comparatively tested against one another as well as against any available traditional methods (i.e., mouthstick page turning).

Data are collected in the areas of electrical/mechanical device performance, patient operation characteristics, and patient acceptance of devices. All devices are initially evaluated in the occupational therapy electronics laboratory. Specifics of these devices are then tested bedside, at home, school, and on-the-job. This report is limited to our findings concerning the high-level quadriplegic population.

A total of 57 persons with high-level spinal cord injury have participated in the evaluation of a total of 31 devices including 11 environmental, 12 mobility, 4 typewriter, and 4 recorder/dictaphone control systems and 4 page turners. The typical participant was a young male of college age with a C-4,5 level of lesion. Age ranged from 16-65 years, lesion levels from C-1 to C-6,7. Most patients were within 12 months post-onset.

Patient preference between devices primarily concerned device performance reliability, ease of operation, and device features. The preferred environmental unit has been the Prentke-Romich ECU-1. A recent redesign of the Prentke-Romich ECU-2 has incorporated auditory feedback with a location marker, which permits total non-visual operation for hearing patients. The ECU-1 may, therefore, become an alternate to the ECU-1, with the deciding factor being one of cost, number of functions, and/or positioning requirements (ECU-1: $590/13 functions/remote display; ECU-2: $430/9 functions/built-in display—total unit must remain in view to see display).

The preferred telephone control has been the Prentke-Romich ADT-5B. The ADT-5B was preferred because of (1) the self-contained design which permits use of the

(continued)

NYU Engineering Program: Electronic Assistive Devices

telephone without a complete environmental system; (2) the option of both confidential handset and handsfree speakerphone listening/speaking; and (3) dialing of all digits.

For control of environmental devices, the highest level lesion patients (C-1/4) have preferred pneumatic controls for both in-bed and out-of-bed use. Slightly lower level lesion patients (C-4,5/5) have generally preferred use of pneumatic controls in-bed and manually operated pressure switches out-of-bed. The lowest level patients have usually preferred pressure switches for all locations.

The overall preferred mobility control system has been an IRM prototype 2-tube pneumatic system which permits total direction control plus continuously variable speed control. The preferred commercial system has been the MED 1-tube Breath Control system. The pneumatic mobility control systems have been preferred over short-throw systems due to cosmesis and greater ease of operation.

Mouthstick and BFP page turning were preferred over electric page turners. The MED/Brusse page turner was preferred over alternate units evaluated; however, application was considered limited to users who had need for considerable 1-direction reading (i.e., literature student).

Patients preferred mouthstick or BFO typing or standard electric typewriters over all of the typewriter systems evaluated. The systems were found to be either slower than traditional methods and/or overly complicated. Typewriters were positioned on inclined stands for mouthstick trials.

The results of psychological testing have indicated that there are no significant differences in psychological test results when comparing users to nonusers of equipment. However, when the activity patterns of both groups are compared, the users were significantly more active, spent more time performing educational activities, and were performing their activities more independently. Individuals exposed to reliable electronic devices during the one to six months post-onset period have a statistically greater probability of becoming users than do those individuals initially exposed to such equipment beyond six months.

A monograph has been prepared which details extensive findings regarding the evaluation of nine environmental units, four typewriter systems, and four page turners. This report, entitled *Environmental Controls and Vocational Aids for Use by High Level Quadriplegics*, is in the final stages of publication and will soon become available for purchase.—*Carol D. Stratford, OTR, Coordinator, Evaluation Project, OT Electronics Lab, RR 310, Institute of Rehabilitation Medicine, 400 East 34th St., New York, NY 10010.*

This work was supported in part by RSA grant 16-P-56801/2-16, Rehabilitation Research and Training Center RT-1 from the Rehabilitation Services Administration, Department of Health, Education and Welfare, WDC.

Physical Disabilities
Special Interest Section Newsletter; Vol. 2, No. 2, 1979

Starting and Financing a Small Business

Before starting a small business or private practice, the entrepreneur must have a very specific idea in mind as to the type of business, i.e. services or product. Writing a program description will help to consolidate ideas. Be as brief and uncomplicated as possible.

The next step is to be honest in analyzing one's motivation. Common motivations are the desire for personal fortune, fame, the desire to be one's own boss or the pure joy of success. Perhaps there are negative elements within the institution where the would-be entrepreneur is presently employed. Dible* identifies eight such elements: 1) inadequate communications, 2) inequity between major contributions and financial reward, 3) promotion and salary policies, 4) questionable employment security, 5) institution politics and nepotism, 6) red tape, 7) questionable relevant educational requirements, and 8) orphan projects, products or programs which are shelved.

The entrepreneur must be sure he has personal resources. Is he extremely competent in his area of specialty? Does he have the three D's: desire, determination, and dedication? Does he have sound knowledge and experience with the service to be offered? Does he have the ability to manage people and resources? Is there a firm and broad base of experience? Does he have

stamina and physical well-being? And lastly, does the entrepreneur have financial resources for such an undertaking?

Beginning with a prototype is highly recommended. Some therapists have started by seeing one or two private patients per week or consulting to one nursing home a month while maintaining their salaried full-time position. This enables one to deal gradually with the increased responsibility of both business and family life.

A well-rounded training program of keeping in good physical shape and maintaining a positive mental attitude will help lead to success. Involve your family, especially your spouse in some aspect of the business. Investigate community resources, college courses, books, and pamphlets regarding management and business. A public speaking course is always helpful. Speak to persons experienced in business such as vendors, bankers, and college faculty members. Entrepreneurs are their own best salespersons. Personality, attitude, and behavior are your best recommendations. Without these selling points your business card left behind for physicians or clients to remember you by, goes unnoticed.

The pro forma or business plan is often the most difficult prerequisite to meet. It is a document which describes in detail the proposed business. It is upon the strength of this document that decisions are made by the entrepreneur regarding the nature of the business and by those providing financial backing. The pro forma must convey optimism while being perfectly accurate. Include documentation of credibility with letters of reference and a letter stating the authority of the entrepreneur in the proposed area of service. What do you provide that no one else can in the present marketplace? State how much money is needed to operate the business for the first four to six months or until a profit is turned. When will a profit be seen? How much money will be turned back into the business? List potential customers or clients and analyze your major competitors. Who composes the staff, i.e. therapist, aide, secretary? Discuss the price of treatment relative to competitors. Decide on the legal structure of the business; sole proprietorship, partnership, or corporation.

A cash flow statement must be included in the pro forma. This is a business forecast for two or three years stating the projected number of treatments or services provided in each month and the charges. The entrepreneur must consider the reliability of the payment source, whether institution, individual, private insurance, industrial insurance, Medicare, or Medicaid. The income is balanced against the out-flow or expenses arriving at a profit and loss statement. This is the "Moment of Truth"!

(continued)

Small Business

To complete the pro forma, include a resume, any articles written by the entrepreneur on related topics, and any other letters of reference.

The final step is to take the pro forma to a financial source. Not everyone has the savings or stocks to start their own business. Some can approach family or friends. OTs have become partners with other OTs or a PT, depending on the laws of that state. Commercial banks and the Small Business Administration are the best resources. This author discourages approaching the referring physicians as it would involve them in a conflict of interest. There are some minority programs which have funds available for women, blacks, or Asians. The Veterans Administration has funds for veterans who meet specific qualifications.

The entrepreneur should read and study a great deal before embarking on such a venture. Don Dible's* text *Up Your Own Organization* is invaluable as well as palatable reading. The life of the entrepreneur is not for everyone and it is important that you be fully honest about your own qualifications and energies. — *Elizabeth Cauldwell-Klein, OTR*

POSITIVES OF PRIVATE PRACTICE

- One can make a higher hourly wage than when working for an institution. Consultants often bill from $25 to $30 per hour.

- More independence.

- Chance of growth with direct reward.

- Flexibility in scheduling working hours.

- Increased responsibility. It is your decision what equipment is purchased and what courses are attended.

- You will learn about the world of business.

Educational Resources For Starting A Private Practice:

1. Business, bookkeeping, accounting, economics, and management courses available at adult education programs, universities and university extensions, MBA programs.
2. General finance workshops provided by larger brokerage houses.
3. Small Business Administration offers workshops.
4. Community resources: attorney, accountant, retired businessmen, other therapists who have done a similar project.
5. Large banking firms have publications on financing small businesses.
6. Read paperbacks, texts, pamphlets, and how-to books on related topics.
7. Dible, Donald, *Up Your Own Organization*, Entrepreneur Press, San Jose, 1976.
8. Manor, Carol, *Activity Programs In Long Term Care Facility*, OT Department, Hyattsville, MD 20782
9. O'Sullivan, Nadine, and Livingston, Fran, *Occupational Therapy Consultancy In The Skilled Nursing Facility*, available from Fred Sammons, Inc.
10. Brasic, Charlotte, *Guidelines For Private Practice In Occupational Therapy*. Available from Occupational Therapy Services, 3858 Reading Rd., Cincinnati, OH 45229 with a check or money order for $4.00.

Physical Disabilities
Special Interest Section Newsletter; Vol. 2, No. 1, 1979

Neurodevelopmental Treatment Approach to Adult Hemiplegia

A Review of a two week workshop offered by Dr. and Mrs. Bobath at Duke University

Bobath treatment approach is based on the assessment of "motor patterns." Abnormal coordination is seen as the main problem for the patient with hemiplegia and, therefore, assessment of his coordination is of the utmost importance. In the spastic patient, abnormal patterning of muscle action is the result of abnormal postural reflex activity; the typical postural patterns being produced by the interaction of various released tonic reflexes. In the hemiplegic patient who demonstrates flaccidity, postural reflex activity is lacking or depressed.

The evaluation of the patient's postural patterns also involves that of his postural tone, i.e. of the strength and distribution of his spasticity. Following are the characteristics of spasticity as described by Bobath: 1. coordinated in definite patterns and produces abnormal and typical patterns of posture, 2. limits joint range of motion by exaggerated co-contraction, 3. increases with voluntary efforts through associated reactions, 4. changeable, 5. interferes with selective functional skills as muscle can act only in mass patterns, 6. prevents normal postural reactions, 7. creates an abnormal sensory feedback, 8. produces apparent muscle weakness.

Keeping in mind the above characteristics of spasticity, Mrs. Bobath tries to reduce spasticity in her treatment approach by: working against patterns of spasticity, breaking up mass patterns and introducing more selective ones, facilitating normal postural reactions in response to being moved as well as facilitating voluntary movements, and avoiding effort and counteracting associated reactions. Through all this she tries to give the patient normal sensory motor experience.

Watching Mrs. Bobath working with a patient is like watching a miracle happen in front of your eyes. She seems to have full control of the situation, putting the patient at ease in front of an audience of 300 or more. She gives the patient constant verbal feedback of right and wrong movements. Mrs. Bobath avoids words like push-pull, or an activity that would increase efforts on the patient's part and therefore increase muscle tone in the patterns of spasticity. While working on the leg, she is constantly observing the patient's posture and affected arm in order to avoid associated reactions. The reverse is true when she works on a patient's arm.

In using the Bobath treatment concept, I have found the following things very effective in my treatment approach:
1. In acute stages, participate in proper positioning along with other team members.
2. Begin the teaching of self ROM (with clasped hands and extended elbows), primarily to improve awareness of the affected side, improving body image through sensory feedback from sound hand, etc. The patient usually needs assistance of the therapist in the early stages.
3. While working on self-care activities, be aware of efforts required to perform activities that cause associated reactions and therefore increases tone in spastic patterns.
4. While concentrating on improving patient's one-handed skills do not keep the affected arm out of sight which would reinforce neglect of the affected side. Whenever possible try to encourage use of the affected arm and hand for assistive and/or supportive purposes.
5. While working on an activity with a patient in a wheelchair, avoid associated reactions and/or positioning of leg in flexion or extension pattern.
6. A work bench can be used instead of a wheelchair during therapy to improve sitting balance, to encourage use of affected arm for support and to include trunk rotation during an activity.
7. The above positioning can be combined and used with perceptual testing and training.

— *Charu Joshi,* OTR, North Carolina Memorial Hosp., Chapel Hill.

Occupational Therapy and the Heart Association— Two Experiences

The chapter of the American Heart Association (AHA) in the area in which I was working established a volunteer rehabilitation team on which I was the occupational therapy representative responsible for evaluating methods of community stroke education. The chapter provided secretarial services and knowledge of whom to contact in the community to support our ideas.

We tried newspaper articles, call-in radio programs, hospital meetings with the rehabilitation team, stroke patients and their families, and rehabilitation team meetings in a local community center for persons in that community interested in coming. Those who attended these meetings found them useful but we felt that too few people were reached through any of these methods to be practicable. Although it may seem irrelevant to list programs which did not work well, we learned a great deal about what not to do for future programs. We also found a great ally in the Heart Association for support of future programs.

Several years later and in another part of the country, I wanted to find some flexible, part-time work as an OT. I contacted the program director of the local chapter of the AHA and suggested we might work together to help the stroke patient in the community. I volunteered to plan a family education program if the Heart Association would provide the local contacts and supportive services. The result of this effort, as yet incomplete, is a program designed as a possible pilot for use by other Heart Association chapters.

Family members of patients discharged within three months and local nursing home personnel will attend one evening a week for four weeks. The program will include basic information about the disease and expectations of performance in transfers, bowel and urinary care, dressing, equipment, occupational and physical therapy services and the names and phone numbers of local rehabilitation and nursing personnel willing to answer specific questions about a particular problem. Hopefully, with improved family education more patients will go home instead of to nursing homes and the time and effort spent on rehabilitation will be preserved after discharge.

Much needs to be done for stroke patients. Community agencies might be willing to help with a little stimulation from occupational therapists.—*Gloria Furst*, OTR.

The Boomerang Club: The Development of a Stroke Club

Stroke patients and their families encounter many problems in management when the patient goes home from the hospital. Many times the patient is self-conscious of his weakness, speech, or emotional liability. All of the combined problems of self-care and socialization are not completely met before the patient is discharged from the hospital or from therapy. It was for these reasons that the Baylor University Medical Center chose to sponsor a stroke club.

It was decided that the club should be held in an informal setting. The advantages of this type program would be that the club would provide an opportunity for patients and their families to share management and home problems with others like them. It would also assist each member in overcoming common problems through sharing similar experiences. It would encourage the redevelopment of social skills for better integration into community life. It would also provide a learning opportunity about the process of strokes, how they happen, and what can be expected in the future.

In order to attempt the development of a program of this magnitude, it was necessary to first request permission from the administration of the Medical Center to sponsor such a program. The next step was to obtain approval and engage personnel from the Department of Physical Medicine. Receiving this backing, the proposal was then taken to the Medical Staff and the Medical Staff Committee on Stroke Care for their endorsement.

After receiving this approval, an executive committee and a steering committee were formed. These committees consisted of professional staff and a selected patient group. A meeting was held by these two committees and it was decided at this time to meet once a month on the third Thursday at 7:00 p.m. in the Occupational Therapy Department. There would be refreshments, a speech of interest to the group, and time for discussion and socialization.

The first meeting was held in September 1971 and the idea and purpose of forming a club was presented to a group of former patients and their families. Following the introduction, the group divided into several smaller groups to discuss the type of program that would be of most interest to them and to gather any other helpful information or suggestions. The attendance at the meeting, about 65 persons, was much greater than expected.

As the Boomerang Club began to develop, other stroke clubs in the country were contacted in order to gather information about their function and membership. A total of 25 clubs were contacted, covering the entire United States. The information received indicated that the structure of the Boomerang Club was much like the other clubs; and that our membership was larger than most. The information also indicated that it was one of the few totally hospital-sponsored clubs, but that the interests and activities appeared to be very much the same.

The Boomerang Club has now been in existence for eight years and has a membership roster of 275. The programs have been varied, consisting of the annual Christmas party, talks by almost all of the medical disciplines, public affairs, travel information and slides, celebrities visiting Dallas, protection of self and property, insurance claims and benefits, etc. The Boomerang Club has far surpassed the original expectations and has become an integral part of the community life of Dallas and the metroplex.—*Virginia G. Chandler*, OTR, Director of Occupational Therapy, Baylor University Medical Center, Coordinator, Boomerang Club, Dallas, TX.

Physical Disabilities
Special Interest Section Newsletter; Vol. 2, No. 1, 1979

Homonymous Hemianopsia—A Patient Family Education Program

St. Luke's Hospitals, Fargo, ND, utilizes the total care team approach for rehabilitation of the stroke patient. It was realized there was an important need to educate patients and their families about their illness. It was believed a better rehabilitation result would be gained through increasing the patient's and family's understanding of specific deficits caused by the stroke.

Several teaching programs were designed in collaboration with appropriate rehabilitation disciplines. Occupational therapy and nursing were the primary disciplines involved in the Homonymous Hemianopsia education program.

The Homonymous Hemianopsia teaching program consists of a teaching packet which includes: 1. A twenty minute audiovisual; 2. Flipchart on stroke; 3. Cardboard glasses; 4. Teaching checklist; 5. Statement of learning objectives; 6. Teaching guidelines for the patient and family.

The learning objectives are: 1. To state in personal terms the definition of Homonymous Hemianopsia; 2. To relate visual deficit to a specific cause; 3. To anticipate the predicted course of the visual deficit; 4. To demonstrate awareness of the visual deficit; 5. To compensate for visual field loss; 6. To recognize, after hospital evaluation and training, activities and situations that are unsafe; 7. To transfer hospital learning to home environment.

Additional patient family education programs for the stroke patient developed at St. Luke's Hospitals include: 1. Aphasia; 2. Anti-coagulant Therapy; 3. Body Scheme Disturbance (in the final stages of development).

These programs can be purchased from St. Luke's Educational Department. For

The teaching checklist is utilized by Nursing and Occupational Therapy:

TEACHING PLAN	TEACHING COMPLETED (date and signature)
NURSE	
1. Definition	1. _____
2. Cause	2. _____
3. Audiovisual "Homonymous Hemianopsia" shown (Dial Learning Resources.)	3. _____
4. Observe and reinforce compensation	4. Patient _____ Family _____
a. Eating	a. _____
b. Ambulating	b. _____
c. Reading	c. _____
5. O.T. Referral (Need Doctor's Orders)	5. _____
OCCUPATIONAL THERAPY	6. _____
6. Initial Contact	
7. Assessment of Self Care Activities	7. Compensates _____ Make Visual Errors _____
a. Feeding	a. _____
b. Dressing	b. _____
c. Grooming	c. _____
8. Assessment of Functional Activities	8. _____
a. Crafts	a. _____
b. Mobility	b. _____
c. Visual Compensation Exercises	c. _____
9. Assessment of Homemaking Activities	9. _____
a. Kitchen	a. _____
b. Other	b. _____
NURSE	
10. Audiovisual Repeated	10. Yes☐ No☐ Date _____
11. Safety Factors	11. _____
12. Post Test (given to patient and/or family)	12. _____
13. Referral	13. _____
a. Prior to Discharge	a. _____
b. Follow Up	b. _____

Family Included:

Comments:

further information please contact Jan Feder, RN, Patient Education Coordinator, St. Luke's Hospitals, 5th Street at Mills Avenue, Fargo, ND 58102.

—*Diane Kaiser*, OTR, Physical Disabilities Liaison, ND.

Physical Disabilities
Special Interest Section Newsletter; Vol. 1, No. 1, 1978

Hands on: A Therapist in Hand Therapy Practice

Georgiann F. Lassiter, OTR, was born in Oklahoma City and graduated from Texas Woman's University in Denton. She is currently president of the Texas Occupational Therapy Association and serves on the standing committee for the Physical Disabilities Specialty section. She is employed by two hand surgeons in private practice and is assisted by one COTA, carrying out treatment for 25 to 30 patients daily. Georgiann considers herself an OT first and a hand therapist second.

The concept of hand rehabilitation as a legitimate sub-specialty is rapidly growing. Many hand surgeons now recognize the valuable contributions well-trained "hand therapists" can make in obtaining optimum functional results in hand surgery cases. Thus, more and more occupational and physical therapists are finding employment opportunities in specialized and rehabilitation settings in medical centers and surgeons' offices.

The concept of a hand rehabilitation unit is not particularly new. In World War II, Bri-

tish and American surgeons realized that patients with severe hand injury or a poor response to injury could be helped by segregation in a controlled educational environment where exercise and functional activities could be encouraged by the therapist and fellow patients with hand problems. The hand surgeon, hand therapist and patient worked together as a team to restore mobility and sensitivity to the hand in order to return the person to his vocational and/or avocational pursuits as soon as possible.

(continued)

Hand Therapy Practice

The modern hand therapist is a specialized occupational or physical therapist who has received further training by the hand surgeon in the details of upper limb anatomy, hand physiology, pathology, surgical technique, wound healing and splinting. Because of this training, the therapist's skills complement those of the surgeon by *reinforcing, not replacing* his pre- and postoperative instructions and explanations. The therapist may be considered an actual extension of the surgeon, carrying out treatment programs in greater detail than his limited time will allow. In addition, the occupational therapist's special skills in motivational techniques, functional activities and splint making add to the surgical treatment to produce optimum results. The patient may also find it easier to relate his special problems or needs to the therapist in the informal atmosphere of the hand rehabilitation unit.

Most ailments or injuries of the hand are minor or transient; even many severe problems may resolve without the need for a hand rehabilitation unit if the patient is highly motivated, young, intelligent and has a favorable emotional and physiologic response to his problem. In some patients however, hand ailments cause a significant alteration in their lives. Their jobs may be threatened, the pain may be overwhelming and stiffness prolonged; independence may even be lost. It is this patient for whom the hand unit is designed. Patients of different ages, races, educational levels, and socioeconomic backgrounds are brought together experiencing one common bond—a hand problem or hand injury.

Treatment sessions, although carried out in group settings to give psychological support and to provide motivation through peer pressure, are highly individualized. The frequency of treatment in the hand unit also varies with the needs of each patient. He may come once a week or once a month. Depending upon his progress, he may stay for thirty minutes, half a day, or all day. Many programs begin with application of a heat modality such as paraffin baths or Hydrocollator packs, with elevation to relax and make the patient's hand more comfortable prior to the exercise program. The whirlpool bath is used only to assist in debridement of open wounds such as burns. Its use as a heat modality for pain relief is ill-advised since the dependency and heat routinely produce swelling in the hand. Heat modalities may be followed by distal to proximal hand massage to decrease edema and hypersensitivity to touch in those patients with such problems. Following this, the patient himself performs his individualized active or passive exercise regimes, monitored by the therapist to assure that the patient is performing correctly. As most patients are expected to be carrying out these exercise programs at frequent intervals throughout the day while *not* in the hand unit, the importance of their correct and diligent performance is constantly reinforced and encouraged.

All aspects of the patient's hand rehabilitation program (edema control, exercise, splinting, functional activities and sensory re-education) are monitored and changed in accordance with the patient's progress and response to his treatment program.

In the performance of the exercise and splinting program in all hand problems, *pain* is carefully avoided. The concept of forceful passive manipulation of joints by the therapist is strongly condemned! Pain with passive motion is a warning sign of joint and soft tissue reinjury which causes more swelling, fibrosis and stiffness. The patient must learn that all active and passive exercises must be gentle enough to avoid pain and tissue reaction, but frequent enough to gently stretch, not tear, adhesions. Pain is not gain.

The patient must understand that the problem with his hand is primarily his, not the surgeon's nor the therapist's, and he, to a large part, is responsible for his result. This key principle is continually emphasized by the surgeon, therapist, and even other patients. The idea that the patient goes to therapy to "get my hand worked on by the therapist" is actively discouraged.

Teaching the patient about his hand and its treatment is an important function of the hand rehabilitation team. Because the patient's understanding, cooperation and follow-through with his hand rehabilitation program are so essential, patient education is initiated at the first visit and is a continuous process throughout the course of treatment. This is done both formally and informally by the surgeon, hand therapist and his peers. The intensity or depth of the patient's education program varies with each individual, but the key is finding some way to get each patient to first understand the "why" of his hand rehabilitation program. Then the patient must learn "how" and "when" he must perform his exercises and other aspects of the program.

Based on these principles, the primary responsibility of the patient becomes that of "self-therapist". The hand therapist in turn assumes the role of educator, evaluator, coach, cheerleader and program co-ordinator.

Along with specific exercises, most patients are involved in the performance of some functional activity. It is not enough to regain a certain number of degrees in range of motion, or to simply improve tendon excursion. This must be combined with actual functional use of the hand by performing some type of purposeful activity with tools or materials. The emphasis is on "ability" not "disability". It is strongly believed that "it is not what you have, but what you do with it!" that counts. At first, it is usually necessary to modify the tools so that the patient can use them with the injured hand.

Often the first "break" in the motivation of the patient comes when he sees that he can use the injured hand for some productive purpose. With patients injured on the job, who are eligible for workmen's compensation, the prospect of litigation and monetary settlement often inhibits the recovery process. In such cases, the performance of functional activities can help demonstrate to the patient that his injury does not prevent the performance of his work. Later, a portion of the patient's job activity can actually be carried out in the hand rehabilitation unit to improve strength, endurance and speed.

Workmen's compensation cases may present another special problem particularly in patients hurt on jobs they do not particularly enjoy. It is very difficult to get this patient rehabilitated while he is being paid to be disabled. The hand rehabilitation unit approach to this problem is simple and direct: "If you cannot work because your hand is hurt, then *you* must spend your time *working on your hand* so that you can return to work." Occasionally, the patient is actually made to "punch in" at 8:00 a.m. and stay until 5:00 p.m. in the hand unit. During this time he is closely observed by the therapist to be sure he both understands the exercises and performs them regularly. Other more motivated patients with similar or even more severe injuries exert peer pressure to encourage the patient to return to work. The work ethic is not inate to most of us. It must be learned and continually reinforced. It is often helpful for such a patient to see his friends and fellow patients return to work and be happy about it.

Patients with rheumatoid arthritis also represent a special group who may receive help from the therapist in the hand rehabilitation unit. After being initially evaluated by the hand surgeon, the patient visits the hand unit for further re-education in specific details of arthritis' effect on the hand. Joint protection skills, intrinsic stretching and "tricks" to improve the function of the disabled hand are taught. Should the patient need a surgical procedure (particularly if the surgery requires a significant effort on the part of the patient to achieve its good result), the patient education is detailed. This often includes a visit with a patient who has recently had similar surgery in order to observe the splinting, exercises required, and the result that may be expected. Often patients who would be poor candidates for surgery may be recognized in this manner.

The reflex sympathetic dystrophy patient is also a special person for whom the hand unit can be helpful. Other patients who have had similar pain and stiffness but are further along in their improvement course can encourage the newcomer to elevate his hand and perform exercises properly. Functional activities are especially useful in dystrophy patients.

(continued)

Physical Disabilities
Special Interest Section Newsletter; Vol. 1, No. 1, 1978

An Effective Exchange— How to Ask for the Information You Need

The PDSS Newsletter will provide a space called *Information Exchange*, where therapists can share information. This will be similar to the Occupational Therapy Newspaper's *Hotline* but focusing on information in relation to physical disabilities.

Many therapists have complained about requests that are printed in the *Hotline*, saying that they are general, vague, and show little or no thought. For example: "We need information on program development, evals, reimbursement, developing contracts with schools, and pros and cons of hospital based programs versus school based programs." . . . In other words; "Come set up my program for." . . . "I am a student doing research on _____. I need therapists' experiences with this approach, descriptions of patients, activities, progression, results, and any other pertinent information." . . . The implication seems to be, "Please do my research for me, I do not have time to write a questionnarie." . . . "I am interested in reality orientation, sensory awareness, remotivation, and consultation to nursing homes. Please contact." . . . Translated that would be; "I am too lazy to do a review of the literature" or "Please write, I love to get mail."

As the above examples show, some writers appear quick to request information without demonstrating any initial investigation of available resources and materials.

Perhaps the writer does not realize the impression that he or she gives is to be "spoon-fed."

Other *Hotline* request were well written, characterized by:

- Stating needs clearly and specifically—"I need information on normal grip strength (measured by dynamometer) for children ages 3-12 years." or "Does anyone know a source for a good self-feeder device for a bilateral trachial dephlegic patient?"

- Willingness to share information—"We would like to hear of the success or failure of such methods and to share our resources." or "Am compiling information, will share." or "I am working in Peace Corps teaching OT, anyone wanting to know more about it, please write."

- Facilitating patient education—"Do you know of families or spouses who would be interested in communicating (written) with wife of a client with this rare disease." or "Would like information, developed or proposed, on patient instruction AV slide presentations for rheumatoid arthritis. Specific areas are. . . ."

- Offering to pay expenses.—"We will forward cost to obtain bibliography and procedure." or "Please call collect at. . . ."

Evaluation forms were the most often requested information printed in previous *Hotlines*. Carole Hays, AOTA Director of Practice, is collecting evaluation forms. They will be compiled in a monograph titled, "Sample Forms"; target date for publication is August 1978.

The second most frequent request was for information to develop programs for specific disabilities. Each state PDSS liaison person will have a computerized print out of state facilities with occupational therapy and basic programs provided, (i.e., motor function, cardiac). Refer to the article "Specialty Section Liaison Person." If national resources are needed, contact PDSS chairperson. Requests for unique program ideas would be best serviced through "Information Exchange."

The effective exchange of information includes both giving and receiving. Remember this space is not limited to requests. You may use this space to informally present treatment ideas, approaches, or equipment that you have found helpful.

Your questions or requests may be of interest and concern to other therapists. So, we would appreciate you summarizing the responses you receive and submitting copy of them to the chairperson so that they will be included in following newsletter. Send your items for this column to: Alice Bowker, OTR, 5217 Sherwood, Little Rock, AR 72206.

Physical Disabilities
Special Interest Section Newsletter; Vol. 1, No. 1, 1978

A Member Speaks Out

Open Letter on Special Interest Groups-A Personal View—by Louise Elfant, OTR, Mt. Auburn Hospital, Cambridge, MA.

Last October, I had the opportunity to attend the Annual Conference of AOTA in Puerto Rico. During the course of the conference activities, meetings were held for members of the five special interest groups to discuss the organizational framework under which these new groups would operate. I attended the Physical Disabilities Group and found particularly interesting the recommendations for developing specialty subgroups. The desire was expressed to formulate a minimum number of subgroups and to avoid any tendency for subgroups to splinter off into their own specialty groups. Yet when suggestions for these subgroups were elicited, no less than 20-30 diagnos-

(continued)

A Member Speaks Out

tic categories, treatment modalities, age groups, body parts, and so on, were listed. The brainstorming session was useful but brought several concerns to my mind.

1.—*Need for Specialization:* In the formative years of the profession, lacking its own theoretical base, occupational therapists have begged and borrowed from other disciplines in the process of defining and delineating professional boundaries and establishing our own frame(s) of reference. The practice that resulted from these sometimes arbitrary boundaries covered many and varied areas of human functioning. It became impractical to learn all areas well, and areas of specialization were defined. In the interest of treating the whole person, however, we have maintained basic education in all specialities.

2.—*Danger of Overspecialization:* As we develop special skills to enhance the quality of treatment, we may sometimes trade off treating the whole person for treating the parts more effectively. We must set our

limits to avoid treating one system to the ignorance of related or causual factors and general health.

3.—*New Directions:* Defining specialty subgroups should reflect the direction in which we want to grow as well as the reality of practice today. I work in general medicine, treating many diagnoses and using many different techniques and theories. I do not wish to belong to a dozen subgroups, each addressing a different diagnostic category or treatment modality (we are not listing in-service topics!) nor do I wish to specialize only in CVA or arthritis.

4.—*Utilization of Resources:* We arrive at the question of resources. How much time and effort are we willing to invest in developing and operating subgroups in addition to national, state, and local organizations that already exist? How do we avoid duplication of services, as most regions have existing vehicles for addressing concerns of practice, clinical and academic education, legislation, etc.?

I suggest that we set our priority the first year as follows: Establish working special interest groups in each state; Include and address specialty concerns within the larger groups; Align the blossoming specialty subgroups such as hand rehabilitation with the larger groups, avoiding unnecessary splintering off or isolation from the general practice; and Evaluate the type of specialty subgroups needed following one year of operation.

We may find that few subgroups are needed and that we prefer to remain specialized only to the extent of the current breakdown. If not, we may still remember that many of us do not choose further specialization and need not be coaxed into narrow categories of practice. Perhaps specialty subgroups should ultimately include only 10-20 percent of the special interest group membership. Clearly, we should consider in what form these groups may best serve us and how we might utilize them to grow professionally.

—*Louise Elfant, OTR.*

Physical Disabilities
Special Interest Section Newsletter; Vol. 1, No. 1, 1978

Statement on Research

The Steering Committee of the Physical Disabilities Specialty Section, with input from members, has established the promotion of research in occupational therapy as a major goal. Wilma West referred to the "tripodal support base" of any professional discipline being service, training, and *research.** She identified the lack of a *national commitment* to research, which unfortunately, still exists today.

Why is reasearch important? The practice of occupational therapy is based on a little-tested body of knowledge. Members of the profession are generally quick to defend the efficacy of their practice on subjective grounds, by and large without objective evidence.

There are several reasons for undertaking research. First, one of the most important is to add to our knowledge base with the result being better patient care. If hypotheses about what treatment is most effective are not tested, each therapist essentially goes through a trial-and-error process as part of treatment implementation in order to determine the best approach to a particular patient. The occupational therapist readily agrees with the need to "share" treatment information, but has balked at the need to do and share research.

Underlying the consensus to share information is the recognition to improve oc-

cupational therapy practice. The commitment to a *scientific* investigation of our treatment is, however, sorely lacking. Many reasons have been suggested for the reluctance of the therapist to pursue research. Had a major commitment to research been made by the profession, some of the "barriers" to research might already have been alleviated/eliminated, or at least a plan established toward the end. Occupational therapists expect recognition as *true* professionals, yet are unwilling to accept the responsibilities, among which is critical examination of their practice in a scientifically accepted manner.

The second rationale for research dovetails with the first. If third party payors can be shown objective evidence of the efficacy of our treatment, occupational therapy might be more likely to get an equitable share of the health care dollar. Members of other, more research-oriented disciplines may also be more likely to support and recognize occupational therapy efforts if results were documented using the tools of research that provide a common ground on which to communicate.

A trend towards occupational therapists abandoning the use of activities has been noted. Therapists clamor for a definition of occupational therapy and the best way to explain what they do to the public and their

colleagues. These may be indicators of a lack of confidence and trust in our treatment and an effort to adopt more accepted treatment techniques, even if they are not germane to occupational therapy. The public becomes confused and colleagues in other disciplines question and respond strongly to these actions. If occupational therapy is to gain increased respect and recognition, would it not be better for occupational therapists to do research and develop its own unique body of knowledge?

And finally, researchers from other fields—sociology, psychology, etc.—are investigating the effects of handicapping conditions on activities of daily living. In fact, there is a trend to measure the results of medical practice in terms of improvement in functional performance. These are the issues occupational therapists deal with daily. Why aren't *we* doing the research? If occupational therapists could seize this opportunity and do the necessary research, the main thrust of occupational therapy would be identified publicly with occupational therapy.

At the last meeting of the chairpersons of all the specialty sections, a resolution was prepared for presentation to the Representative Assembly. The resolution recommends the following action: That the advocacy posi-

(continued)

Statement on Research

tion be extended for an additional year with a change in emphasis to the promotion of research efforts by individual members, university faculties, practitioners, or other appropriate bodies. Functions inherent in this position would be:

- Development of mutual support systems and research networks,
- Serving as a central resource to members on research issues,

- Extensive effort to be accessible and available to expedite the development of research,
- Work with the specialty section, Commission of Education, Commission on Practice and National Office to mobilize resources.

In addition, the Physical Disabilities Specialty Section will have one member of its Steering Committee identified as a liaison on research. Members were also strongly urged to participate in the 1978 AOTA Conference Institute "F"—Everything You Always Wanted to Know About Research But Were Afraid to Ask"—on May 5.

For more information about the status of research and an analysis of the issues surrounding this topic, the reader is referred to proceedings of the 1976 Research Seminar described in the September 1976 issue of *AJOT*.

* Wilma West, "Nationally Speaking—Research Seminar" *AJOT* Vol. 30 (Sept., 1976), No. 8, p. 477.

5

Sensory Integration
Special Interest Section

Sensory Integration
Special Interest Section Newsletter; Vol. 6, No. 2, 1983

Tactile Defensiveness: Historical Perspectives, New Research—A Theory Grows

Anne G. Fisher, MS, OTR, and Winnie Dunn, M Ed, OTR, FAOTA, CSSID Faculty

Historical Perspectives

In 1964, Ayres first defined tactile defensiveness (TD) as "feelings of discomfort and a desire to escape the situation when certain types of tactile stimuli are experienced." Defensive reactions are characterized by a certain type of hyperactivity and distractibility manifested by (1) abnormal increases in skeletal movement and verbalization and (2) "a tendency to respond to stimuli not relevant to the test situation." A tendency to extinguish (rub or scratch out) light tactile stimuli when applied to the arms, hands or face is common. "Feelings of discomfort" and the "desire to escape" emotionally are expressed verbally and/or physically as fight or flight reactions. Such defensive reactions may also be associated with depressed scores on certain tactile tests, especially Graphesthesia (GRA), Localization of Tactile Stimuli (LTS), and Double Tactile Stimuli (DTS).

In 1964, Ayres postulated (1) dual afferent tactile pathways "—a protective system which responds to stimuli with movements, alertness, and a high degree of affect (often negative) and a discriminative system which enables intepretation of the temporal and spatial nature of stimuli for cognition. (2) Under certain circumstances, the two systems lose (or never attain) their natural balance, the protective system predominating. (3) When the protective system predominates, the hyperactivity syndrome is aggravated, affect and somatic discomfort are heightened, and perceptual-motor development is retarded." The syndrome does not interfere with academics per se, but the behavior/over arousal may interfere with learning.

The theory of TD and the above postulates were based upon theories of pain reported in the literature prior to 1964. In 1920, Head postulated a peripheral dichotomy for sensation based on receptor specificity. Peripheral receptors were of two types: protopathic (phylogenetically old; produced diffuse persistent, unpleasant, but also, sometimes pleasant sensations; emotionally charged) and epicritic (phylogenetically newer; responded to gentle contact or thermal stimuli; discrete, precisely localized; affectively neutral; permitted perception of objects and discrimination). The protopathic system was normally suppressed by the epicritic, but manifested itself in pathological states.

Because discrete pain receptors that projected directly to known pain receptors in the brain were never identified, subsequent investigators postulated a central dichotomy with modality-specific pathways in the central nervous system. The dorsal column-medial lemniscal (DC-ML) system, thought to be phylogenetically newer, carried information concerning primarily touch-pressure and joint position (discriminative touch) along somatotopically organized, precise, direct pathways. The anterolateral (AL) system, thought to be phylogenetically older, carried information concerning primarily pain, temperature, itch, tickle, and crude touch along indirect pathways with large receptive fields. Since the large A-beta fibers commonly associated with mechanoreception/touch-pressure and that projected to the DC-ML system seemed analogous to the epicritic receptors postulated by Head, the DC-ML system was sometimes referred to as the epicritic pathway or system. Similarly, because smaller A-delta and C fibers associated with pain, temperature, and crude touch and that projected primarily to the AL system seemed analogous to the protopathic receptors postulated by Head, the AL system was sometimes referred to as the protopathic pathway or system. As with the epicritic and protopathic receptor dichotomy, the epicritic and protopathic pathway (central) dichotomy postulated that the DC-ML system normally suppressed the AL system. However, like the peripheral dichotomy, the central dichotomy was criticized because research had failed to demonstrate discrete pain pathways, and there was a known interaction between the DC-ML and the AL systems.

In 1965, Melzack and Wall developed their Gate Control Theory of pain. This theory accounted for receptor and pathway specialization, but also considered that there was some degree of interaction between the DC-ML and AL systems. Experimental lesions of the AL system were found to modify but not abolish pain, and experimental lesions of the DC-ML system were found to modify but not abolish discriminative touch. This theory also accounted for experimental evidence of (1) the spatial and temporal patterning and encoding of tactile input, (2) higher level and psychological influences on pain, and (3) spatial-temporal summation and spread of pain, none of which were necessary or possible with a theory postulating a central or peripheral dichotomy.

The Gate Control Theory postulated that a neural mechanism in the dorsal horn (substantia gelatinosa) acted as a gate to increase or decrease the flow of neural impulses to the central nervous system. The amount of sensory transmission was controlled by the relative activity of A-beta fibers, and A-delta and C fibers, and by descending influences from the brain. Large A-beta fibers closed the gate; small A-delta and C fibers opened the gate. Opening the gate resulted in the summation and spread of pain.

An important component of the theory was the role of cortical influences (e.g., anticipation, anxiety, experience, attention) on the modulation of pain. Melzack and Wall hypothesized a source of higher-level inhibition that was activated by a central cortical control trigger. Primarily somatic but also visual, vestibular, proprioceptive, and auditory inputs to the midbrain reticular formation descended to spiral cord levels via the reticulospinal tracts. Cortical projections also descended indirectly via the reticular formation and reticulospinal tract, and directly via the corticospinal tract. The theory postulated that (1) these inhibitory, descending cortical influences were triggered by the rapidly ascending cortical projections of the DC-ML system, and that (2) these descending influences projecting to the substantia gelatinosa could influence or modulate information coming in over slower tactile pathways.

Current Theory

Subsequent to 1964, the Gate Control Theory was incorporated into the theory of TD and served as a theoretical basis for treatment. Now, instead of "the application of tactile stimulation as a means of bringing a better balance between the protective and discriminative systems, thereby enhancing tactile perception and reducing tactile defensive behavior"[1] the application of the same epicritic tactile stimulation (e.g., touch-pressure) was hypothesized to close the gate by altering the relative balance beween protopathic and epicritic tactile inputs.

Although subtle, there is an important difference; unfortunately, this difference is often minimized and/or ignored. Tactile defensiveness can no longer be considered a basis for impaired somatosensory perception and low tactile scores per se. Similarly, the hypothesis that the reduction of TD results in improved somatosensory perception per se is no longer valid. Instead protective and discriminative

(continued)

Tactile Defensiveness

abilities must be considered as separate but related functions of the somatosensory system. Ayres found that many children with impairment of one function also demonstrate impairment of the other ($r = .54$). However, either TD or impaired somatosensory perception can occur in isolation; some children demonstrate TD but obtain normal scores on the tactile tests, and some children obtain low scores on the tactile tests but show no evidence of TD. Furthermore, many children with TD demonstrate low scores on some but not all of the tactile tests. Those tests most likely to elicit TD (i.e., GRA, LTS, and DTS) are those tests most frequently affected. It is logical to speculate that, if a child is having an adverse reaction to the tactile stimuli applied during these tests, that child will be unable to attend to the discriminative aspects of the task.

New Research

Although the Gate Control Theory provides a hypothetical model for understanding TD, recent research in pain mechanisms has failed to support the presence of a discrete mechanism within the substantia gelatinosa for the gating of tactile inputs.[9]

Support for the concept of a gating mechanism for the modulation of tactile inputs would have made the tactile system unique among the sensory systems. Perhaps, therefore, it is not surprising that recent research suggests that such modulation and inhibition of pain is accomplished by way of descending pathways that originate in major ascending relay nuclei such as are known to exist in other sensory systems.

The ascending pathways of the AL system include (a) the neospinothalamic and paleospinothalamic tracts that project to the thalamus and constitute only a small pecentage of the AL fibers; and (2) the spinoreticular, spinobulbar, and spinoannular tracts that project to the tegmental reticular formation, subcoeruleus nucleus, raphe nuclei, the central grey core (which extends from the periaqueductal grey area to the periventricular grey and medial thalamic areas), the hypothalamus, and the limbic system. Both groups of AL-ascending pathways have projections to SI and SII of the somatosensory cortex.[6,7]

Sites of origin of descending pathways involved in the inhibition of pain include: SI, ventral basal thalamus, lateral hypothalamus, cerebral peduncles, raphe nuclei, lateral reticular formation, and periaqueductal grey and the periventricular grey areas. Pathways descending from cortical levels can be separated from those descending from brain-stem levels both anatomically and functionally. These pathways project not only to the substantia gelatinosa (lamina II and III), but also to lamina I and V to X and to the inter-mediolateral cell column.[6,8]

Experimental lesions of those higher centers provide insight into their roles in pain perception and modulation of pain. Cutaneous touch and sharp pain sensations are lost with lesions to the ventral basal nucleus of the thalamus. When a lesion is placed in the intralaminar nucleus of the thalamus, chronic deep pain can be relieved, but cutaneous pain is still present. These observations imply that separate functions may continue to be localized at this level. The somatosensory cortex seems to have a role in the appreciation of localized and sharp pain (neopathways), but chronic dull pain is not relieved with the ablation of SI and SII. These results imply that the thalamic projections are important in the process of pain perception.[7]

The sensorimotor, somatosensory, and limbic cortices may also modulate pain processes by exerting influence on other important central nervous system structures. These centers influence the hypothalamus, periventricular grey, and periaqueductal grey. In turn, it appears that these pathways subserve the emotional expressions associated with pain and serve to modulate pain input according to the emotional state of the individual. Projections to the hypothalamus and the limbic system also seem to play a role in responses associated with autonomic nervous system activity, and with aggressive and adversive behavioral responses to somatosensory input.[7,8]

The perception of pain can apparently be differentiated from tactile perception. When patients who have undergone frontal lobotomy experience noxious tactile stimule, they fail to perceive the stimuli as noxious, although they recognize that they were touched. Similarly, electrical stimulation to the periaqueductal grey, periventicular grey, and lateral hypothalamus results in inhibition of pain afferents. Pain is not perceived, but conscious perception of other characteristics of the sensory event is not altered.[2,3,7,8]

Although the inhibitory influences of higher centers on the modulation of pain are known to exist and this inhibitory control is known to be a critical part of normal functioning, the neural pathways are complex and knowledge of them remains obscure. However, clinical descriptions of "lack of inhibition" in children who display TD seem to be compatible with the concept that higher level influences are not adequately modulating tactile inputs. As a result, tactile stimuli normally perceived as nonnoxious are perceived as adversive. Furthermore, treatment might well be directed toward enhancing these descending cortical influences, by employing techniques to decrease arousal (i.e., touch-pessure, slow linear vestibular stimulation, neutral warmth, etc.).

Current research is also being directed toward the investigation of the role of neurotransmitters in the modulation of pain. Opiate receptor sites have been identified in several brainstem structures. These include portions of the posterior horn of the spinal cord, midline brainstem structures (the periventricular grey and periaqueductal grey), and the intralaminar nucleus of the thalamus. Poorly localized pain seems to be processed by these pathways. Since this type of pain is relieved by the administration of opiates (morphine), it appears that a neurochemical balance is necessary for the normal perception of pain. This is supported by research indicating that inadequate levels of serotonin (5-HT) result in heightened sensitivity to mechanical stimuli that would ordinarily be innocuous.[2,3,8]

Clinical Implications

Before the development of the Gate Control Theory, Ayres recommended using touch-pessure to decrease TD. Touch-pressure (epicritic input) was hypothesized to balance painful (protopathic) stimuli. When the Gate Control Theory was developed, treatment techniques for TD did not change markedly. Only the hypothesis about why touch-pressure input seemed to reduce TD changed; touch-pressure input was hypothesized to close the gate. Now, recent research suggests that clinicians must again modify the theoretical explanation for reducing TD through the application of touch-pressure. Presumably touch-pressure, proprioception, and other sensory inputs, which clinically have proved effective in reducing TD, enhance the descending inhibitory pathways and/or the level of neurotransmitters at receptor sites. Clearly, the exact mechanism remains obscure. There is a need for both neurophysiologists and clinicians to investigate the effects of sensory inputs on pain perception.

REFERENCES

1. Ayres, A.J. Tactile functions: Their relation to hyperactive and perceptual motor behavior. *American Journal of Occupational Therapy*, 1964, *18*, 83-95.
2. Kerr, F.W., & Casey, K.L. Pain. *Neurosciences Research Progress Bulletin*, 1977, *16*, 1-207.
3. Liebeskind, J.C., & Paul, L.A. Psychological and physiological mechanisms of pain. *Ann. Rev. Psychol.*, 1977, *28*, 41-60.
4. Melzack, R. *The Puzzle of Pain*. New York: Basic Books, Inc., 1973.
5. Melzack, R., & P.D. Pain mechanisms: A new theory. *Science*, 1965, *150*, 971..
6. Mountcastle, V.B. (Ed.) *Medical Physiology* (14th Ed.). St. Louis: C. V. Mosby, 1980.
7. Noback, C.R., & Demerest, R.J. *The Human Nervous System*. New York: McGraw-Hill Co., 1981.
8. *Society for Neuroscience Abstracts*, 1982, *8*, Pain: Modulation I, 767-771 and Pain: Modulation II, 804-806.
9. Vierick, C. Somatosensory system. In R. B. Masterson (Ed.), *Handbook of Behavior Neurobiology: Vol. I, Sensory Integration*. New York: Plenum Press, 1978.
10. Wall, P.D. The gate control theory of pain mechanisms: A re-examination and restatement. *Brain*, 1978, *101*, 1-18.

Sensory Integration
Special Interest Section Newsletter; Vol. 6, No. 2, 1983

Sensory Registration, Autism, and Tactile Defensiveness

Winnie Dunn, MEd, OTR, FAOTA, And Anne G. Fisher, MS, OTR, CSSID Faculty

Definition Of Terms

Recently, Ayres has indicated that the role of sensory registration is an important construct for clinicians to understand. Sensory registration is a process hypothesized to occur within the central nervous system in preparation for a response.[5,8,11] Pribram and McGinnis also referred to this phenomenon as the "orienting reflex." Vinogradova defined the orienting reflex as a "reaction to novelty which does not depend upon stimulus qualities, but appears with any detectable change of a stimulus." The identification of a stimulus as novel may depend upon the ability of the organism to have memory of previously experienced stimuli.

Vinogadova (1970) described four requirements that must be met before sensory registration can occur: (1) the ability to perceive the stimulus, (2) the ability to scan through one's memory store, (3) the ability to compare new input with old information that may be relevant to the present situation, and (4) the ability to "decide" whether registration is to occur. The channels of registration are opened when the oganism identifies the stimulus as unique — that is, the organism cannot find an exact counterpart in memory and, therefore, "registers" the sensory experience. The channels of registration are closed when the organism identifies the stimulus as the same — that is, the organism finds an exact counterpart in memory, and, therefore, "decides" to block the channels of registration because the stimulus is familiar.

Pribram and McGinnis (1975) reviewed the literature on attention, and identified three basic attentional control processes that may assist the clinician in grasping the concept of sensory registration. These three processes are termed (1) *arousal,* (2) *activation,* and, (3) *effort.*

Arousal is a "phasic physiological response to input" that occurs when ANY change in ANY parameter of the stimulus is present. Arousal appears to be a reflexive response that habituates or adapts readily; arousal asks the question "What is it?"

Arousal seems to be related to the response that opens the channels of sensory registration; when a change in ANY parameter occurs, a unique stimulus is present, one that is not found in the memory store[7]. Sokolov (1960) referred to these patterns of memory, which are used to determine the uniqueness of a stimulus, as "neuronal models." He stressed that ANY mismatch with these "neuronal models" will produce orienting. When a stimulus

becomes established (i.e., when a "neuronal model" is developed; adaptation occurs), the arousal response decreases. When ANY change occurs in the stimulus, arousal again occurs.

An example of this process is exhibited in a lack of arousal to familiar tactile stimuli. Under normal circumstances, an individual pays little attention to the tactile stimuli elicited by clothing. However, if the expected pattern or timing (i.e., feel) of tactile input changes (e.g., a stiff label or a weed stuck in the fabric "scratches" the skin; mismatch with the "neuronal model"), an arousal response is exhibited.

Activation is a tonic physiological readiness to respond. Activation differs from arousal in that activation maintains a behavioral set to continue ongoing perfomance. Activation habituates slowly, and appears to be involuntary[5,8] it asks the question "What is to be done?" Interestingly, there is increased cortical desychronization during activation.

Activation appears to contribute to the construction of "neuronal models" in two ways: (1) It controls the somatomotor system that provides the sensory input upon which appopriate motoric responses are built. (2) It assesses the feedback available from the outcomes of behavior.[5,8] These two functions highlight the importance of sensory processing and sensory feedback in the construction of accurate "neuronal models."

Effort is seen as the coordinator of arousal and activation. Effort appears to be a voluntary mechanism; energy is expended from the system due to a change of state in central control systems.[5] As with all functions of the central nervous system, it is very important that this type of modulation be manifested so that any one function does not predominate. If modulation of arousal and activation does not occur, the individual is aroused by sensory feedback from movement as well as by changes in sensory input. As a result, the individual is continuously activated to move because of the arousing input from preceding movement. This description of constant arousal and repeated activation bears a marked similarity to the behavioral picture of hyperactivity and distractibility frequently seen in the child with TD.

Central Nervous System Structures Implicated in Sensory Registration

Several structures within the central nervous system have been hypothesized to carry out the function of arousal, activation and effort:

The amygdala is a forebrain structure

where information from sensorimotor systems involved with the momentary cessation of behavior (i.e., when arousal occurs, ongoing activity is suppressed and the individual orients toward the mismatched stimulus) converges with input from central nervous system structures involved in concomitant emotional reactions (i.e., interest in the stimulus).[4]

The hippocampus appears to be involved in the sensory registration process by providing tonic inhibitory influence upon the reticular formation as follows:

1. When MATCH occurs, the stimulus has been found EXACTLY as presented in the memory store; therefore, *novelty is absent.* In this case, the hippocampus seems to inhibit the reticular activating system so that arousal does not occur. There is no reason for the individual to be aroused because the stimulus is familiar.

2. When MISMATCH occurs, the stimulus has not been found in its exact form in the memory store; therefore, *novelty is present.* In this case, the inhibitory control of the hippocampus is blocked. Because inhibition is not imposed upon the reticular formation, arousal is initiated, which in turn leads to sensory registration of the unique stimulus.

Hence, the hippocampus seems to play a dual role in the sensory registration process. First, it compares the stimulus with the memory store ("neuronal models"), and second, it blocks (inhibits) or deblocks (disinhibits) the reticular activating system.

Other brain mechanisms also seem to be involved in the complex processes of arousal, activation, and effort. These include the basal ganglia, limbic structures, and portions of the frontal lobe.

Sensory Registration and Autism

When Ayres discussed sensory registration at the Second Annual CSSID Symposium in Cincinnati (1981), she did so in reference to the autisticlike child. In a similar manner, Gold and Gold (1975) and Damasio and Maurer (1978) theorized about the neurological processes involved in childhood autism. Their hypotheses were drawn from theoretical literature, and they attempted to apply the avoce constructs to possible explanations of a difficult clinical problem. They hypothesized a possible malfunction in the basic alerting and attentional mechanisms in autistic children. In examining attentional models, Gold and Gold concluded that incoming information (sensory input) is pro-

(continued)

cessed inappropriately; rather than being perceived as novel or MISMATCH, the system tends to perceive incoming information as nonnovel and insignificant (i.e., resistance to MISMATCH that normally would cause registration to occur). Therefore, the messages that reach the cortex are disregarded rather than registered.

If autistic children demonstrate such malfunction in basic alerting and attentional mechanisms, the dysfunction may account for some of the behavioral manifestations observed by clinicians. As originally described by Rutter (1966), the autistic child demonstrates disturbances in five areas: (1) motility, (2) communication, (3) attention/perception, (4) ritualistic and compulsive behaviors, and (5) development of social relationships.

Damasio and Maurer (1978) suggested that disturbances of motility, which included characteristics such as dystonia of the extremities, bradykinesia, hyperkinesia, involuntary movements, rigidity or hypotonia, and inability to simultaneously perform two motor tasks (all motor disturbances associated with basal ganglia and frontal lobe disorders), are indicators of central nervous system involvement in autism.

Disturbances of communication seem to be related to functions of the mesial aspects of the frontal lobes and the neostriatum (part of the basal ganglia structures)[2] Communication disturbances of autistic children seem to be related to aspects other than the construction of thought in language form. Damasio and Maurer indicated that nonvebal communication is usually seriously impaired. Gestures are not used to compensate for inability to communicate verbally; autistic children also fail to attend to appropriate stimuli in the environment that would facilitate the communication process. "These defects seem to derive from a lack of initiative to communicate and from a lack of 'orientation' towards stimuli and are suggestive of an underlying impairment in higher motor or perceptual control." These characteristics are also seen in patients known to have damage to the mesial aspects of the frontal lobe.

Attention and perception are critical behavioral disturbances in the autistic child. As with disturbances of communication, Damasio and Maurer (1978) hypothesized that autistic children demonstrate less sustained orientation to stimuli that is compatible with a disorder in attention. "Orientation towards a given object will only be carried out after the organism has determined that the object is of impor-

tance for future behavior.... The response of an organism to a given stimulus depends on the set of 'goals' of that organism and on a hierarchically organized 'executive control' that will modulate the response according to the 'goals'." Perhaps the sensory registration process, discussed above, provides the ability to set "goals" through the use of the "neuronal models" to determine whether sensory events are appropriate for the "goals" of that individual. If "neuronal models" are not being developed due to difficulty with sensory registration, then attention may appear random and less purposeful.

Damasio and Maurer (1978) hypothesize that ritualistic and compulsive behaviors reflect an adaptive response of a dysfunctioning nervous system to the demands of the environment. Since autistic children do not have the resources available that would normally allow appropriate responses, they do what they know how to do. Resistance to change, then, is viewed as a method of communicating the "catastrophe" of facing new stimuli without the proper resources to "create a new and appropriate response." Although clinicians normally would have difficulty looking upon such inappropriate behaviors as "adaptive," consideration of the dynamic interaction of the central nervous system with the body in which it is housed, and with the environment in which it lives, enables the clinician to realize that perhaps autistic children perform what they "can perform adequately."

Although difficulty with social relationships is often considered a primary disturbance characteristic of the autistic child, Damasio and Maurer (1978) considered this to be a secondary characteristic due to disturbances in all the other areas and similarly related to frontal lobe, limbic system, and basal ganglia circuitry.

Sensory Registration: Autism vs. Tactile Defensiveness

Although the link between TD, autism, and sensory registration may seem to be obscure, it is possible to speculate that both TD and autism are disorders of different aspects of sensory registration. A primary component of sensory registration is the orienting reflex that is the orienting "toward" a stimulus because of its novelty. In contrast, TD can be viewed as an "away from" response to an adversive stimulus. The primary disturbances seen in the autistic child have been attributed to a failure to orient and a resultant lack of sensory registration. TD might be viewed as over arousal and repeated activation due to

an impairment in the modulation of these two functions by effort. Failure to register appears to be less amenable to therapeutic intervention. Ayres and Tickle (1980) found that sensory integrative therapy was more effective in those autistic children who registered sensory input, but failed to modulate it, than in those who were hyporesponsive, or who failed to orient to sensory input. Viewing orientation as a "toward" response and TD behavior as an "away from" response motorically is analogous to extension toward an object to grasp and explore and flexor withdrawal, respectively. Interestingly, McMillan and Moudy (1982) found that perception of pain and nociception were suppressed by active flexion or extension of a limb more than when it was relaxed, but that the greatest suppression occurred during active extension. This suggests that TD may be greatest when the child is relaxed or sitting still and may help to explain their hyperactivity. Furthermore, that active extension, and to a lesser extent, flexion, reduce pain may explain why activities involving cocontraction and proprioception have clinically been shown to reduce TD.

References:

1. Ayres, A.J., & Tickle, L.S. Hyperresponsivity to touch and vestibular stimuli as a predictor of positive response to sensory integration procedures by autistic children. *American Journal of Occupational Therapy*, 1980, *34*, 375-381.
2. Damasio, A.R., & Maurer, R.G. A neurological model for childhood autism. *Archives of Neurology*, 1978, *35*, 777-786.
3. Gold, M.S., & Gold, J.R. Autism and attention: Theoretical considerations and a pilot study using set reaction time. *Child Psychiatry and Human Development*, 1975, *6*, 68-80.
4. Isaacson, R.L. *The Limbic System.* New York: Plenum Press, 1974.
5. McGinnis, D., & Pribram, K. The neuropsychology of attention: Emotional and motivational controls. In E. Wittrack (Ed.), *The Brain and Psychology.* Academic Press, 1980.
6. McMillan, J.A., & Moudy, A.M. Effects of limb position on pain perception in human subjects. *Society for Neuroscience Abstracts*, 1982, *8*, 771.
7. Pribram, K.H. *Languages of the brain: Experimental Paradoxes and Principles in Neuropsychology.* Englewood Cliffs, NJ: Prentice-Hall, 1971.
8. Pribram, K., & McGinnis, D. Arousal, activation, and effort in the control of attention. *Psychological Review*, 1975, *82*, 116-149.
9. Rutter, M. Behavioural and cognitive characteristics of a series of psychotic children. In J.K. Wing (Ed.) *Early Childhood Autism: Clinical, Educational and Social Aspects.* Oxford, England: Pergamon Press, 1966.
10. Sokolov, E.N. Neuronal models and the orienting reflex. In M.A.B. Brazier Ed.) *The central nervous system and behavior.* New York: Josiah Macy Jr. Foundation, 1960.
11. Vinogradova, O.S. Registration of information of the limbic system. In H. Hinde *Short-term changes in neuronal activity*, 1970.

Sensory Integration
Special Interest Section Newsletter; Vol. 6, No. 1, 1983

Sensory Integration Groups—An Effective Treatment Modality in Child Psychiatry

By Paula Kramer Goldstein, MA, OTR

Children with sensory integration dysfunction are often seen in child psychiatry programs because of their concomitant emotional problems, one of the most common being poor or inadequate self-image. These emotional side effects may interfere as much with the child's ability to interact with peers as does the primary deficit.

Dr. John O'Brien, a child psychiatrist, states that the main psychological problem for these children is poor self-esteem. They sense that something is wrong with them, that they are not like other children. They seem always to be in trouble with their parents, their teachers and themselves. They can't even get their bodies to work the way they want them to.

Clinically, children tend to fall into two categories. The first is the child who is depressed and isolated, responding to feelings of inadequacy and teasing from peers by withdrawal. The second is also a depressed child, but one who is more aggressive and irritable. Such children respond to teasing by fighting back or at times by warding off teasing by poking fun at themselves, becoming the class clown. Both of these groups of children feel that they are very different from their classmates and that they are the only ones who have such problems.

OT intervention using sensory integration techniques has been implemented on a one-to-one basis with these children. When dealing primarily with emotional issues, an activity or task group approach is usually employed. The combination of sensory integration principles, used in a small group, may effectively deal with both physical performance deficits as well as deficient peer interactions.

Banus describes one-to-one treatment as most effective because it allows the children to direct their own programs while the therapist subtly intervenes. She suggests that older children may be embarrassed in front of peers, but concedes that group therapy can be of benefit to depressed, lethargic and poorly motivated children.

Paula Kramer Goldstein, acting coordinator of the OT Program at Kean College of New Jersey, maintains a small private practice. She is certified by the Center for the Study of Sensory Integrative Dysfunction in the administration and interpretation of the SCSIT. Goldstein is also a doctoral candidate in OT at New York University.

S. F. Slavson has stated that the child's group must (a) deal with activity rather than interview, (b) present the activity in a safe, protective setting where behavior and interaction are not allowed to become destructive, and (c) allow for the child to have some degree of choice. It would seem that combining Slavson's ideas with a sensory integration approach would provide optimal effectiveness and melding of treatment goals.

There may be some advantages to group sensory integration treatment. It tends to reduce feelings of isolation, and provides the children with an actual peer group, possibly for the first time. They can see that they are not alone, that others are having similar difficulties. They have an opportunity to develop an awareness of strengths amidst weaknesses that are so acutely apparent. They may see that they can perform one activity better than others. The children may be more motivated to attempt something in front of peers rather than when each is alone with the therapist. The group experience promotes a healthy interaction where the therapist may skillfully reduce the children's withdrawn or aggressive reactions by encouraging involvement among children about specific task or activity. Finally, the group provides a forum for dealing with feelings. Once the children feel comfortable and trust the therapist and other group members, they may be able to express some feelings about themselves and their abilities.

A therapy group should be set up with care, having all children appropriately evaluated and treatment goals set. The group should be as homogeneous as possible, with children experiencing similar types and levels of dysfunction. It is preferable that they be of the same sex and close in age. Four children should be the maximum number in a group to allow the therapist to monitor their stimulation and activity. It may be beneficial to have an aide, volunteer or student involved to assist in monitoring the group.

The therapist should seek a balance of temperaments among the children in a group. Clear limits and expectations set by the therapist must be stated and repeated as needed so that children understand them. Most importantly, they should be consistently upheld. Activities should follow the same guidelines as those used in individual treatment, providing controlled stimulation to help bring about an adaptive motor response.

The therapist functions as the leader of the groups, structuring activities and providing the necessary hands-on stimulation. Several activities aimed at treatment goals for the group should be suggested, allowing the members to choose and thus help direct their treatment. The therapist should facilitate appropriate interaction, maintain physical and emotional safety, and provide support for all participants. It is important that the therapist know the children well in order to facilitate the necessary development of each one.

Avoiding direct competition is important. When using team games, teams should be rotated frequently. Although some mild competitions may be stimulating, the children should be encouraged to compete with themselves so that they can improve over time and with practice. It may be helpful to have a child, or the whole group, chart progress in one activity from week to week.

Groups are not beneficial to every child. They may be contraindictated when sensory integrative deficits are very severe, especially with tactile defensiveness and postural insecurity. Children with these problems may feel particularly threatened in a group situation. Children with emotional problems so severe that they are out of touch with reality and exhibit psychotic behaviors probably would not benefit from group sessions. For children 5 years of age or younger, a group may not be advisable, since children this age usually need much more attention and supervision than can be provided.

In some cases, the group experience may be more useful than individual treatment. At other times, it can be used to supplement one-to-one sessions. This depends on the severity of the sensory integrative and emotional dysfunctions, as well as the judgment of the therapist.

The use of groups may present an interesting and effective method for dealing with both the emotional and sensory integrative problems of the child within the child psychiatry setting. It incorporates the theory and dynamics of OT and can be cost effective and enjoyable for all involved.

BIBLIOGRAPHY

Ayres AJ: *Sensory Integration and the Child,* Los Angeles: Western Psychological Services, 1980.

Banus BS et al: *The Developmental Therapist Edition 2,* Thorofare, NJ: Charles B. Slack Inc., 1979.

Battle J: Self esteem of students in regular and special classes. *Psychological Reports* 44: 212-214, 1979.

Gardner RA: *MBD: The Family Book About Minimal Brain Dysfunction,* New York: J. Aronson, 1973.

(continued)

Sensory Integration Groups

Kessler J: *Psychopathology of Childhood*, Englewood Cliffs, NJ: Prentice-Hall, 1966.

Lowrey LG, Slavson SR: Group Therapy Special Section Meeting. In *Group Psychotherapy and Group Func-*

tion, M. Rosenbaum and M. Berger, ed. New York: Basic Books Inc., 1963.

O'Brien JD: The psychoanalytic psycho-therapy of the minimal brain dysfunctional child. In *The Treat-*

ment of the Emotionally Disturbed Child. GD Goldman, ed., Adelphi Univ. Press, In Press.

Farnopol L: Introduction to neurogenic learning disorders. In *Learning Disorders in Children*, L Farnopol, ed. Boston: Little, Brown & Co., 1971.

Sensory Integration
Special Interest Section Newsletter; Vol. 6, No. 1, 1983

Sensory Integration Intervention in a Pediatric Mental Health Clinic

By Geraldene Larrington, MA, OTR

This paper is intended to share informally some clinical perspectives from a sensory integration-based OT program at the Children's Mental Health Out-patient Service, Olive View Medical Center, Sylmar, CA.

Pediatric OT services were implemented in 1971 to deal with a number of patients loosely identified as "organic" and not considered prime treatment candidates in the program's psychoanalytic frame of reference. The children's "organicity" was reflected in presenting problems of learning disability and hyperactivity. Management consisted of medication and monthly parent contacts. The OT role was to start sensory integration testing and treatment of this core case load, provide testing for selected incoming cases, treat new cases as needed, participate in twice weekly patient staffing, and meet weekly in a supervisory hour with the chief psychiatrist.

The OT program with this core group was only partially successful. However, as sensory integration testing was incorporated into the intake process, the cases in treatment became more appropriate and greater progress was shown.

Since the case load developed slowly, OT service began t—accept medical outpatient referrals and thus developed two separate case loads: one mental health, one medical. Over the years it became apparent that each case load was distinctly different, based on sensory integration assessment. Children in the age range of 5 to 12 years had different types of sensory integration problems depending on which service made the referral. The mental health case load was heavily Vestibular Bilateral Integration (VBI), whereas the medical cases were heavily apraxic or had noticeable speech or language problems.

Geraldene Larrington, MA, OTR, a former staff member of the Olive View Medical Center, Los Angeles County Hospital, is on the faculty of the Center for the Study of Sensory Integrative Dysfunction.

The geographic and socioeconomic status of these two groups overlapped, although there were initially more middle-class families in the mental health group and more lower-income families in the medical service. Later, these differences equalized as more middle-income families sought specialized services through the medical service. Children in both groups tended to have normal or above average intelligence and did not have medical diagnoses such as cerebral palsy.

The difference between cases referred from the two services are understandable, based on the visibility of the children's problems. The children with VBI dysfunction had subtle problems, with minimal physical involvement. Therefore, physicians had not been able to identify a physical source for their problems, assumed the problems were emotional/behavioral, and eventually referred the children for mental health services.

Apraxic children, on the other hand, had noticeable motoric involvement so that the physicians could make a referral for therapy based on the need they saw.

Family relationships tended to be different between the two groups. Children from the mental health case load with VBI tended to have more strained family relationships. Told repeatedly that their children's problems were emotional/behavioral and to change child rearing patterns, parents had increased stress. Very few home programs were attempted in this population. As the children made changes, their problems were better understood and guilt was relieved. Relationships did improve but direct participation in the treatment at home was not a part of that healing. Some parents were used as helpers in the OT clinic in some treatment sessions so that the therapist could model behavior for the parent, continue to communicate the nature of the problems and the purpose of treatment activities, and still keep the treatment session fun and stress-free for both the parent and child.

Initially, treatment was once a week.

Both apraxic and VBI children made good, although slow, progress. The course of treatment was often predictable in that behavior changes associated with treatment frequently occurred in about 3 months. Eventually, treatment was increased to two times per week. The changes were dramatic. The course of treatment was speeded up significantly with behavior changes manifesting themselves as early as six weeks.

Children were treated for 50-minute sessions. An environment appropriate to the sensory needs of the child was provided with a preselection of possible activities and games to ensure participation. The sessions were child-directed, however, in that the child's preferences, aversions and reactions were noted and respected. Jean Ayres' chapter on the Art of Therapy in *Sensory Integration and Learning Disorders* describes best the type of guidance and interaction the therapist provided. The parallel between sensory integration treatment and psychotherapy was doubly meaningful because of our setting in which the child-led therapy session had precedence in this psychoanalytic milieu.

Initially, all treatment was one-to-one, with the therapist providing the play partner to the child. With experimentation and the addition of an aide, it was found feasible and effective to treat two or three children simultaneously when there was a one-to-one ratio of therapist/aide to child. This provided exciting play partners for part of the sessions, as needed for models, motivation and fun, and also allowed for the responsible therapist/aide to be responsive to the child's needs and abilities and do individual programming within the therapy session.

The behavior changes that occurred as treatment progressed were of great interest. The children frequently became obnoxious, opinionated, bossy and in other ways let themselves be known to their world. Related to this was a new level of

(continued)

physical interaction with their world. They frequently became more propulsive, forceful and expansive in their spontaneous motor play. They appeared to believe that they were Supermen and that laws of gravity did not apply to them. More than a few children all but flew into the therapy room and from halfway across the room threw themselves through the air for a full body landing in the sand table. They would begin to propel themselves in the net with new-found strength and abandon. Considering that most of them still looked like motor disasters, one feared for their safety during this time, yet none actually harmed themselves.

The whole tone of this period was that they truly felt alive—"I feel, therefore I am"—that they felt some control over themselves and their world. One might suggest that their egos had experienced a new lease on life. It is exciting to find the psychoanalytic circle looking at the possible relationship between the ego and the vestibular system. More research demonstrating our effectiveness in this domain is needed.

Many parents required some help in coping with their children during this time. We supported them with the knowledge that it would not last. Within one to three weeks the children usually settled down but with a new, more positive, assertive interaction with the world. Therapy continued to shore up and strengthen newly developing sensorimotor abilities and help the children acquire more subtle automatic responses and lay the foundation for the voluntary development of new skills.

Treatment usually lasted one year; rarely more than one-and-a-half years. At this stage the children became bored with the activities despite the variation provided, which appeared to indicate that they had benefited maximally from what we had to offer.

The following case illustrates a number of ideas about mental health population: (1) Improved academics is not the only or most important goal of sensory integration therapy; (2) Sensory integration problems interfere greatly in a variety of human activity spheres such as dressing, feeding, play skills, sibling relations and, most importantly, ego development; (3) Sensory integration treatment, based on good assessment, can ameliorate successfully problems in activities of daily living and ego functions.

The presenting complaints for this 8 year-old boy were educational; he was not learning despite a good IQ. His family was intact and was very supportive.

Evaluation with the Southern California Sensory Integration Tests and clinical observations suggested vestibular and bilateral integration problems, but with suspicions of some right hemisphere dysfunction. Sensory integration treatment was underaken with a guarded prognosis, particularly academically.

As treatment progressed, the family began to share the extent to which his everyday living had been affected. At 8 years of age, he became independent in self-dressing. Independence came with strong, self-reliant defiance. One morning in treatment as he automatically headed to his mother to get help in removing a pullover sweater, he suddenly turned away and said almost defiantly, "I'll do it myself!" And he did. His mother whispered, "We've been getting a lot of that lately!" It was learned that he had required much help, especially with getting clothes on correctly and tying shoes.

This was an exciting time in his treatment. Many skills came together in rapid succession or more accurately "all at once." It was revealed that, because he was such a messy eater, he had always had to eat breakfast in his pajamas or else he would have to redress each morning. The pajamas went into the laundry daily and his table, chair and floor space had to be cleaned up after each meal. As this messy eating was resolved, so were extra chores and scheduling problems.

Mastery over spatial elements was seen in larger arenas. One day the parents were called out of the house by an enthusiastic voice, "Come see *me*!" The parents realized the voice was coming from the towering pine tree in their yard. Their son who had tended never to take his feet off the ground was high over their heads.

Difficultly with bike riding was a deficient play skill. Occasionally, he would try briefly and timidly to ride in the garage and driveway. Imagine the mother's surprise to realize that the object streaking down the lane was her son on his bike. What's more, he was using only one hand as the other waved frantically at her while he shouted, "Hey Mom, look at me!"

He began to assert himself in his relationships with his two older sisters who had constantly picked on him, defending himself and asserting his existence in their world. He was fortunate to have parents who could accept his assertiveness and who were willing to guide it into acceptable modes of behavior. They were disappointed, however, that commensurate academic gains were not made.

This case illustrates an important value in sensory integration treatment. The quality of this boy's life was dramatically improved. He feels good about himself in more realms; he can feel his existence and worth as a human being. He did make some gains academically but there were still reading deficits that were not improving with sensory integration therapy.

There are probably similar populations of patients in other children's mental health outpatient clinics who, because they do not manifest overt neurophysiological problems, are undiagnosed and struggle through critical years with interventions that are less effective. (There were several children in our OT program who had had a year of psychotherapy and served as their own control in assessing the effectiveness of the two methods and controlling for the effect of individualized attention.)

Sensory integration therapy for these children seems worthwhile. They may have good intelligence and the potential to contribute to society. Yet their lives are significantly disrupted by the interference with spatial and organizational abilities, which, in turn, interfere with activities of daily living and educational performance. But, most important, they lack the sense of self that makes them feel confident and fulfilled.

Treatment directly involving the primary senses (tactile, vestibular and proprioceptive) appears to offer an avenue to this important aspect of mental health. Ashley Montagu suggests that tactile and vestibular input is critical to the human experience of love required for development. Robert Frick, in a psychoanalytic journal, is suggesting a sensory basis for the ego. The primary sensory inputs we provide in sensory integration therapy may be directly subserving the developing ego function—the feelings of having mastery over self and space, of being functionally effective, of being worthwhile, of being loved and of being alive!

REFERENCES

Ayres AJ, PhD: *Sensory Integration and Learning Disorders.* Western Psychological Services, 1972

Frick RB, MD: The ego and the vestibulo-cerebellar system: some theoretical perspectives. *Psychoanalytic Quarterly* II, 1982

Montagu, A: *Touching: The Human Significance of the Skin.* New York: Harper & Row, 1972.

Sensory Integration
Special Interest Section Newsletter; Vol. 6, No. 1, 1983

Identity Crisis?

A letter received recently at AOTA from Aetna Life Insurance Company has stirred concern about how occupational therapists may be identifying their services when billing third-party payers. Aetna asked for clarification of and guidelines for sensory integration therapy and questioned its acceptance by the medical profession. A response to their inquiry was formulated and sent to them that we hope will give information to support reimbursement for services.

However, it is strongly advised that your services be billed as *occupational therapy* when requesting payment from insurance companies. Third-party payers may reimburse for OT but may deny payment for a specialized approach they do not understand or recognize.

As occupational therapists, we bring a rich and varied background to our clinical settings. Although we may emphasize certain techniques or work with a selected patient population, we cannot lose sight of our generic base and the wealth of skills available that allow us to function in many settings. By identifying ourselves as therapists specialized to evaluate and treat only certain disorders, we create confusion outside of the profession and may distort the recognition of our various abilities. In these times when competition for health care dollars is increasing, we need to be keenly aware that we must strengthen our position and refrain from any actions that create confusion about our professional identity. Occupational therapy has become a recognized reimbursable service by many third-party reimbursers and every effort is being made to continue and expand the coverage for our service.

Sensory Integration
Special Interest Section Newsletter; Vol. 6, No. 1, 1983

The DSM III, Sensory Integration, and Child Psychiatry—Implications for Treatment and Research

By Lela A. Llorens, Ph.D., OTR, FAOTA

Child psychiatric disorders have been redefined and reclassified in the *Diagnostic and Statistical Manual,* 3rd edition (DSM III).[1] The new major classifications are: I. Intellectual, including Mental Retardation; II. Behavioral, including attention deficit disorder and conduct disorder; III. Emotional, including anxiety disorders of infancy, childhood or adolescence and other disorders of these age groups; IV. Physical, including eating disorders, stereotyped movement disorders and other disorders with physical manifestations; V. Developmental, including pervasive and specific developmental disorders and Other Diagnostic Categories that are specific such as Affective Disorders; Schizophrenia; Organic Mental Disorders; Substance Use, Schizophreniform, Anxiety, Somatoform, Personality, Psychosexual, and Adjustment Disorders; and Major Depression.

A review of the diagnostic criteria for many of the new classifications reveals behavior descriptions that suggest sensory integration dysfunction. This in turn suggests the need for evaluation of sensory integration to be considered routinely in the treatment and rehabilitation of children with the following diagnoses:

Lela A. Llorens, Ph.D., OTR, FAOTA, is a professor and graduate coordinator at San Jose State University.

Attention Deficit Disorders[2]
Conduct Disorders
Anxiety Disorders, particularly Avoidant Disorders
Reactive Attachment Disorder of Infancy
Schizoid Disorder of Childhood
Oppositional Disorders
Identity Disorders
Eating Disorders
Stereotyped Movement Disorders
Pervasive Developmental Disorders, and
Specific Developmental Disorders (Axis II)

> Developmental Reading, Arithmetic, Expressive Language, Receptive Language, Articulation, Mixed Specific, and Atypical Specific Developmental Disorders.

Routine sensory integration evaluation to determine the quality of sensory integration function and dysfunction would provide a baseline for understanding and charting the functional integrity of the child's neurophysiological/neuromotor system. Such routine evaluation would facilitate the therapist's ability to begin intervention at a level commensurate with the child's ability to assimilate and integrate sensory stimuli from purposeful, goal-directed activities.[3]

Since many children with psychiatric disorders may not respond well to standardized sensory integration tests, objective clinical observations[4] may be the most useful technique for gathering baseline evaluation data. Such a baseline would make it possible to chart and periodically re-evaluate treatment progress and outcomes. Outcome data are essential in determining the effectiveness of OT intervention.

The new DSM III classifications, sensory integration theory, and the therapist's skill in observing functions related to sensory integration are an effective combination for increasing the precision with which therapy can be planned, administered and measured. Determining the effectiveness of therapy is a task that can be enhanced by utilizing research methodology. The Case Study method lends itself to the structure of practice and generates data useful both for practice and research.[5]

REFERENCES

1. American Psychiatric Association. Diagnostic and statistical manual of mental disorders, 3rd Edition. Washington: American Psychiatric Association, 1980.
2. Silver LB: Treatments for attention deficit disorders. *Sensory Integration Special Interest Section Newsletter* 4(4):1-3, 1981.
3. Ayres AJ: Sensory integration and the child. Los Angeles: Western Psychological Services, 1979.
4. Southam M: Directions for administering clinical observations. San Jose: San Jose State University, Department of Occupational Therapy, 1981.
5. Cox R: The case study method of research — introduction and part 2. *Sensory Integration Special Interest Section Newsletter* 4(1):1,3-4, 1981.

Sensory Integration
Special Interest Section Newsletter; Vol. 6, No. 1, 1983

The Effects of Vestibular Stimulation on Verbalization and Attending Behavior of an Autistic Child

By Kristine Karsteadt, MHS, OTR

Abstract

The effects of vestibular stimulation on the language and attending behavior of an autistic child were studied. An eight and one-half-year-old male subject participated in two types of OT activity sessions on alternate days over a period of 12 days.

Kristine Karsteadt, MHS, OTR, is presently employed at the North Central Florida Community Health Center, Gainesville, FL. This project was submitted in partial fulfillment of the requirement for a Master of Health Science degree at the University of Florida, Gainesville, 1982.

One type of session involved activities that provided vestibular stimulation, while the other type of session involved fine-motor table activities. Immediately prior to and after the activity sessions the subject worked with a tutor on school-related activities. The behavior of the subject was recorded during each of the three daily sessions in terms of his ability to attend to tasks and the number of verbalizations he produced either spontaneously or in response to a prompt.

Data were compared on a daily basis utilizing information from the pre- and post-treatment tutoring sessions to determine the effects of the two types of OT interventions on the subject's performance.

Results indicated a marked increase in spontaneous verbal language during vestibular stimulation activity sessions as compared to fine-motor activity sessions. The subject's obvious enjoyment of vestibular stimulation activities, particularly swinging, was expressed through laughter and increased effect.

Although other results gathered from the data regarding changes in language production and attending behavior as a result of vestibular stimulation were inconclusive, observations of the subject before, during and after the study indicated that vestibular stimulation appeared to be a useful treatment technique in this case.

Sensory Integration
Special Interest Section Newsletter; Vol. 5, No. 4, 1982

Occupational Therapy Services for Hearing-Impaired Children

By Helen M. Madill, BOT, MEd, OT(C)
The University of Alberta
Consultant Occupational Therapist
Alberta School for the Deaf, 1974-1980
and
Olivia C. Gironella, PhD
The University of Alberta
Consultant Pychologist
Alberta School for the Deaf, 1971-1981

In 1974 occupational therapy services were requested by the administrators of the Alberta School for the Deaf. Teachers were concerned about ten elementary school children between the ages of five and ten years who demonstrated the following kinds of deficits:

"D. is poorly coordinated, clumsy, cannot climb the rope in gym or execute a hand-over-hand sequence to go along a bar; he misses the chair, except for a bit of the corner when sitting down."

"P. is tense, unsure of himself, withdrawn, socially inept; he becomes angry and frustrated when he cannot perform as well as other children."

"J. has a very short attention span for most things going on in the classroom. While walking down the hallway he appears quite unsteady and on occasion trips over his own feet with no other obstacle in his path."

"S. tends to swing her legs while attending to the teacher. The degree of difficulty for her from any given lesson can be measured by the degree of rigour of leg-swinging. She cannot learn somehow to put letters together in a finger spelling sequence to form the correct words."

The above are excerpts from psychologist's referral data. These summaries are similar to reports of behavior of hearing children who demonstrate different types of learning disabilities, the only difference being that the referred children were all severely to profoundly hearing impaired. Their learning difficulties were secondary handicaps.

In 1975 Jensema reported the results of achievement tests completed by multiply-handicapped hearing-impaired children. He indicated that the numbers of those children were increasing and that "each specific kind of additional handicap tends to exert a unique degree of influence on academic achievement."Although our referring teachers were not in a position to indicate the degree to which their childrens' difficulties were influencing their performance, they were aware that these children had learning problems that were not typical of their hearing impaired peers.

The first problem facing the occupational therapist was to locate an adequate

evaluation instrument. The use of the clinical observations using total communication supplemented by demonstration proved to be quite adequate. Several common difficulties were found: poor muscle tone and cocontraction, poor equilibrium responses, difficulty assuming "unusual" positions (i.e., reflex inhibiting position ATNR), motor impersistence, poor bilateral motor coordination, reliance on visual monitoring, and abnormal responses to being touched.

There seemed to be sufficient clinical signs to indicate that these children likely experienced sensory integrative deficits in addition to their hearing impairment. As total communication was used throughout the junior department, it appeared possible to use this method of communication with the SCSIT. By signing and speaking the instructions simultaneously and ultimately making use of the "phonic ear," a certified therapist should be able to administer the battery.

The vocabulary level had to be carefully checked, therefore the first total communication format was reviewed by the psychologist and senior teacher. (This was later revised by two occupational therapists, H.A. Yuschyshyn and G. Watson,

(continued)

responsible for programming at the School 1979-81.)

Nine males and one female student had been referred to occupational therapy for assessment and remedial programs. These students were matched with peers by age, sex, cause of deafness, and residential status who were also selected from a teacher-referred group. They were considered to function quite adequately in academic and social areas. The SCSIT was administered to both groups, augmented by the total communication instruction format.

The following results were obtained. All the children in the peer group demonstrated score profiles that were within the expected limits (scores between +1.0 and −1.0). There were only two tests that were consistently poorly executed by this group: bilateral motor coordination, and standing balance.

One child in this group demonstrated greater difficulty performing motor tasks. Although he ultimately achieved success, it was with considerable effort. He was slower to complete items on the motor tests, particularly imitation of postures.*

The children with difficulties who were initially referred by their teachers for assessment and programming demonstrated score profiles that were similar to those gained by learning-disabled children. A high incidence of generalized dysfunction was demonstrated, for example, motor planning and bilateral coordination difficulties associated with signs of vestibular-based deficits (poor muscle tone, equilibrium reactions). Bilateral motor coordination and standing balance tests were again consistently poorly executed.

Remedial programs followed those generally described by Ayres (1972) and were continued for one academic year. There was general improvement in motor performance. Teachers reported that hyperactivity and distractibility decreased, tactile defensiveness decreased, and fine motor skills also showed improvement. The results of this small pilot study were reported at the Canadian Occupational Therapy Conference (Saskatoon, 1976) and the Australian Occupational Therapy Conference (Sydney, 1978).

Three pilot studies were then executed by senior occupational therapy students and returning therapists (diploma graduates completing bachelor of science degree requirements) in the Department of Occupational Therapy at The University of Alberta between 1977 and 1979. Each of these unpublished studies attempted to answer research questions that arose from the pilot project briefly described above.

The purpose of sharing results of small, unpublished studies with colleagues is to assist therapist who may be contemplating

designing similar small research studies. By sharing our successes and partial successes (some would call these failures), we hope that you will avoid similar pitfalls.

A small study was designed to test the hypothesis that a sensory integrative approach to therapy would positively affect the vestibular functioning of a sample of hearing-impaired children as measured by the Southern California Postrotary Nystagmus Test (SCPNT). Nine students identified with sensory integrative dysfunction and hyporesponsive reactions on the SCPNT served as the experimental group. Nine controls (matched as far as possible by cause of deafness, age, and residential status) who also demonstrated hyporesponsive reactions on the SCPNT were selected. A four-month remedial program was provided for the experimental group.

Results of this small study showed that the experimental group scores on the SCPNT demonstrated a trend in the direction of increased nystagmus, but this increase was not statistically significant. Those children whose deafness was caused by exogenous causes exhibited lower durations of nystagmus than those with unknown causes of deafness, but this was not statistically significant. Several limitations must be considered. Aside from the small sample, there were twelve out of the eighteen children for whom the cause of deafness was unknown. No record of academic achievement was kept. One of the problems with working with hearing-impaired children of elementary school age is that no achievement data are available. These children frequently arrived at Alberta School for the Deaf with little or no vocabulary or communication skill if they had not been able to attend the Association for the Hearing Impaired Preschool. Teachers therefore must give priority to the development of language and communication skills. It is not possible to obtain achievement scores until these children enter the senior programs.

The SCPNT appeared to be useful as an initial indicator of vestibular dysfunction but not as an indicator of change (Poetker, 1977). Monitoring functional change in such areas as muscle tone, concontraction, equilibrium, motor persistence in the manner outlined by Wood (1982) is indicated.

Stodalka (1978) established normative data for the students at Alberta School for the Deaf on the postrotary nystagmus test (N=158). These norms were significantly lower than those established by Ayres (1975) for the hearing population. There was greater variability in the performance of our sample, no nystagmus was recorded for several subjects and, upon retesting after an interval of some months, those scores remained unchanged.

Yuschyshyn and Waddell (1979) estab-

lished normative data for the students at Alberta School for the Deaf on the standing balance tests from the SCSIT (N=158). Comparison of the data obtained to that of Ayres (1972) demonstrated a significant reduction in static balance skills in this sample of hearing-impaired students. The following is a summary of the important factors relating to this sample:

1. Improved performance on SBO was observed in conjunction with increasing age. There was no age effect on SBC.
2. Sex of the child was not related to performance on either task.
3. A significant positive relationship was found to exist between performance of either SBO or SBC and the duration of postrotary nystagmus.
4. No significant main effects were observed for degree of hearing loss or time of onset of hearing impairment.
5. The exogenously deaf subjects showed significant deficits in SBC tasks. Etiology did not relate significantly to SBO.
6. As mental ability improved, so did standing balance (eyes open) improve, but this trend was absent with standing balance (eyes closed).

(Yuschyshyn & Waddell, 1979)

In January 1982 the Department of Occupational Therapy agreed to provide assessment and programming to hearing-impaired students at the Association for the Hearing Impaired Preschool. Fourteen children between three and five years of age were assessed using the clinical observations, VMI, and Goodenough-Harris Draw-A-Man Test. A teachers' behavioral checklist was also compiled. This was completed on all the children in the preschool so that some comparison could be made between the skill development of children without secondary problems and those referred.

Again it was found that the clinical observations using total communication supplemented by demonstration performed adequately. A review of findings indicates that these young hearing-impaired children demonstrate poorer muscle tone, equilibrium, bilateral coordination, and rhythm than one would expect of their hearing peers. Some difficulty was encountered in the assessment of ocular pursuit: even these very young hearing-impaired children watch the faces of those who work with them very intently and it is not easy to redirect their gaze from your face to an object. (Small molded plastic figures that fit over the end of a pencil provide a more interesting target for ocular pursuit.)

Both of the pencil and paper tests provided limited information with this group

(continued)

Hearing-Impaired Children

of children. In the early stages, hearing-impaired preschoolers are involved in a lot of dramatic play and creative free play is encouraged. Teachers use every available "teaching moment" to relate the object or event to the appropriate sign and sound to build language and communication skills through total communication. Structured activities are in the minority, therefore lack of experience has a major effect upon the final product. It is possible that the Miller Assessment for Preschoolers may prove to be a useful assessment tool with young hearing-impaired children.

It took longer to establish rapport with these young hearing-impaired children than it does with hearing children of similar age. For this reason during the initial assessment periods children were accompanied by staff members. Later in remedial sessions children generally attended in pairs—somehow leaving the classroom with a friend was an adventure, but going alone was a frightening experience.

Programs were designed for ten of the 14 children, and these generally involved activities that incorporated vestibular and proprioceptive input to increase muscle tone. activities designed to normalize postural reflexes, and reactions to tactile input. Activities designed to assist with bilateral coordination and motor planning were also included. Programs were left with preschool staff to be monitored by the occupational therapist from the Alberta School for the Deaf.

For additional information, contact:
Occupational Therapy Support Services
Alberta School for the Deaf
6240 - 113th Street
Edmonton, Alberta T6H 3L2

* This child was referred for programming at the commencement of the next academic year. It appeared that he was able to keep pace with the rest of his class at the lower level, but, when promoted, the strategies he had developed to cope with his motor planning difficulties were no longer sufficient.

REFERENCES

Ayres, A.J. *Sensory Integration and Learning Disorders.* Western Psychological Services: Los Angeles, 1972.

Ayres, A.J. *Southern California Postrotary Nystagmus Test Manual.* Western Psychological Services: Los Angeles, 1975.

Jensema, C.J. A note on the achievement test scores of multiply handicapped hearing impaired children. *American Annals of the Deaf,* 1975, Vol 120:1, 37-39.

Poetker, K.M. *Sensory Integration Therapy and the Deaf Child.* Unpublished paper, Department of Occupational Therapy, The University of Albert, April 1977.

Stodalka, H. *Norms of Nystagmus Duration in a Hearing Impaired Population.* Unpublished paper, Department of Occupational Therapy, The University of Alberta, April 1978.

Yuschyshyn, N.A. and Waddell, K. *Standing Balance in a Hearing Impaired Population: Norms and Implications.* Unpublished paper, Department of Occupational Therapy, the University of Alberta, April 1979.

Wood, P.A. Designing clinical record forms for research data collection. *Australian Journal of Occupational Therapy,* in press.

A list of selected references from the Poetker and Yuschyshyn papers follows:

Arnvig, J. Vestibular function in deafness and severe hardness of hearing. *Acta Oto-Laryngologica,* 1955, 45, 283.

Auxter, D. Learning disabilities among deaf populations. *Exceptional Children,* 1971, 37, 8.

Bordley, J.E., Hardy, W.G. Etiology of deafness in young children. *Acta Oto-Laryngologica,* 1951, 40.

Case, S., Dawson, Y., Schartner, J., Donaway, D. Comparison of levels of fundamental skill and cardio-respiratory fitness of blind, deaf, and non-handicapped high school age boys. *Perceptual & Motor Skills,* 1973, 36, 1291-1294.

Davis, H. *Hearing and Deafness.* Holt, Rinehart, Winston: Toronto, 1966.

Dublin, W.B. *Fundamentals of Sensorineural Auditory Pathology.* Thomas: Illinois, 1976.

Fraser, Wolstenholme, G., Knoght, J. *Sensorineural Hearing Loss: A CIBA Foundation Symposium.* Churchill: London, 1970.

Frost, J.O., Miller, M. Prenatal rubella frequently does cause impaired vestibular function. *New York State Journal of Medicine,* 1971, 71, 971.

Gacek, R. The pathology of hereditary sensorineural hearing loss. *Annals of Otology, Rhinology & Laryngology,* 1971, 80, 289-298.

Hardy, W.G., Bordley, J.E. Problems in diagnosis and management of the multiply handicapped deaf child. *Archives Oto-Laryngologica,* 1973, 98.

Koningsmark, B.W. Hereditary congenital severe deafness syndromes. *Annals of Otology, Rhinology, and Laryngology,* 1971, 80, 269.

Long, J.A. Motor abilities in deaf children. *Teaching, College, Contributions in Education,* 1932, 1, 514.

Myklebust, H.R. Significance of etiology in motor performance of deaf children with special reference to meningitis. *American Journal of Psychology,* 1946, 59, 249.

Myklebust, H.R. *The Psychology of Deafness.* Grune & Stratton: New York, 1960.

Van Zyl, F.J., Ives, L.A. Visual perception and eye-motor coordination in a group of young deaf children. *Developmental Medicine and Child Neurology,* 1971, 13.

Vernon, M. Meningitis and deafness: the problem, its physical, audiological, psychological, and educational manifestations in deaf children. *The Laryngoscope,* 1967, 77 1856-1874.

Wright, M. *The Pathology of Deafness.* Manchester University Press: Manchester, 1971.

Boyd, J. Comparison of motor behavior in deaf and hearing boys. *American Annals of the Deaf,* 1967, 112, 4, 598-605.

Carlson, B.R. Assessment of motor ability of selected deaf children in Kansas. *Perceptual & Motor Skills,* 1972, 34, 1, 303-305.

Geddes, D. Motor development profiles of preschool deaf and hard of hearing children. *Perceptual and Motor Skill,* 1978, 46, 1, 291-294.

Jaffe, B.F. *Hearing Loss in Children.* University Park Press: Baltimore, 1977.

Jensema, C., and Mullins, J. Onset, cause, and additional handicaps in hearing impaired children. *American Annals of the Deaf,* 1974, 119, 6, 701-705.

Koningsmark, B.W. Hereditary congenital severe deafness syndromes. *Annals of Otology, Rhinology, and Laryngology,* 1971, 80, 269.

Levine, E.S. *The Psychology of Deafness.* Columbia University Press: New York, 1960.

Lindsey, D., O'Neal, J. Static and dynamic balance skills of the 8 year old deaf and hearing children. *American Annals of the Deaf,* 1976, 121, 1, 49-55.

Rahto, T., Aantaa, E. Equilibrium disturbances caused by hearing aids in hard of hearing children. *Journal of Laryngology and Otology,* 1977, 91, 4, 357-359.

Rapin, I. Hypoactive labyrinths and motor development. *Clinical Pediatrics,* 1974, 13, 11.

Rosenblut, B., Goldstein, R., Landay, W. Vestibular responses of some deaf and aphasic children. *Annals of Otology,* 69, 747.

Shein, J.D. Deaf students with other disabilities. *American Annals of the Deaf,* 1975, 120, 1, 37-39.

Upfold, L.J. Deafness following rubella in pregnancy. *Medical Journal of Australia,* 1970, 1, 9, 420-424.

Zausmer, E. Congenital rubella: pathogensis of motor deficits. *Pediatrics,* 1971, 47, 1, 16-26.

Sensory Integration
Special Interest Section Newsletter; Vol. 5, No. 3, 1982

Sensory Integration Deficits in Retrolental Fibroplasia

By Linda Baker Nobles, MS, OTR

Retrolental fibroplasia is a condition which is most often seen in premature infants who receive oxygen therapy. When an infant receives high levels of oxygen, spasms in the retinal blood vessels can result. The spasms are followed by edema of the peripheral vascular system which can lead to stretching of the retina and to partial or total retinal detachment. These changes in the retina are generally observable at one month of age and may progress for some time. This condition which occurred frequently in the 1940's and 1950's has become rare until recent years when advancements in neonatology have allowed premature infants with very low birth weights to survive.

Children who have suffered retrolental fibroplasia can demonstrate a variety of other deficits besides the visual impairment. Whether the cause of these deficits

(continued)

Retrolental Fibroplasia

is due to prematurity, organic impairments, or lack of environmental stimulation is undetermined. Visually impaired children of many etiologies are frequently slower in development because the lack of visual stimulation prevents them from normally exploring their environment. However, the child with retrolental fibroplasia often demonstrates more overt perceptual and sensory integrative deficits. Many of these problems are observable in the classroom. This child may have such difficulties with projects which require spatial and temporal reasoning. He frequently demonstrates problems using both hands together in tasks requiring exploration, manipulation, and construction. Fine motor skills are generally poor and the child may have a great deal of difficulty learning to read and write Braille. It is often difficult for the child to perform self-care skills such as feeding and dressing. The child may have a great deal of difficulty moving freely and dressing. The child may have a great deal of difficulty moving freely through space and becomes

easily lost, causing poor acquisition of mobility skills. He may also demonstrate a reluctance to participate in large motor activities. He often prefers to sit and rock or engage in other self-stimulatory behaviors.

When tested in occupational therapy for sensory integration deficits, children demonstrate a variety of responses. On the Postrotary Nystagmus test, they will often indicate either a desire to continue the spinning or they will have difficulty tolerating ten rotations. (The evaluation of the nystagmus response in the visually impaired is contraindicated because an interpretation of standardized scores is inappropriate.) The children are often unable to maintain the extensor position when required to life only the head, arms and shoulders. They can usually assume the flexor or ball position for only a few seconds. Hypotonic muscle tone is often observed. Proprioceptive responses are generally very inadequate. When an arm or leg is placed in space, returned to the side of the body and the child is asked to return it to the same position, he or she

may place the limb in a difference plane or use the opposite limb.

This child often appears to be earthbound; unable to momentarily stand on one foot, jump or hop. Often he or she is unable to run. Bilateral integration deficits are also in evidence and can be observed when the child is performing gross motor activities.

The child with retrolental fibroplasia that displays any or all of these difficulties is a good candidate for sensory integration therapy. Initial improvements usually seem to occur in the child's ability to better integrate vestibular-proprioceptive information. This integration appears to benefit the child in several ways. There is usually a decrease of rocking and other self-stimulatory behaviors. The child seems less fearful of movement and will generally display more confidence in moving through space. This may be the most critical step for the visually impaired child to achieve, because it is only when he can begin to make some sense of his body and its relationship to space that he can begin to truly explore his environment.

Sensory Integration
Special Interest Section Newsletter; Vol. 5, No. 3, 1982

Early Intervention With The Visually Impaired Infant

By Linda Baker Nobles, MS, OTR

The infant that is born into a world without vision or with only partial vision is missing a critical sense that contributes to normal development. It is important to intervene early with this child to help prevent problems that may develop later and to encourage as normal development as possible. Early intervention is only successful if the parents can be integrated into the home programs. It is often most beneficial to work with the parents and the infant in the home situation because it allows the parents to feel they are the critical factor in the development of their child.

The most important point in working successfully with this child and his parents is to develop a sense of the bonding between the parents and the infant. Bonding with a visually impaired child can be delayed because the infant is slow to respond to the parents. A sighted infant spends time gazing at his mother's face which encourages smiling and beginning speech. This response in turn stimulates the mother to continue talking and playing

with the infant. The visually impaired infant often does not seem to respond to the mother, so the mother does not respond to the infant. Bonding can be encouraged by explaining to the parents the importance of talking and playing with the infant. The parents should be encouraged to have the infant's place their hands on the parents' faces. The infant will begin to explore the face and eventually learn to identify the parent by tactile cues as well as auditory cues.

Another area that is often slow to develop in the visually impaired infant is the extensor muscles of the neck, back and legs. The primary reason for this delay seems to be the lack of visual input. The sighted infant in the prone position begins to raise his head because he is receiving visual input that stimulates him to continue lifting his head. The visually impaired infant does not receive this visual stimulation and does not continue to lift his head. This position soon becomes a frustrating position and the child refuses to tolerate it. This position can be en-

couraged by having the parents provide gentle vestibular input in the prone position, either by rocking the child in their arms or rocking them forward on a bolster. In addition, because it is often difficult at an early age to determine the amount of vision present, the parent can use flashlights or other colored lights while the child is in the prone position to stimulate the child to lift his head and look towards the light source. Once the child begins to tolerate the prone position, it becomes easier to encourage the development of the extensor muscles.

The visually impaired infant often begins to achieve developmental levels such as the sitting and quadruped positions within normal limits, but then the development appears to stop. For example, this child will be able to assume the quadruped position, but instead of creeping, he will proceed to maintain this position and rock, because the lack of visual input prevents the child from moving towards an object. Research indicates that until the child is

Continued On Page 2

Visually Impaired Infant

because the lack of visual input prevents the child from moving towards an object. Research indicates that until the child is able to localize sound, he will not move. It is imperative that he learn to identify the source of sound and light. This can be encouraged by using toys that have texture and sound. Flashlights and penlights with bells or noisemakers attached are also useful items. The parent can be encouraged to first allow the child to become familiar with the toy. Then the child is placed in different positions (sitting, prone, supine) and the toy is removed just out of reach from the child. The light and/or sound is then activated. If the child does not make a movement with his hands or feet to locate the object, he is supplied with a tactile cue as well as a sound cue. These activities are continued until the

child can locate the object by sound or by light without the tactile cue. The same sequence can then be used to encourage the child to move towards an object.

The child's crib can also be a very stimulating environment. It is recommended that a crib gym be attached as early as possible. The child will hit it with his hands and feet accidentally and begin to develop the cause and effect relationship. This is also a very good toy to begin developing bilateral skills because the child uses both sides of the body to activate the toy. Another good item to place on a young infant's crib is a string of Christmas lights. This assists the child in learning to use what vision he has and this will be important later. Aluminum mirrors are also good toys because they reflect light and allow the child to see his own face if he has

more vision. Although cribs and playpens are important environments, it is important to encourage the parents to allow the child to spend time on the floor so that he begins to feel secure in all environments.

There are other general techniques which encourage normal development. Probably the most important is that the parent must talk constantly to the child and involve him in all aspects of his life, since the child will only learn what he experiences directly. It is also important that the child receive a great deal of vestibular, proprioceptive and tactile input. The parents will need to initially provide this and then help the child learn ways of providing it himself. It will become critical later that he has an adequate perception of his body in space and its relationship to his environment.

Sensory Integration
Special Interest Section Newsletter; Vol. 5, No. 3, 1982

Case Study: Mandie By Lynne Hall, OTR

At age four Mandie was referred by the Intermediate School District for a summer of private occupational therapy. An evaluation indicated a partial visual impairment, poor balance, delayed righting and equilibrium responses and mild hypotonia throughout her body. Using the Denver Developmental Screening Test, gross and fine motor skills were at approximately the 18 to 20 month levels. Personal social skills were at about 2 1/2 years and language was approximately at age level. This child was extremely fearful in space, becoming very upset whenever her equilibrium was even slightly disturbed. Mandie manipulated and controlled all situations through her language, her strongest area of development. She reportedly started to sit alone at six months, crept at 20 months though did not crawl according to her mother. She began walking at 3 years 4 months and started using full sentences at 3 1/2 years.

A therapy program was begun for one hour weekly. Because the child was so fearful in space, most of the time was spent on the floor. Treatment goals were to further improve balance, equilibrium responses, gross and fine motor skills through a sensory integration approach. Emphasis was placed on providing controlled sensory input in all sensory systems, especially the tactile, proprioceptive and vestibular systems. A variety of activities were tried, but it soon became obvious that her favorite was proprioceptive

and vestibular related, i.e., sit-bouncing on a large inner tube. She was also quite responsive to music, which we still use to stimulate other types of activity. As Mandie was extremely resistive to change, we stayed with her favorites until she was familiar with our environment and comfortable with our routine. Mandie enjoyed therapy sessions, sometimes displaying tantrum behavior because a session was over. Therapy was continued past the initial summer. Currently she has occupational therapy one hour a week, nursery school three mornings a week and goes to a public school program two afternoons a week. A visual impairment consultant from the Intermediate School District visits her home once a week. The school system feels she is not yet ready for kindergarten.

Gradually over the last one and a half years Mandie has progressed to sitting in a hammock swing, rolling prone over a carpeted barrel, rolling inside a carpeted barrel for ten feet and now we are working toward sitting on the bolster swing. Her balance is such that she can now jump with two feet from a 6 inch mattress to the floor. Equilibrium responses are much improved but still somewhat slow. As she has made these progressions, she has gone from crawling up the stairs to walking up the stairs in a reciprocal pattern. She also began to explore her environment, moving more freely with much less fear in space.

At school, she will reportedly seek out the balance beam. Where previously she would sit in one place, she now reaches out and moves to explore items in the treatment room. Her mother reported a similar exploration pattern in their backyard.

During a recent five week break in therapy, Mandie's mother noticed increased head rolling activity. By providing controlled vestibular stimulation in various planes this type of behavior seems to be minimized.

While Mandie still controls her environment with her language, she is making progress in the development of other areas. Using the Denver, Mandie, who is now just six, demonstrates fine and gross motor skills at approximately the 30 to 36 month level. Her personal social skills are at approximately the 33 month level. Her mother reports that gross motor skills are her favorite now. While progress is slow, it has been consistent. Mandie's own resistance to change must be dealt with constantly. At times when she must complete a task in order to do something she likes, she will do it quite rapidly. Other times, she does not seem to care.

While evaluation levels can give us approximate gains, watching this child perform activities which were previously impossible tasks is a delightful experience. More than anything, a sensory integration

(continued)

Case Study: Mandie

therapy program has given the child a freedom of movement which congenitally blind children have a great deal of difficulty developing. Being more comfortable in space should enable her to perform other life tasks with greater ease in the future.

Lynn Hall, OTR, is in private practice in Kalamazoo, MI.

Sensory Integration
Special Interest Section Newsletter; Vol. 5, No. 3, 1982

Case Study: J. By Mary E. Zemlick, OTR

Client J. was a 28-year-old male whose total blindness was diagnosed at birth as resulting from Retrolental Fibroplasia (RLF). He was referred to The Michigan Rehabilitation Center for the Blind for a 20-week Personal Adjustment program emphasizing training in Mobility, Adapted Kitchen Skills, and Personal Management. Information regarding previous education and training was unavailable. His IQ was determined, by previous testing, to be 59. Visual acuity was described as Hand Motions, bilaterally.

Activities of Daily Living

J. was independent in basic self-care skills but could not tie his shoes. J's personal management program focused on tasks requiring sequential organization, and motor planning, such as laundry, room organization and cleaning. Though J. was unable to tell time, he was usually able to independently attend class within 5 to 10 minutes of the scheduled time. A talking digital clock, with alarm set to tell the hour and half hour was considered. Training in money skills emphasized the paying for goods to the next dollar, as J. was unable to count, or properly make change.

Communication

J. was unable to write with pen, or hold a stylus properly to write Braille with a slate. He could not use a Braille writer or typewriter. J. was able to operate a cassette tape recorder, could insert tapes and batteries but was unable to use a telephone jack with his recorder to solicit aid or follow information given over the phone.

J. demonstrated mispronunciation of many common words (for example saying *v*raille for *B*raille) but appeared able to auditorily discriminate between similar and dissimilar words. He could repeat three and four part sentences, but his Mobility instructor reported J. to have difficulty repeating and following simple sequential route directions given him verbally. J.'s difficulty with spatial concepts and laterality and directionality appeared responsible for the mobility deficits.

Mobility

J. was dependent in travel. His instructor reported J.'s goal to be the ability to travel with a sighted guide properly in new environments, solicitng this assistance in the community, and to use the handivan for limited travel. He has no functional cane technique.

Sensory Integration

In the participation of Sensory Integration activities, J. was observed to focus with his eyes at bean bags tossed to him. He seemed to be able to avoid objects without the use of protective techniques while walking through the gym. In Crafts class, he was observed sorting tiles by color and could locate tiles by color and could locate tiles and beads visually. Subsequent Low Vision Evaluation and training suggested J. had more vision than previously documented—near vision being, with the right eye 10/400 and with the left eye 10/600. Visual testing was difficult as J. was unable to name the symbols he saw, or describe the direction of letters presented him. It became apparent that J. had some vision, but that his visual perception was nearly absent. Teaching goals were altered to include the improvement of visual perceptual skills.

Initially, "visual" activities frustrated J. and he frequently excused his difficulty by stating that he could not see. As he became increasingly more successful, and was praised for his performance, J. abandoned such remarks.

Sensory Integration evaluation revealed severe deficits in performance on all subtests of the Southern California Kinesthesia and Tactile Perception Tests. Observations determined J. to have an inability to cross the mid-line of his body, lack of hand dominance, poor knowledge of body parts with difficulty isolating them for purposeful movement and hypotonicity. Primitive postural reflexes were intact. J. had poor equilibrium reactions and poor proprioception. J. was unable to walk a balance beam, or stand on either foot independently. Spatial concepts were poor, performance of fast or slow unilateral and bilateral alternating movements was poor. Curiously, J. was able to

stand on his head up to three minutes, but demonstrated definite deficiency in co-contraction of arms, shoulders and neck.

Sensory Integration Treatment was conducted on an average of 4 times per week for 50 minute sessions, during a total of 20 weeks. The focus of the treatment was to: Integrate primitive postural reflexes, improve tactile-motor planning, improve the ability to isolate body parts for purposeful movement, improve muscle tone, improve processing of sensory input — especially the improvement of Visual-Motor skills, improve space and form perception and improve equilibrium.

Many treatment techniques used are described by A. Jean Ayres in *Sensory Integration and Learning Disorders and Activities for the Remediation of Sensorimotor Dysfunction in Primary School Children.*[1] Scooter board, jogger trampoline, platform swing, hammock swing, and nystagmus board were used extensively to provide vestibular input, to improve muscle tone, and to improve postural and bilateral integration. Equilibrium reactions, motor planning, laterality and bilaterality were emphasized through the use of the T-stool, tilt boards, balance beam, barrel rolling, obstacle course, and especially trampoline activities. Proprioception was influenced by weighting J.'s extremities during many activities. Re-evaluation of Sensory Integration function determined J.'s performance to have improved significantly on all of the SCSIT Kinesthesia and Tactile Perception tests. Initially, J. was unable to respond correctly to any of the items on the Manual Form Perception Test. Upon re-evaluation, he was correctly able to identify 7 of 12 forms presented, though his response time was delayed. On the evaluation of Graphesthesia, he was correctly able to reproduce 6 of 12 shapes drawn on the backs of his hands. J. demonstrated less cortical and more smoothly executed movements. He was able to maintain reflex inhibiting postures. Balance improved and J. was able to maintain balance

(continued)

Case Study: J.

on T-stool during kick ball activities and could walk a balance beam without assistance or anxiety. Standing balance eyes open, which previously was impossible, was 13 seconds on the right foot, and 23 seconds on the left foot upon re-evaluation. Standing balance with eyes closed was 11 seconds on the right foot and 20 seconds on the left. Trampoline activities, with upper extremities weighted, which initially produced awkward and rigid movements, resulted in fluid arm swing and normal walking gait while on the trampoline.

J. learned to tie his shoes, and demonstrated the ability to participate in and enjoy craft activities requiring bilateral hand use, and sequential steps. He was able to identify some colors by name, and common geometric shapes when incorporated into activities. He was able to hold a pen and chalk in his right hand and print his

initials. He was able to trace shapes, letters and numbers, and had begun discriminating them visually. He demonstrated improved problem solving and judgemental skills in situations which he previously refused to attempt.

Conclusion

Though J. is extremely unique in his presentation of vision but lack of visual perception, his deficits in sensory integration function are common among the blind population. Sensory integration most noticeably improved J.'s equilibrium reactions, postural security and bilateral integration. Visual perceptual skills improved. Other staff members spontaneously reported J.'s improved confidence and tolerance of new activities, as well as improved ability to follow sequential directions for cooking and cleaning and craft tasks. Spatial concept development and motor planning improved along with hand

dominance, with resultant ability to use a pen to write or a cooking utensil more appropriately. Visual-motor skills improved.

The improved emotional functioning is difficult to record and control. However, in this case it may have been more socially acceptable for J. to describe his sensory integration deficits, which were apparent in his performance of any simple task, as functions of his blindness. As integrative functions improved, and J. was able to learn new tasks more easily, he completely eliminated his previously continuous remarks, to the effect that he could not perform because he could not see. He even encouraged other students to persevere as he had.

REFERENCES
1. *Activities for the Remediation of Sensorimotor Dysfunction in Primary School Children.* Title III ESEA Project. Goleta Union School District, 5689 Hollister Avenue, Goleta, CA 93017.

Sensory Integration
Special Interest Section Newsletter; Vol. 5, No. 3, 1982

Adapting Evaluation Procedures for the Blind   By Mary Pat Gilbert, OTR

The following are suggestions for an observational assessment of sensory integrative function within the blind population:

1. *Muscle Tone and Reflexes* — all components are taken from Ayres' Clinical Observations of Neuromuscular Development. They include a general muscle tone assessment; cocontraction; postural background movements; supine flexion; prone extension; Schilder's arm extension posture; protective extension; rolling; ATNR and reflex inhibiting posture; and STNR.

2. *Balance, Equilibrium Reactions, and Gross Motor Skills* —
A. Balance beam
B. Hopping — right, left and bilateral, both moving and in place
C. Galloping
D. Skipping (omitted if individual indicates he/she is unaware of how to do so.)
E. Jumping Jacks — can be described verbally and subject can be given hands-on assist if unaware of how to perform; observe motor planning.
F. Standing Balance — eyes open *and* closed for those who have light perception or better vision.
G. Jumprope — optional
H. Angels in the Snow — adapted from Purdue Perceptual Motor Survey. Watch for motor planning and overflow.

I. Prone Beach Ball — put subject on large sturdy therapy ball with feet off the ground to look for gravitational security and tilting reactions when the ball is moved.
J. Chair Jumping — have subject step up on standard armless chair (or stool, if frightened of the height). Hold hand and have him jump down. Watch for fear and motor execution.

3. *Proprioception and Kinesthesia* —
A. Ayres' Kinesthesia Test — for observation *only*
B. Pathwalking — designed for observation of movement through space without object orientation. Holding subject by shoulders, move him forward three steps, make 90 degree turn, walk another three steps, turn 180 degrees and ask subject to retrace path. Take individual through first path physically to be certain directions are understood. Can path be imitated? Are turns made consistently and without error? Observe quality of turns. May also add paths with two turns.
C. Passive Placement of the Arms in Space — Place upper extremity in desired position such as 90 degree shoulder flexion, using goniometer to measure. Allow subject three seconds to experience that position; place arm back at side. Subject then returns arm to ex-

pected position. Remeasure, expected position within 15 degrees of original. Consider all upper extremity joints.
D. Matching Arm Placement — Place one upper extremity in desired position and ask subject to match with other extremity. Again measure — expect match to be within 15 degrees.

4. *Spatial Awareness* —
A. Awareness of Body Part Relationships — Ask a series of questions (we use 10) prefaced by: "Which is closest to the top of your head?" . . . (i.e. "Your waist or your hips?") If level of understanding is questioned, ask subject to point to various body parts.
B. Orientation of Objects — subject is placed between four objects, one in front, one behind, one to right, one left (each approximately three feet from subject). We use chair, stool, small table and small bench. Orient twice to objects. State which object the subject is facing. Ask "Which object is on this side?", "Which is behind?", etc. Turn a quarter turn, and repeat. We ask series of ten such questions. Another 10 items involve movement between objects. "Sit down in chair.", "Find a block on the bench.", etc. Ask several multistep questions. Observe ability to relate body to

(continued)

Adapting Evaluation Procedures for the Blind

object; object to object; quality of turns and movement between objects.

5. *Hand Skills* — Several suggestions include: bead stringing; shoe tying; pegboard making horizontal and vertical lines and/or simple design reproduction; making a person from clay; and matching shapes with parquetry blocks. We use set of 12 vertical dowels that are affixed side by side in thick piece of wood (total length approximately 2 1/2 feet, with tallest dowels 18 inches). Wooden spools are used for a variety of activities — right hand placement to right side and to left (to look at crossing midline); same with left; placement of one spool on each dowel with right hand and with left (sequencing); simultaneous placement with right and left; and reciprocal placement.

6. *Tactile Functions* — Ayres' Tactile Battery is used, again, for observation *only*. MFP shapes can be named or described. Ability to manipulate blocks is important assessment. May ask subject to identify

coins or like objects; choose the larger of several objects; distinguish textures, etc.

7. *Postrotary Nystagmus Test* — For observation only. Look for nystagmus; do not draw conclusions from it. Observe head control, maintenance of body position on board, dizziness, vertigo and general tolerance.

8. *Auditory Sequential Memory*, as included in Clinical Observations, is also utilized.

General Considerations:

1. Observe extraneous movements — rocking, swaying, etc. which may be related to the vestibular system. Ask subject if he sought out movement stimulation, i.e. twirling in just one direction.
2. Watch for reflex and overflow patterns during walking and other movements.
3. You will be relying heavily on verbal directions. Don't assume understanding of basic concepts such as right, left, facing, diagonal, etc. Hands-on assistance can be given if feasible.

4. If subject has light perception or better vision, occlude vision for tactile, proprioceptive and spatial awareness tests. May want to repeat latter with visual input.
5. Don't expect balance to be comparable to a sighted individual — vision plays an important role in static and dynamic balance.
6. If proprioception is poor, carefully analyze findings on tactile tests where difficulty experienced may be result of deficient proprioception rather than deficient tactile discrimination (esp. FI and GRA).
7. This evaluation has been used with adults and children ten years and up. With younger children and lower functioning adults, portions or adaptations may be used.

Mary Pat Gilbert is a therapist at the Rehabilitation Institute, Kansas City, MO.

Sensory Integration
Special Interest Section Newsletter; Vol. 5, No. 2, 1982

Sensory Integration—How to Program for Deaf School Children

By Arlene C. Finocchiaro, OTR, Margaret S. Sterck School for the Hearing Impaired, Delaware

Hearing-impaired and deaf children with sensory integrative dysfunction present many similar problems as observed in children with learning disabilities. However, for the deaf, the impact of the dysfunction further limits the compensation strategies which are needed to accommodate to a major sensory loss.

Compensation skills would normally develop through other sensory systems, especially vision, but if these are inefficient, a child's total learning and performance capacities are significantly altered. Etiological factors related to the origin of the hearing impairment may underlie mild to moderate neuromotor deficits accompanying the sensory loss and the sensory integrative dysfunction. When interpreting clinical observations and sensory integrative test data and planning therapeutic goals for these children, the special demands of their academic environment need to be considered.

As an example, at the Margaret S. Sterck School for the Hearing Impaired in Delaware, a total communication approach incorporates the use of sign language. Starting from infancy, deaf students must

develop prolonged visual attention and visual concentration to attend to combined verbal and sign language communication.

Additional visual skills are required for perception of sign language. Receptively, differentiation between signs requires visual spatial analysis of sequentially moving stimuli integrated with language concepts. To add some confusion, everyone has a different style for signing, just as people have different handwriting, and some are easier to read than others. Thus, form constancy is an essential component for language conceptualization.

As there is generally a prevalence of visual abnormalities among deaf students, efficient dependence on visual skills is at risk. Within the Sterck School population, 62% of 85 students from nursery through high school levels demonstrated eye movement inefficiencies.

Expressively, sign language requires fine motor stability, bilateral integration and complex fine motor planning, all integrated with sequential language concepts. Thus, vestibular-cerebellar integration, underlying aspects of bilateral integration, movement stability, and rhythmic se-

quencing of fine movement, provides a basic foundation for sign language movements. Integrity of vestibular integration must be discussed with the audiologist and the speech therapist as voice quality and speech production may be influenced by the quality of 8th cranial nerve function.

Efficient visual skills are needed in other academic areas, especially reading. Visual spatial perception and visual sequential memory are important components in reading, as phonetic clues may be limited or absent for word differentiation. Even learning the alphabet may be difficult, because it requires memorizing a sequence of 26 visually unrelated symbols. Students demonstrating sensory integrative dysfunction may reverse letter or number sequences, inappropriately copy sequences of letters or numbers, or have difficulty with spelling and memorizing math facts.

Interpreting vestibular responses presents a particular challenge due to the frequency of vestibular problems associated with deafness. Rarely is information

(continued)

Sensory Integration—Deaf School Children

available in Delaware regarding caloric or electronystagmographic testing, and the quality of functional vestibular responses is determined by the occupational therapist. Postrotary nystagmus testing should be approached cautiously because some deaf children are extremely sensitive to rotation. After rotation, some children show depressed nystagmus because they may have developed exceptional visual concentration and quickly refocus as would an ice skater. When there is support for damage to the labyrinths or the vestibular portion of the eighth nerve, integrity of the visual and proprioceptive systems should be closely scrutinized for their compensatory and therapeutic value.

As postrotary nystagmus may vary widely in this population, other tests of balance combined with clinical observa-

tions may provide more consistent reliable information regarding functional vestibular responses. As balance problems would be expected within this population, 49% of the 85 students referred for sensorimotor screening did demonstrate such problems. Also, 38% demonstrated inadequate postural reflex integration and antigravity postural control, and 13% demonstrated choreoathetoid-like movements.

For many of these students, sensorineural deafness accompanied or resulted from a disorganizing neurological condition such as rubella, cerebral palsy, meningitis, childhood Meniere's disease, or high risk birth factors. They may be educationally placed according to the major handicapping condition of hearing impairment, but their sensory integrative and neuromotor dysfunctions may be just as

significant.

Since some states provide public school services for the deaf from birth through age 21, which is the case in Delaware, occupational therapists have the opportunity to significantly affect many phases of educational programming.

References:

Barrett, S. S.: Assessment of vision in the program for the deaf. *American Annals of the Deaf,* 1979, 124, 745-752.

Ingalls Holderbaum, F. M., Ritz, S., Hassaneim, K. M., & Goetzinger, C.P.: A study of otoneurologic and balance tests with deaf children. *American Annals of the Deaf,* 1979, 124, 753-759.

Pennella, L: Motor ability and the deaf: research implications. *American Annals of the Deaf,* 1979, 124, 366-372.

Poizner, H., Battison, R., & Lane, H.: Cerebral Assymmetry for American Sign Language: the effects of moving stimuli. *Brain and Language,* 1979, 7, 351-362.

Sensory Integration
Special Interest Section Newsletter; Vol. 5, No. 2, 1982

Sensory Integration and the Hearing-Impaired Child

By Dorothy Jirgal, MA, OTR, Occupational Therapy Consultant, Project HOPE, San Diego County Department of Education

My first interest in the sensory integration needs of the hearing impaired child developed when a little girl was referred to the Occupational Therapy Department at Children's Hospital and Health Center in San Diego some years back due to her obvious incoordination problems and very poor balance. With therapy, her motor proficiency improved. So also did (to everyone's amazement) her expressive language. She had gained three years in one year's time in the area of expressive language on the I.T.P.A. (It is to be noted, however, that she was receiving hearing education concurrent with her occupational therapy.)

After this case, other children with hearing losses and *suspected* sensory integrative dysfunction were referred to occupational therapy routinely for evaluation and, if indicated, therapy. An "informal" criteria was developed which helped to delineate the children who would most likely benefit from occupational therapy services. Children were referred who demonstrated some or all of the following characteristics:

1. Their inability to acquire language skills commensurate with the degree of loss after hearing aids had been fitted and after they had been started on a hearing education program.

2. Their inability to acquire sufficient language commensurate with intellectual potential.
3. Known learning problems—either in the reading-language domain or in the mathematical computation domain.
4. Behavioral problems not felt to be primarily environmentally induced, and that were manifested by poor coping ability, which often was shown by any combination of the following behaviors:
   a. frequent temper tantrums
   b. unusual stubbornness
   c. inflexibility
   d. lack of social relativeness and poor peer interactions
   e. over-activity with a need for constant movement (This was often accompanied by poor sleep patterns)
   f. lack of purposeful play
5. Poor attending ability in general and the inability to attend both auditorily and visually at the same time or the inability to process two sensory modalities simultaneously. (These children often appeared visually and/or auditorily distractible.)
6. Poor motor coordination and balance, unusual clumsiness, poor muscle tone, lack of good central stability and inadequate postural adjustments. (With some of the "over-active" children there ap-

peared to be a predominance of extensor tone.)
7. Difficulty with motor planning with accompanying frustration at attempts to learn new motor skills—such as hopscotch, jumping rope, or riding a bicycle and difficulty performing children's art and crafts projects involving cutting, coloring, pasting and folding.
8. Poor oral-motor functions with any or all of the following:
   a. poor muscle tone around the mouth
   b. difficulty controlling saliva
   c. inability to suck, chew or swallow adequately
   d. poor motor planning of the tongue for speech sounds
   e. absent or hyperactive gag reflex
   f. fussy eating habits, especially related to certain textures of foods
   g. poor articulation

(Criteria list taken from a paper by this author presented to the Second International Conference on Auditory Techniques—Pasadena, California—1979)

Assessment of young hearing impaired children utilizing standardized tests such as the Southern California Sensory Integration Test series was often quite difficult due to the communication barrier and the

(continued)

Sensory Integration and the Hearing-Impaired Child

frequent attending problems of many of the children. The exception was the Southern California Post-rotary Nystagmus Test that children often "craved" and which often provided valuable information on how the children were or were not processing movement input. Probably of greater value was the use of an extensive sensorimotor and play history filled out by the parents and further expanded upon in the parent-therapist interview. Close attention was paid particularly to tactile and vestibular integration. Observation of the child at play in the Occupational Therapy Clinic was often most helpful. Sometimes these sessions could be structured in part to gather more clinical data, i.e., introducing activities in different positions on the scooterboard, or placing the child in a net-swing.

In those cases in which therapy appeared to be the most successful, probably the most significant change was the ability

of the child to attend—to both look and listen simultaneously. Because this was sometimes so dramatic, the author "was convinced" there had been a change in hearing thresholds. In most situations this was not so, although the child often attended better during the audiological testing procedures. Since sensory integration treatment is directed towards subcortical functions, it is reasonable to presume that both attention and auditory processing have potential to improve, and since before structured language education can be wholly successful the child must be able to attend and process, the children were often more successful in hearing education therapy.

The second area in which the parents often reported a positive change was the child's overall behavior. There appeared to be a decrease in temper tantrums and frustration with a concurrent improved ability to cope better—particularly in group

situations: i.e., "Now I can take my child to the grocery store or to a family gathering without him falling apart." This must have facilitated a more relaxed and enjoyable relationship between parents and child. As the hearing impaired become more organized so often did their play and there was less of a need to be just running around.

In conclusion, the auditory system is a very complex system with sub-cortical centers that provide for sound analysis and integration. Joan Wilentz, in her excellent book *The Senses of Man*, states that "no other system of the body makes as many stop offs enroute to the cortex, splits and branches as extensively so as to supply information from each ear to both sides of the brain." Occupational therapy, utilizing a sensory integration approach can, in carefully selected cases, facilitate a child's ability to maximize his potential.

Sensory Integration
Special Interest Section Newsletter; Vol. 5, No. 2, 1982

Sensory Integration Programming for Hearing-Impaired Children

By Shoshana Spiegel

Kendall Demonstration Elementary School is a part of Gallaudet College and is located on its campus in Washington, DC. It is a day school which serves hearing impaired children from 0-14 years of age who live within a 40 mile radius of the school. Being a demonstration school, Kendall has frequent American and International visitors. Materials that are developed on campus are widely disseminated as part of the mission of the college. There is also a high school on campus that serves local pupils and those from other states and countries.

Kendall's communication policy is "total communication." This means that oral and manual communication, along with other modes such as pantomine, gestures, and drama are used as necessary with the goal being successful reception and expression of language by each child. The communication issue is a major one, in deaf education, with some schools stressing an oral approach and others encouraging the development of manual communication. While not central to the role of occupational therapy, the subtle implications of communication method will be mentioned later.

School enrollment is nearly 200. Classes are small with approximately six students in each. The Instructional Division has six departments:

1. Preschool serves children from 0-2 at home and those from 2-4 at school.
2. Primary includes 5-8 year olds.
3. Elementary is responsible for 9-11 year olds.
4. Middle School teaches 12-14 year olds.
5. The Special Opportunities Program, new in the fall of 1981 serves all ages of the multiply handicapped and gifted.
6. Diagnostic and Support Services provide special assistance to all age levels. In addition to OT there are nurses, counselors, psychologists, audiologists, a social worker, a speech/language pathologist, an audio technician, and a consultant PT, opthamologist, pediatrician, ENT specialist, and psychiatrist. The coordinator of parent programs and the coordinator of sign language programs for families are also in DSS.

Occupational therapy came to Kendall

in the Fall of 1979. The need had become apparent the previous school year when nearly 20 pupils were referred to the Diagnostic Prescriptive Teachers due to "perceptual-motor" difficulties. At that time there were three DPTs, one of whom had worked closely with an OT in a previous job. She recognized the need for an OT. This was substantiated when the OTs at Cripped Children's Services screened the identified children and it was determined that the majority had sensory integrative dysfunction.

The main emphasis of the therapy program has consistently been treatment of children with consultation to teachers having secondary emphasis. The reason for this is that the degree of SID in most of the children warranted direct OT intervention.

In the first year of the OT program, efforts were made to educate teachers about what OT did and what symptoms could suggest appropriate candiates for referral. A videotape entitled "Introduction to Sensory Integration" was developed and demonstrated some screening

(continued)

items and treatment activities. At that time, before the existence of the Special Opportunities Program, there were fewer multiply handicapped pupils. Most of the children who needed OT had SID and usually had the subtle signs typical of the learning disabled hearing population. An additional clue was sometimes the quality of the motor production of signs or fingerspelling.

The second year of the OT program, Kendall began using a Child Study Team format to routinely review each child in the school and to refer those with possible problems to the specialists. The purpose of this strategy was to facilitate better communication of teachers and specialists through a teaming effort with the end result being a better program for each child. Meetings for each department were held twice a month for two hours each time. The session was divided into routine reviews and referral of the children who seemed to have pressing needs that could not wait until they came up for the routine review.

This approach replaced a random referral arrangement which lacked a central coordinating group to monitor or prioritize referrals. Staffings were held only when a situation reached crisis proportions for a particular child. One advantage of the CST system was the opportunity for the OT to use the meetings to further educate the faculty members on a less formal basis than the inservices she had presented.

Also during the second year, collaboration with one PE teacher occurred. More multiply handicapped children were enrolled at the school and it was necessary to adapt activities for them. The idea of a developmental approach was encouraged by the OT and to some degree was carried over into other PE classes by one of the two PE teachers.

Another focus of the second year was an effort to inform parents of the therapy program through an inservice. The presence of the OT at IEP conferences led to suggested home programs for the summer.

The process for assessment has remained the same since the initiation of the OT program. As children were referred, they were screened using an adapted version of the clinical observation format by Jan Johnson with some items from the Purdue Perceptual Motor Survey added. This includes testing of reflex residuals, muscle tone, balance, eye, hand, and foot preference, eye movements, bilateral motor coordination, tendency to cross the midline, and ability to imitate movement patterns. Having several years of experience, this therapist found the use of clinical observations to be an adequate screening instrument. This is particularly true since most of the children referred

had symptoms of the VBI syndrome which is easily identified using this tool.

Due to the communication difficulty, it was not feasible to use the Ayres battery. However, in December 1981, with permission of Western Psychological Services, a videotape of signed instructions for the SCSIT was made by Galluadet TV studio. This was the end product of the collaboration of a deaf linguist and this therapist. It is intended for use as a teaching tool for therapists with some knowledge of sign language.

Most of the children referred for OT had a history of meningitis, rubella, or some other type of illness. The typical picture included poor balance, hyporesponsiveness to rotation, low muscle tone, and reflex residuals. These symptoms were accompanied by academic difficulties such as poor handwriting or reading skills which had usually prompted the referral. As the teachers became more sensitive to subtle signs, occasional referrals were received on children of deaf families who seemed to have symptoms more typical of dyspraxia. These observed tendencies suggest the need for further investigation of the correlation of etiology and dysfunction. This aspect does not seem to be given must attention in deaf education and could be significant. The majority of the OT caseload of 33 pupils are primary aged children. The one OT is seeing nearly one half of that age group (20). There is a waiting list of other children who have been referred. Most are new admissions who have arrived since the beginning of the school year. The OT has not been involved in the intake process. This is due to time constraints and the reliability of others to appropriately refer. The development of the Special Opportunities Program has led to the admission of children whose need for OT has been previously demonstrated. It also has increased the need for use of NDT.

Once the assessment is completed, treatment has been scheduled in half hour sessions. The reason for this time span is that most teachers would be reluctant to have their pupils pulled out of class for longer time periods. It also has enabled the therapist to take on a larger caseload. However, a severe drawback has been a lack of intensity of treatment. It is harder to see progress with such limited therapy. Only a few children have been seen twice weekly.

Most children were seen individually at least at the beginning. Pairs of children with similar dysfunction were grouped together with usually positive peer interaction. The youngest preschoolers were seen in class groupings of three or four children. The teacher or class aide assisted and then was able to bring ideas back to the classroom for carry over.

The equipment used for therapy is typi-

cal of a clinic treating SID. Due to a healthy budget at the start of the OT program, it was possible to purchase a wide assortment of hanging equipment. This is ideal for use with the hearing impaired children, most of whom seem to crave the movement stimulation. The platform swing is particularly helpful since pairs of children can be stimulated simultaneously. The children love to "fly" using the four suspended loops, also by Southpaw. The SDE airspot trainer, an inflated cylinder measuring 36 x 64", is invaluable.

Progress varied with the children. Several have shown remarkable changes that seemed related to OT treatment. Feedback from teachers and some parents has been used to decide whether a child should continue in therapy or be terminated.

Improvements in reading, handwriting, and fine and gross motor skills have been described. The PE teacher has been particularly helpful in observing physical progress. Previously, in a setting where the oral approach was used, children who were not progressing in auditory training were referred to OT. After sensory integrative treatment, many were able to make better use of their residual hearing. Since the oral approach alone is not strongly stressed at Kendall, this outcome has not been observed.

While implementation of sensory integration treatment with the hearing impaired is similar to using the approach with any other child, there are some special issues. Learning sign language has been a challenge, sometimes frustrating. It gives one a better understanding of motor planning! It has also been a very beautiful experience to have access to a new mode of expression and another group of people. Luckily, it was possible to use demonstration during therapy before manual communication became fluent. A definite milestone was the ability to use sign langauge smoothly enough to reprimand clients! Actually a major concern is safety. Visual attention is necessary for communication and is often difficult to attain, especially when the child is on hanging equipment and in motion. Warning the child of impending danger becomes a problem even for the fluent signer.

Behavior management becomes a greater challenge with the hearing impaired who can shut out the therapist completely by closing their eyes.

Another concern is the implication of awkwardness in movement for a person who relies totally on manual communication. This creates a need to look at the developmental process involved in learning to sign. It is a particular problem for a CP child with athetoid movements that

(continued)

Sensory Integration Programming for Hearing-Impaired Children

also prevents the development of legible handwriting.

An important theoretical consideration is the significance of the vestibular system. In the early seventies, the neurophysiological connections between the two branches of the eighth cranial nerve began to be examined. If there are common pathways, it is possible that one system can influence the other. Perhaps this is why the use of residual hearing became more efficient in the "oral" children who received

vestibular stimulation. Another relationship of particular importance to the hearing impaired is that of language development and the vestibular system. If indeed there is a correlation, then perhaps vestibular stimulation can facilitate this crucial aspect of function. Although many clients had delays in language development, they were not referred to OT because of this dysfunction.

The use of sensory integration therapy with the hearing impaired requires the

same knowledge of theory and practice but adds a unique challenge.

For information regarding loan of the videotapes, the author may be contacted at 2213 Cocquina Drive, Reston, VA 22091.

Shoshana Spiegel, MHS, OTR
Kendall Demonstration
Elementary School
Gallaudet College
Washington, DC

Sensory Integration
Special Interest Section Newsletter; Vol. 5, No. 1, 1982

The Balcones Sensory Integration Screening—Revised Edition

Occupational therapists working in the educational setting are well acquainted with the relationship between the lack of academic achievement and the presence of sensory integrative dysfunction. If therapists are successful in explaining to educators the concepts and theories regarding this relationship and the possible remediation techniques which occupational therapists utilize, they may be inundated with referrals for occupational therapy services for the learning disabled/ sensory integrative dysfunctioning child. The conceptual problem has been hurdled but the therapist is now faced with a multitude of "mechanical" problems including large numbers of children to evaluate and treat, inadequate space, not enough therapists, and, above all, not enough time.

The Balcones Special Services Cooperative in Austin, Texas, sought answers to all these mechanical problems. The director of the co-op, Dr. Ruth Haak, and the staff were strongly committed to the "whole" child concept and also to broadening the understanding of the learning-disabled child through the use of sensory integrative and neuropsychological concepts. After attending a lecture given by Dr. A. Jean Ayres, Dr. Haak thought that sensory integration had a place in the evaluation procedures used in the co-op. She felt that sensory integration theory filled many gaps in lower brain function not addressed by classic neuropsychology.

In 1976, Dr. Haak received a Title IV-C, ESEA grant the goal of which was development of a program for zero eject of learning-disabled adolescents. Cynthia Jones, occupational therapist with the co-op, developed the original Balcones Sensory Integrative Screening Protocol as one

of several projects on the grant. The intent was for the Screener to provide a screening base for the most basic brain stem and associated area responses. It was designed to be used alone as a screening instrument or as a component of a more detailed neuropsychological battery. In its use as a screener, it identified students who would benefit from formal sensory integrative/sensorimotor evaluation and programming. Information gained from the screening was helpful in identifying special problems in neuro-behavioral, behavioral, and/or classroom performance. It was to aid the therapist in consulting teachers about appropriate expectations to set in the classroom.

Because of time constraints, the original instrument had nine subtests that were each drawn from a prenormative data base—the items all came from previously accepted or original batteries. Some of the tests used include the Purdue Perceptual Motor Survey, the McCarron Assessment of Neuromuscular Development and the Southern California Sensory Integration Tests.

The Balcones Sensory Integration Screening Test (BSIST) is composed of 11 subtests. With some experience, the entire battery requires 20 minutes to administer and score. An additional 5 minutes is needed to develop the profile, which will be discussed later. The only piece of equipment would be a dynamometer but, because the score for this item is based on comparative hand strength, an adapted blood pressure cuff/sphygmomenometer would work. A minimum of space is required—a hallway would suffice! Each item is scored on an objectively defined scale from 1 to 4. A total score as well as

standard scores can be tabulated. In addition, comparisons of right and left performances can be done. It is recommended that the therapist using the test have experience with sensory integrative theory, evaluation, and treatment techniques, although certification in the SCSIT is not necessary for use of the Balcones.

In 1979, the Screener was revised to include two tactile-based subtests. It was then administered to two first grade, two second grade, and two third grade classes in two public schools. The total sample tested was 130. The age of the subjects ranged from six to nine years. Racial distribution of the sample was that of the population at large in Texas. The items were then factor analyzed and eight major components were identified. These eight factors were used to make up the Sensory Integration Screening Profile. Some of the factors identified were designated Tactile Feedback, Vestibular, Proprioception, and Ocular Motor Control.

After test administration, raw scores from the test items are placed next to the appropriate factor on the Profile form and totaled. The total raw score is then plotted on the scale line for that factor, which will convert it to a standard score. By connecting the plotted points, a profile or graph is constructed.

A weakness of the test lies in the standardization. The items on the test are rated on a four-point scale and there was not enough spread in the resultant numbers to allow for a true distribution of the scores to be determined. The scores are too compressed. There are some factors for which it is not possible to achieve a score below

(continued)

Balcones Sensory Integration Screening

—1.0 standard deviations below the mean, or above +2.0 standard deviations above the mean. It is felt by the authors, therefore, that in many instances a negative standard score of even —1.0 may be indicative of dysfunction. A last point regarding the problems with standardization is that the items tested represent neuromotor functions that are not present or absent in degrees. A child either is able to do the activity or is not. In spite of the four-point scale, "grades of ability are not seen as frequently as one might think."

The BSIST has proved extremely useful in developing "monitoring" service delivery programs for the public schools. This approach as used in the TOTEMS course advocates a method of providing services that fall between regular (i.e., daily or weekly) hands-on treatment and consultation. Children are screened using the BSIST, and additional testing can be done for children demonstrating the need and remediation programs can be established by the therapist. Motor "labs" using sensorimotor activities appropriate for small

groups of two to three children, grouped according to their profile, are carried out daily by school personnel other than the therapist. These motor lab programs have been quite successful in three different Texas school districts under three therapists. It is important to state that in all these programs, the key ingredient to the success was the occupational therapist who monitored the program. When therapist involvement lagged or was dropped, the program did not continue. The ethical issue regarding sharing our expertise with those outside occupational therapy is of concern. In these three cases, it is agreed by the therapists that, regardless of the interest and time spent with the implementation of the motor lab, continuation of the program did not occur without the therapist's theoretical background.

In addition to the public schools, useful applications of the BSIST were found in centers for the mentally retarded, adolescent psychiatric settings and general psychiatric settings. Some data gathering from these three settings is being done in the

hope of expanding that data base.

In the fall of 1981, the BSIST-Revised Edition was published by the Texas Occupational Therapy Association, Incorporated. It is available from them in test kit form (except stopwatch and dynamometer) with the proceeds going to the Association. Three workshops were held by the authors of the Revised Edition in three Texas cities. The objective of the workshops was to teach uniform administration and scoring methods. The BSIST is a screening test and will remain so. Its use in the public schools where therapists are expected to treat large numbers of children gives the therapist a "handle" and some objective justification for further testing and program development.

Additional information regarding the BSIST is available from: Texas Occupational Therapy Association, Inc., PO Box 2042, Austin, TX 78768, (512) 479-8792.

Submitted by Mary Ann Monkhouse Kleuser, OTR Fort Worth, TX

Sensory Integration
Special Interest Section Newsletter; Vol. 5, No. 1, 1982

Vibration as a Therapeutic Tool

Notes From A Workshop Presented By Josephine C. Moore, PhD, OTR

In working with autistic and mentally impaired children who actively sought vibratory stimulation, I was curious about the need these children were demonstrating and the possible effects of such input. When given the opportunity, subjects applied hand-held electric or battery-operated vibrators primarily to the face and head, especially the mouth, nose, ears and/or chin. Dr. Josephine Moore's discussion of phylogenetic considerations and neural components of vibration facilitated a better understanding of the childrens' need for and possible benefits from this source of stimulation.

Vibration is the product of pressure and/or sound wave forms traveling over time, having two identified components: *frequency* and *amplitude*. *Frequency* describes the wave speed or number of waves passing a given point in one second of time. This component is expressed in Hertz (H_z) or cycles per second (CPS). Figure 1 illustrates this concept.

The Manufacturer of a particular vibrator should be able to tell you the frequency

if the package insert or a stamp on the vibrator does not indicate this. (Many electric ones have a frequency of 60 H_z.)

Amplitude describes the intensity or height of the wave form, as illustrated in Figure 2, and is measured in millimeters (mm). You can actually measure the amplitude by holding the head of the vibrator against a ruler and noting the amount of displacement from midline that occurs as it operates.

Both frequency and amplitude can be described as high or low, these being terms relative to the conditions described in any particular study conducted on vibration. "Because of the relative use of these terms, it is wise to state the H_z and amp. of the vibrator in two ways: (1) . . . when the vibrator is 'free standing', i.e. not touching anything, and (2) . . . when applied to the

(continued)

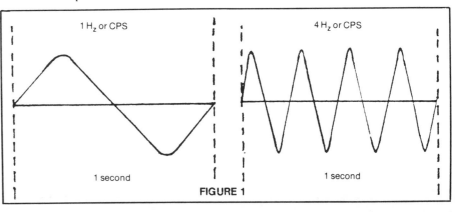

FIGURE 1

Vibration as a Therapeutic Tool

body." Under both circumstances amplitude remains constant, however, the frequency may decrease (depending upon the amount of applied pressure) when the vibrator is applied to any surface. Most studies have found that high frequency, low amplitude vibration is most effective for facilitation. "In spite of different statements in the research literature the optimal vibratory stimulus for a therapeutic response in man appears to be in the range of 100-200 H_z with an amp. of 1.0 mm to 2.5 mm." Under experimental conditions (on animals where one parameter is tested), 200-300 H_z may be best for stimulating the muscle spindle, especially when placed on stretch. Be sensitive to individual differences and try variations within these ranges on yourself and your clients to find what works best.

Low frequency-high amplitude (1-30H_z and greater than 2.5 mm.) vibratory stimulation should be avoided in patients with CNS dysfunction because this tends to alert through the sympathetic nervous system and can lead to disorientation. Examples of natural events where such conditions exist include earthquakes, thunder, volcanic eruptions and tornadoes. All demand arousal of the organism for protection from danger.

Phylogenetically, touch-pressure receptors or touch-vibratory receptors are believed to be the original basis for vibratory sense, an essential component in the development of time and space orientation. Two major types of vibratory sensors are found in humans: (1) *Flutter* or low frequency (5-50H_z) vibratory receptors believed to be located primarily in the epidermis and dermis, including hair follicles and Meissner's corpuscles; (2) *Vibration* or high frequency (50 or 100 to 300 H_z) receptors located in subcutaneous and deep tissues. The latter category includes:

a. Muscle spindles (especially Group Ia afferent of the nuclear bag);
b. Pacinian corpuscles, especially in the hands and feet;
c. Pacinian-like corpuscles found in muscles, tendons, joint capsules, periosteum, peritoneum, pericardium and heart, external genitalia and mammary glands, and interroseous membranes;
d. Bones (skeleton and ossicles) and teeth. Conduction through solid material travels at a more rapid rate than through air;
e. Fluid-filled chambers surrounded by membranes and/or bones. This includes the vestibulocochlear apparatus, eyes, subarachnoid space and CNS ventricular system, pericardial and abdominal cavities;
f. Soft membranes which receive and resonate vibratory impulses, including tympanic membranes, and round and oval windows of the ears.

This helped to explain the craving for stimulation about the face and the head by the children, and encouraged the thinking that input to the vestibular receptors might be enhanced by this application. However, vibration of the jaw, face, bony prominences of the head, and teeth, especially with low frequency stimulation, may create nausea, vertigo and other sympathetic reactions. Use this wisely, allowing the individual to be the guide based on his/her own needs while monitoring responses indicative of sympathetic over-activation.

A number of factors have been found to enhance vibratory stimulation, increasing facilitation of the tonic vibratory reflex (TVR), a proposed mechanism which is excitatory to Group Ia fibers of the muscle spindle. Some of those factors are mentioned here. Better results are obtained when the individual is actively involved, both in voluntary muscle contraction and in applying the vibrator to a site on the body. Birth to approximately 50 years seems to present the optimal ages at which responses can be obtained. As persons get older, there appears to be a decline in receptors and/or their response to stimuli. Vibration of an agonist is facilitatory to itself and its synergists (autogenic excitation) when properly used and inhibitory to its antagonists (reciprocal inhibition). When applied closer to the bone or bony prominences, vibratory stimulation can spread to the antagonists, creating inhibition in the agonist and/or withdrawal. Tendons, especially long, thin ones, provide the best site for application, with stimulation of the muscle belly being somewhat less effective. The myotendinous junction may also be an ideal site for input in producing a response. Resistance against the vibrated muscle is more facilitatory than using vibration alone. Placing the muscle in lengthened range (or stretch) also helps facilitate the TVR. Medications may have varying effects, depending upon the site where they have an influence. For example, muscle relaxants tend to decrease the TVR, whereas sympathetic stimulators can make it more sensitive to input.

A maximal TVR response can normally occur in 10 seconds, although in some individuals the effect may take up to 60 seconds to achieve. It is important to know your subject well! Short, repeated periods of vibration, for example 20 seconds on, 10 seconds off, has been found more effective than 1 long stimulation period. The amount of pressure applied is an important variable in achieving the desired result. Firm, gentle pressure has greater effect than firm deep pressure which could result in a loss of frequency. Excessive pressure can reduce the frequency by as much as one-half of its value. When using a 60H_z electric vibrator under such conditions the frequency could be cut to a dangerous range (30H_z)! If the application is too light, it can result in discomfort from a tickling sensation and lead to withdrawal. A loosely applied vibrator, especially if low frequency/high amplitude, held in one place on the skin can lead to thermal changes causing irritating and/or burning sensations. Individual differences, mood and override of cortical influences (trying too hard, concentrating on the stimulus, etc.) are additional factors that can enhance or depress the TVR and must not be overlooked.

Vibration, when used in combination with other types of stimulation, can be an effective and useful therapeutic tool.

Reported by Gretchen Dahl Reeves, MA,
MOT, OTR
with permission of Dr. Moore

Suggested References

Bishop, B., "Vibratory Stimulation I. Neurophysiology of Motor Responses Evoked by Vibratory Stimulation." *Phys Therapy*: 54 (23): 1273-82, December 1974.
Bishop, B., "Vibratory Stimulation Part II. Vibratory stimulation as an Evaluation Tool." *Phys Therapy*: 55 (1): 28-34, Jan. 1975.
Bishop, B. "Vibratory Stimulation. Part III. "Possible Applications of Vibration in Treatment of Motor Dysfunctions." *Phys Therapy*: 55 (2): 139-143, Feb. 1975.

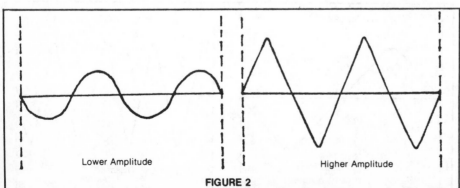

Lower Amplitude   Higher Amplitude

FIGURE 2

(continued)

Vibration as a Therapeutic Tool

Eklund, G. and K-E Hagbarth, "Normal Variability of Tonic Vibration Reflexes in Man" *Experimental Neurology*: 16: 80-92, 1966.

Hagbarth, K.-E. "EMG Studies of Stretch Reflexes in Man." *Electroencaphalogramy and Clinical Neurophysiology*, Suppl. 25: 74-79, 1967.

Hagbarth, K.-E. "The Effect of Muscle Vibration in Normal Man and in Patients with Motor Disorders" in *New Developments in Electromyography and Clinical Neurophysiology*, 3: 428-443, 1973.

Hagbarth, K.-E. and G. Edlund, "The Muscle Vibrator—A Useful Tool in Neurological Therapeutic Work," *Scandinavian Journal of Rehabilitation Medicine* I: 26-34, 1969.

Sensory Integration
Special Interest Section Newsletter; Vol. 4, No. 4, 1981

Treatments for Attention Deficit Disorders

as discussed by Larry B. Silver, M.D.
National Institute of Mental Health, in "Child Development Notes", CIBA—Geigy Corporation

CHILD DEVELOPMENT NOTES (CDN): Dr. Silver, let's begin by defining what we are talking about, because everyone tends to have a slightly different concept of children with Attention Deficit Disorders (ADD).

Dr. Silver: In the sixties and seventies we began to study these children and adolescents more carefully and noted that the common theme was that most seemed to have one or more types of learning disabilities. In addition, 20 to 40 percent seemed to be hyperactive, distractible—or both. And, third, most of them developed secondary social, emotional and family problems.

Recently, the decision was made to split the clinical picture into two groups. In one category are the specific developmental disabilities, including learning disabilities. The other category focuses on what (some) felt was the most critical issue in that area—that is, the attentional deficit. And so they labelled it Attention Deficit Disorders (ADD)—with or without hyperactivity.

There is still controversy over this label. Clinically, we see children who are hyperactive but not distractible.... Also, it defeats the purpose of trying to alert clinicians that learning disabilities and hyperactivity are so commonly related that if you see one you must look for the other.

The importance of this becomes painfully clear in terms of what is seen clinically and what you read in the literature about the outcome of various therapies. You'll see a report of 20 hyperactive children who have been put on psychostimulants and who, after a period of time, are not doing any better in school. They may both ask whether or not the child has learning disabilities and whether anyone is doing anything about that. Stimulant medication will help hyperactivity or distractibility but it will not cure a learning disability. So the child becomes even more frustrated because he or she is now available for learning but still just as unable to learn as before.

There are follow-up studies in which children on psychostimulants are followed into adulthood. The researchers discover that, even though these children are calmer as adults, they still cannot hold down jobs, they're underachievers, and so on. No one asks the key question, "Did they also have learning disabilities, and did anyone ever do anything about that?"

If primary-care physicians don't ask how the hyperactive or distractible child is doing in school—and if he is not doing well, try to find out why—they may miss a very critical part of the diagnosis. When children are not recognized as having learning disabilities, they may be left behind in school, get increasingly frustrated, and subsequently develop behavior disorders.

At that point, they are too often referred to mental health professionals. However, unless the mental health professional knows that there is a difference between an emotional problem that causes academic difficulties, the child may be misdiagnosed as primarily emotionally disturbed. You cannot get rid of a poor self-image with one hour a week of psychotherapy, if a child is getting twenty-five hours a week of failure in school. It's a losing battle.

CDN: Bearing in mind all of these points, as well as the need to consider each component in this cluster of findings, just what do you feel is acceptable treatment?

Dr. Silver: The acceptable treatment, as I see it, must relate to all three aspects of the clinical picture. First, learning disabilities in the school—the acceptable treatment is special education. The specific learning disabilities need to be identified and an individualized education program developed. Outside the school, the most important therapeutic intervention is to make the parents and the child aware of the child's learning disabilities. Unless they know their child's strengths and weaknesses, parents have no way of understanding their child and helping him or her maximize successes rather than magnify weaknesses.

For example, the parents, unaware that their son has visual motor and fine motor disabilities but normal gross motor skills may constantly send the boy out to baseball, basketball or football—which often will be a failure. But if the parents know where the strengths are, they can build on them. They can get their son into soccer, bowling, or swimming—where he might have some success. They must run interference, selecting activities that build on strengths but do not expose weaknesses.

The second level of treatment has to do with the hyperactivity or distractibility. Here, the important thing is to make a differential diagnosis between a behavior you observe and an actual diagnosis. Let's take hyperactivity for example. All children who are overactive are not "hyperactive." There are at least three reasons why a child might be hyperactive. An anxious child may walk and pace, be very nervous, and appear to be hyperactive. This child will not respond to a psychostimulant. There is also the child who is depressed; he or she may be very restless and have trouble focussing. These children also may not respond. But in the specific group of children who have what we feel is a neurophysiologic deficit, the stimulants will work quite well.

Often the history will be helpful. In neurophysiologically based hyperactivity, you will usually get a history of lifelong hyperactivity. On the other hand, you will often find that anxiety-based hyperactivity relates to very specific life-spaced experiences. For example, the child is only

(continued)

hyperactive at school, but not at home; only hyperactive after 6:30 p.m., when daddy comes home; only hyperactive after the first grade, but not before. In the depressive type, you often find that the hyperactivity begins around a situational crises such as the death of a parent, birth of a sibling or a divorce. The same differential thinking is needed in distinguishing between a child who cannot concentrate and a distractible child. You see the same type of temporal differential with distractibity.

I think you should not use a psychostimulant unless you truly believe that there is neurophysiological deficit and that a psychostimulant will help to compensate for it.

CDN: You mentioned the third level of treatment. I assume you're referring to social, emotional and family problems.

Dr. Silver: In this area, determining the acceptable treatment is most critically centered around making the right diagnosis. If you feel that these problems are secondary to learning disabilities, hyperactivity and/or distractibility, then your first approach is to minimize these problems by 1) working with the school to get appropriate school programs going; 2) educating the parents; and 3) using psychostimulant medication when that is indicated. After that, you can take a closer look.

My own personal experience is that after four or five sessions, or what I call "preventive family counseling"—educating the mother, father and siblings, as well as the patient—the behavioral problems will usually begin to minimize or disappear. If they don't, I begin some form of psychological intervention but only in conjunction with a total multimodal approach. to put these children into psychotherapy without first looking at the cause of the emotional stress is not only nonproductive, but often catastrophic. . . ."

CDN: Can you describe some controversial approaches to treating ADD?

Dr. Silver: I find that they fall into two broad categories, essentially. One I call neurophysiological retraining, which means that you do some sort of activity outside the body that, hopefully, will reflex up to the brain and alter or improve brain functioning. The other involves ortho-molecular medicine.

In terms of neurophysiologic retraining perhaps the most common and most controversial is the patterning technique of Doman and Delacato. Their theory is that in the ADD child, the body has failed to progress through a sequence of developmental stages in terms of motor, language, visual or auditory competency. They claim

they can correct this by going through a pattern of exercises that retrains the brain by pouring in new affective sensory stimuli and thus increasing its ability to organize and function.

The bottom line is that the American Academy of Pediatrics, the American Academy of Cerebral Palsy, and the Canadian Association for Retarded Children have reviewed the literature and concluded that there is no evidence to suppot the validity of the Doman-Delacato method.

Another controversial treatment relates to the developmental optometrists who have certain programs and will improve learning disabilities. There are several reasons why I usually do not use optometrists. None of the reasons relates to the validity of the concepts or whether or not they do a successful job.

One concern is that optometrists, in screening mainly the visual and visual-motor areas, may not pick up on auditory or language disabilities. The first advice I give to parents is to have a complete special educational evaluation that looks at all aspects of learning. If they find that learning disabilities relate only to the visual and visual-motor tracts, they then may choose to see an optometrist.

The third controversial model of neurophysiologic retraining is the sensory integrative therapy of Jean Ayres. Her techniques are applied mostly by the occupational therapist. As with optometry, the controversy is not on whether the techniques are valid—here, the research is excellent and the results suggest that this therapy is valid. It is more a question of how it's used than anything else.

Ayres believes that the capacity of the neocortex to react to auditory and visual processing is dependent upon the brainstem's ability to organize such sensory inputs. Based on this idea, techniques have been developed that involve vestibular or tactile stimulation of various areas of the brain in order to make them work more productively.

As with the optometrist, my concern is that if a parent should go directly to an occupational therapist, the therapist may pick up difficulties in those areas, but miss auditory-language and/or other types of disabilities. So my advice again is to go to someone who does a complete evaluation. If the difficulties are in the motor areas, an occupational therapist may be helpful. As I mentioned before—children are much more likely to benefit from an approach used within the context of their disability. Therefore, occupational therapists who work as part of a special educational team in a school environment are, in my view, more likely to be successful.

CDN: Dr. Silver, evidently there could be some validity to some of these neuro-physchological retraining methods. What about orthomolecular medicine?

Dr. Silver: Orthomolecular medicine was a label coined by Linus Pauling for the treatment of mental disorders by providing the optimal molecular environment to the mind. There are several categories of controversial orthomolecular treatments for ADD.

The first concept was the use of massive doses of vitamins to treat various emotional or cognitive disorders, particularly schizophrenia. However, neither the theory nor the treatment approach has been shown to be correct.

In 1967, megavitamin therapy was proposed for learning disabilities. I feel that studies have produced no evidence that megavitamins help with learning disabilities, hyperactivity or distractibility.

Another orthomolecular model focuses on the idea that these ADD children have deficiencies in trace elements such as copper, zinc, magnesium, manganese or chromium. Again no studies have supported this theory: in fact, there is no evidence that trace elements play any role in improving learning disabilities, hyperactivity or distractibility.

A third theory is that allergic sensitivities cause the central nervous system to react in a less functional way. Many pediatric allergists report that in their practice they encounter a higher than expected incidence of allergies in children with learning problems, hyperactivity or distractibility. All I can say at this time is that some of the research is very promising but we still don't have all the answers. We are at a state of the art rather than a state of the science.

Still another theory suggests that glucose is the main nutrient of the brain and that learning disabilities, hyperactivity and distractibility are caused by hypoglycemia. A review of the studies done on this suggests that there are no documented data yet to support this theory and no evidence that being on a hypoglycemic diet has been successful.

CDN: How do you feel about the latest controversial approach, the Feingold diet?

Dr. Silver: Several three- to five-year studies were undertaken in different academic settings. The results do not support Dr. Feingold's claim that 48 to 50 percent of hyperactive children show a dramatic improvement in behavior when placed on a diet that eliminates salicylates and artificial food colors and flavors.

(continued)

Attention Deficit Disorders

The current evidence indicates that a few hyperkinetic children (on the order of 2-3 percent) may experience an adverse reaction to one, or several, of the large number of artificial food colors and flavors with a rapid onset of hyperactive behavior lasting about 20-30 minutes. What I think often happens is that 100 children may try the diet, 2 or 3 get some benefit—sometimes a very marked benefit—and the parents are so convinced, they join the Feingold Associations.

It appears that, for most of the children, the changes in family dynamics (placebo effects) resulting from the entire Feingold therapeutic regimen are most beneficial than the actual diet modifications. Any important potential benefit, however, must be weighed against the long-term harmful educational impact of communicating to a child that his or her behavior is controlled by what he or she eats—rather than communicating what is actually true in terms of central nervous system function.

Dr. Larry Silver is Associate Director of the National Institute of Mental Health. He is also Clinical Professor of Psychiatry at Georgetown University School of Medicine and Secretary of the American Academy of Child Psychiatry. Dr. Silver began publishing in the hyperactivity/ attentional deficit/learning disability syndrome in the late sixties and is recognized as the originator of important fundamental concepts in this area.

Reprinted by permission of Dr. Silver.
(Opinions expressed are those of Dr. Silver)

Sensory Integration
Special Interest Section Newsletter; Vol. 4, No. 4, 1981

A.J. Ayers: An Introduction

The following has been excerpted from an introduction of A. Jean Ayres presented by Wilmà West, MA, OTR, FAOTA, at a workshop on "Occupational Therapy for Sensory Integrative Dysfunction" held in Cincinnati, Ohio, on June 26, 1981. The complete text of this introduction has been published in the CSSID Newsletter

"Although it was with great alacrity that I accepted Ginny Scardina's invitation, some months ago, to introduce Jean Ayres today, it was only yesterday that I realized why this singular honor was bestowed on me. Obviously, I am the senior occupational therapy citizen here, and that means that I have known or known of Jean Ayres longer than any of you who have committed yourselves to applications in treatment of the research and theory development which have characterized Jean's professional career. Thus, while all of you have nurtured the many trees she has planted and some have even set out seedlings of their own, those of us at a greater distance from the forest may have enjoyed a wider vista of your collective efforts and deeper insights into their meaning for the future. I can best share that vista with you by summarizing the highlights of Jean Ayres' contributions to occupational therapy and, through our profession, to the total body of medical and behavioral knowledge.

"Jean Ayres' professional experience has spanned three decades and, remarkably for one individual, had great impact on the three essentials of any professional endeavor—namely, practice, research and education. . . .

"Of primary importance among her educational contributions are her scholarly publications, which number 52. The

breadth of these publications is of special note in that, while 21 have been in *The American Journal of Occupational Therapy*, 15 have been published in other professional periodicals and 10 in proceedings and monographs based on national meetings; further, 31 of her journal articles have been republished in four separate book collections. In addition, Jean Ayres has authored two books, written chapters in four books edited by others, produced four professional films, and developed, standardized and had published 18 psychological tests. While this volume of productivity is impressive in and of itself, we also recognize some very special attributes of her publications: 1) the commitment and motivation that led her to find, make, take the time to write and submit for publication on such a regular basis, 2) the disciplined restraint that is required of the professional scientist/reporter, and with which she has always written, and 3) her speaking through other publications than our own, to the broad professional community concerned about both general and special needs of the children to whom Jean Ayres' life and work have been committed.

"The other major medium for Jean's educational contributions has been the many workshops and conferences wherein she has so generously shared her changing and new concepts with practicing clinicians. . . . The inspiration for and the thread of continuity in most of these conferences and workshops was Jean's special contribution in the form of careful reporting of data from her ongoing practice and research. "In fulfilling what has been characterized as the highest goal of research—namely, the sharing of knowledge

through dissemination of results, by teaching as well as writing, Jean Ayres has exemplified the supreme role of the educator to motivate the practitioners and researchers of the future. That she did this so well and for so long, at what must have been great personal sacrifice in terms of her own practice and research, constitutes an educational contribution we may never be able to measure fully.

"The impact of Jean Ayres' teaching has been felt in other areas than individual practices that have been strengthened by new approaches to treatment. First, there was the organization of the Center for the Study of Sensory Integrative Dysfunction, which was a creative and responsive move on the part of Jean's close California colleagues, to maximize her professional and educational contributions through a mechanism for certification in sensory integrative theory and practice. Second, the establishment, growth and development of a strong Sensory Integrative Specialty Section within our national professional organization has given impetus to the sharing of knowledge that has multiplied Jean's earlier practice and research. And third, there is the ongoing effort between AOTA and CSSID to implement plans for joint certification in sensory integration by these two organizations. All these, and more, I would remind us, have emanated from the educational contributions Jean Ayres has made based on her practice and research.

"Small wonder, is it, that Jean has been the recipient of the two highest awards of The American Occupational Therapy Association; of a post-doctoral traineeship

(continued)

A.J. Ayers

from the National Institute of Mental Health for study at UCLA's Brain Research Institute; been named to the 1971 edition of *Outstanding Educators of America,* and been invited to membership in four national honorary societies, for foreign languages, scholarship, and education.

"To review the achievements that constitute the many rich contributions of Jean Ayres' career is as inspiring as is the opportunity to attend this workshop. May *our* central processing and sensory integrative functions be equal to the challenging thoughts and theories she will be presenting. And please, may we do her the only

honor it is within our power to accord: to strive, to seek, to find full understanding, but never to misuse the information she so generously shares with us."

Sensory Integration
Special Interest Section Newsletter; Vol. 4, No. 3, 1981

From Idea to Finished Product—Or How to Market Your Ideas

By Clark L. Sabine, MEd, OTR

As health professionals having daily contact with people, occupational therapists are in an excellent position to observe human problems and to find and develop new ways to solve or overcome these problems. It may be a new treatment or evaluation approach, a variation of an existing treatment method, a piece of adaptive equipment or an assistive device. In any case, it is important to share your ideas for your own satisfaction and professional development as well as for their contribution to the enhancement of humankind. Treatment approaches and clinical results can be shared through papers presented at state and national professional meetings or published in professional journals or newsletters. Assistive devices and therapy equipment can also be shared by publishing "how to" articles in professional publications. A wider distribution of equipment and devices can often be attained by commercially marketing your ideas. This article will deal with the most advantageous ways of marketing your product ideas.

The First Step

In selling your idea, the first step is to clarify in your own mind what you have to sell. Is it a concept, a "why haven't they done this before?" flash that is untried or untested, or is it a fully developed item that you have been making for years for your patient/clients? Is the product in a finished form or made of a temporary material that would not be acceptable on the commercial market? If so, it may require a lot of redesigning to achieve a prototype. Even when you have some fabrication skills and can produce an attractive product, it may not be manufacturable from an economic standpoint. Many ideas are sent to manufacturers that can be

made but are not marketable because of economics. For example, the product may be elaborately made, overbuilt or require such large financial investments in molds or dies that the market price is driven too high. The product would then never achieve a volume high enough to penetrate the market or to pay for itself.

Other items are marketable but not manufacturable product. Often the product has to be completely redesigned and built from materials at hand, perhaps from a low temperature plastic or other temporary material. It cannot be assumed by the developer, though it often is, that this rough "breadboard prototype" can be instantly translated into a permanent, manufacturable product. Often the product has to be completely redesigned and bears little, if any, resemblance to the original concept. Some ideas are so customized that they have to be individually fabricated to fit each person's needs. Probably the only way to determine whether an item is both manufacturable and marketable is to work with a reputable manufacturer-distributor who can aid in prototype development and market testing of the product.

Selecting a Manufacturer

The best manufacturer to select is one that already produces the category of gadget you have invented. If you have designed a better mousetrap, don't try to get it built by a lampshade manufacturer unless it is made of lampshade materials. The manufacturer should be supplied with enough information about the idea so that he can determine whether or not to express an interest. Inventors sometimes refuse to tell anything about their ideas for fear that they will be stolen, hence they never get marketed. Also, do not assume that a manufacturer will know about the

market for your product. Manufacturers are not necessarily marketers.

Protecting Ideas: To Patent or Not to Patent

Ideas for the health-related fields such as therapy equipment, rehabilitation, and self-help aids are generally low volume items. High volume items are those that every homeowner might buy. If you invent an item that can be sold in the mass market by Sears, General Motors, etc., by all means patent it because you could get rich! Items for the rehabilitation field may also be patented. A chief advantage of patenting for the rehabilitation market is that your patents can be included in your professional resume. In this author's opinion, low volume items for the therapy field are not worth patenting since this greatly increases the cost of the product to the consumer, thereby limiting access to it by many. Patents do not necessarily fully protect you since the initial search and patenting process is only the beginning. Patents might need to be defended by costly legal battles against infringement. It is relatively easy for a determined copier to design around a patented product. Beware of firms that promise to patent and market your ideas. There are those who would give you false encouragement in order to run up large legal and marketing fees but never get the product on the market. Literature on the patenting process is available at a minimal cost from the United States Department of Commerce field offices located in most major cities or state capitols.

Getting Credit for Ideas

In a health profession, the best probable way to gain recognition or credit for an

(continued)

From Idea to Finished Product

idea is to publish the item with illustrations, photos, etc., in a professional journal. Keep in mind, however, that an item that is published, if it has not been sold to a manufacturer or patented, is subject to copy by anyone. Under current patent laws you have one year from the publication date to obtain a patent.

One possible way to protect your idea is to gather original drawings and sketches, a diary of steps in inventing and descriptions and have them dated, signed and witnessed by yourself, a trusted friend and a notary. File these in a safe place. This is sometimes referred to as a "poor man's patent."

In attempting to sell your ideas to a manufacturer, you may wish to protect your ideas by having the manufacturer sign a disclosure form stating that he agrees not to reveal or use your idea if no agreement to purchase is reached. Once an agreement is signed and the product is about to be released to the market, you should publish an article with your name in a professional journal. Not only will this give you credit among your peers, it will also help in the promotion of the commercial version of the product. Don't worry if some people want to make their own from your specifications. The number of those

who do so will be insignificant if the commercial version is well-designed and realistically priced.

Avoiding Pitfalls

Remember to survey the field, examine old professional journals, look in as many commercial catalogs as possible before trying to sell your idea. The wheel does get reinvented everyday.

Very few ideas are really new or original. Most "new" products are simply minor variations on a theme or new combinations of two or more old ideas or slightly varied modifications. Old ideas expressed in new space-age materials may change the shape and look of age-old concepts. Of every 100 ideas submitted for manufacturing, less than one percent probably reach the market.

Making the Most Money on an Idea

If you decide to manufacture the idea yourself and to market it, you may stand to make the most money if you can successfully do both. You may also stand to lose the most. Keep in mind that a substantial contribution of both time and investment

money may be required for building prototypes, buying molds, purchasing materials in quantity to cut costs, manufacturing it yourself or having someone else make the goods, and obtaining promotional and advertising materials. Packaging and shipping orders across the country can be a nuisance when done on a part-time basis. Perhaps a better alternative is to sell the idea or concept outright to a manufacturer-distributor who will then assume all of the financial risks. If the product is well-developed before selling it, a royalty agreement may be negotiated. Your professional assistance in preparing instruction sheets or directions for use on products of a technical nature will probably be appreciated by the manufacturer and will make use of your professional expertise. Keep in mind that you probably won't make a lot of money, but it is satisfying to see your idea on the market and made available to all.

Mr. Sabine has invented a number of orthoses and assistive devices that are currently commercially available. He is presently Marketing Manager for Fred Sammons, Inc., having been a clinician educator and researcher in occupational therapy.

Sensory Integration
Special Interest Section Newsletter; Vol. 4, No. 3, 1981

Manufacturing Therapy Equipment as a Small Business Enterprise—A Case History

By Bob Salo, OTR and Frank Kurkowski, OTR

The following is a description of a part-time business that produces equipment for the treatment of sensory integration disorders and adaptive devices for the physically handicapped. The company was started as a part-time venture by the authors, employed as full-time occupational therapists by a public school district. Bob Salo has four years of experience treating sensory integration disorders in public school children and Frank Kurkowski has much experience designing special equipment for physically impaired students. Both therapists are Maddak Award recipients for equipment they have developed.

Two main factors led to the formation of this company. First both therapists saw a need for equipment that was not currently

available on the market and second, both had many ideas for new equipment from their experiences in treating students. They decided to pool their resources and develop several pieces of equipment to sell, and to act as consultants for the design of special equipment and adaptive devices for the physically impaired. A lawyer was employed to start the incorporation process. The company had its debut at a state occupational therapy association convention where a booth was rented and equipment put on display.

Equipment is designed to meet the needs of therapists and handicapped individuals. For example, a need was expressed by itinerant school therapists for a

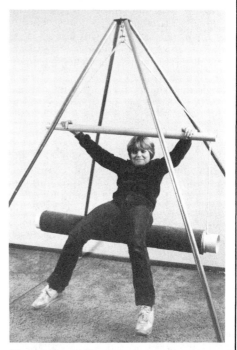

Quad Pod, portable overhead support.

(continued)

portable overhead support to be used for providing vestibular stimulation. Such a device would have to be easily transported by an itinerant therapist from school to school, require little time to set up, and have adequate strength to safely support a swinging child.

Given these requirements, a piece of equipment was designed and manufactured in a home workshop as are all company products.

Success is based on the offering of innovative and unique products that fill real needs of therapists and handicapped individuals.

Bob Salo and Frank Kurkowski are affiliated with Habilitation Products, Inc.

Sensory Integration
Special Interest Section Newsletter; Vol. 4, No. 3, 1981

The Evolution of an Equipment Supply Company

By Michael Brown, Robert Aumann, Woody Eggleston

The development of an equipment supply company followed from a combined effort to make and sell a quality inexpensive gymnastic mat. Many requests for other types of equipment followed and the company grew.

The first encounter with the field of sensory integration came about when an occupational therapist commissioned Michael Brown to design and make protective coverings for the window sills and columns in the area where she treated clients. Following the completion of this, Brown was asked if it was possible to build other equipment needed for OT clients. This first "project" was the redesign of a bolster swing that required only one point of attachment from the ceiling. The swing served the same purposes as another design, but because it requires only one hanging point it is especially useful to therapists who have a limited working space.

In working with occupational therapists, Brown recognized the need for effective therapy equipment. He also felt that much of the existing equipment was unsafe and he learned that there were no national standards of safety required of such equipment.

About this time Michael met Bob Aumann through a mutual interest in rock climbing. As well as being climbing partners, they became business partners along with Woody Eggleston. The trio began to design and construct equipment as therapists requested it. Most of the actual building of the equipment was done in Aumann's living room.

The first large-scale exposure to the field of sensory integration came in 1977 during a conference held in Dayton, Ohio. A flier was distributed at the conference to make therapists aware of their services.

(continued)

Michael Brown Testing The Flexion Disc Swing.

Equipment Supply Company

Before any equipment is made available to the general public, the company conducts its own safety tests and asks several therapists to use and critique the equipment. Any necessary modifications are then made before the equipment is released to the public.

The company's knowledge of the SI field has grown through through participation in seminars and conferences during the past several years. Through personal contact with therapists, the company has been able to explore the existing needs of therapists and to develop equipment to meet these needs.

It has taken several years of hard work and personal sacrifice for the company to reach the level of production it now maintains. The list of equipment now extends far beyond the redesigned bolster swing.

As the demands and needs of therapists change, existing equipment is continually updated and redesigned. The company's aim is to provide the same high quality service to therapists that therapists provide to their clients.

Michael Brown, Robert Aumann, and Woody Eggleston are co-owners of Southpaw Enterprises, Inc.

Sensory Integration
Special Interest Section Newsletter; Vol. 4, No. 3, 1981

Equipment Development

By Winnie Dunn

The role of measurement in the evaluation process in occupational therapy is critical. To assess patient treatment goals and progress towards those goals, the therapist requires as precise a measure as is technologically available. Because of the scarcity of tools that adequately measure patient progress, many therapists design evaluation materials in lieu of relying solely on clinical judgment. The potential for bias is increased since there is more therapist involvement with the client in the therapeutic process and conversely, bias is decreased as measurement becomes quantifiable and objective.

Observation of the integrity of equilibrium responses has been an important area to consider in determining the improvement of postural control. The considerations described above were evaluated in relation to measuring equilibrium responses. A more quantifiable method was developed for use in a clinical project. The goal was to measure the amount of tilt tolerated by individuals before they feel the need to use protective extension responses.

A tool was newly developed to meet our treatment needs. Some of the information gathered in the process of making this piece of equipment available to therapists may be of interest to others similarly involved in designing equipment.

My first step was to call a company I knew that marketed adaptive equipment. After describing my idea to the person with whom I spoke, I was asked to write a letter describing my equipment, enclosing pictures if possible. I then received a call from the company and was provided more information, including:

1. Pros and cons of going through the patent process, i.e., the expense and time involved in the process and its usefulness in dealing with items for a broad consumer market;

2. Methods of protecting the name of the item, such as placing (tm) after the name to designate that you are in pursuit of a trademark;

3. Description of the trademark process, which involves a search to assure that the name you wish to protect has not been used before. You then apply for the registration of that name;

4. Suggestions regarding the copyright of directions for the use of equipment. When directions are copyrighted, persons wishing to "copy" them within legal bounds, must develop different descriptions, thereby creating a more difficult task for themselves.

The role and function of a marketing company was also explained to me. A prototype could be developed by the company that would then be sent to me to test for additional suggestions. Obligations established between the company and the inventor include varied arrangements, depending on how much of the idea is your own and how much is generated by the company people. Financial arrangements also vary, with some ideas bringing a flat fee, others a percentage of each sale. It was helpful to know the company's schedule so that I would have a general time frame by which to set my expectations. For example, new items are placed in the catalogue only at selected times. All of the information was most helpful since I had no ideas about this aspect of the business world.

I proceeded to contact a patent attorney in my area to inquire about patent, copyright and trademark procedures. I was advised that I had been given good and accurate information from the company with which I had spoken. The cautions he gave were the same as those expressed by the original company, with the details of steps to take also coinciding. The attorney's professional fees would be based upon the specific process I requested him to complete, with the historical search being the major portion of the charge.

While the process has been an interesting one, it does take a long time to complete. My first contact was made in the Fall of 1979 and we are not yet finished! But I do feel good about having an avenue for sharing one of my ideas with other therapists. That is something that I could not have done alone!

Winnie Dunn is employed at St. Luke's Hospital, Kansas City, MO. She is also a CSSID Faculty member. Her recent piece of equipment, the Dunnometer (tm), is soon to be available.

Sensory Integration
Special Interest Section Newsletter; Vol. 4, No. 2, 1981

Comments from the Chair, Gretchen Reeves

As we mature professionally, continuing to develop our knowledge base and our skills, we bring a constantly enriched repertoire of abilities to the practice of occupational therapy. In applying any approach which may facilitate change, we seek to improve the quality of life for persons with dysfunction and hope that others will recognize ours as a valuable and necessary contribution to health care. While this may often be the case, unfortunately it is not always the rule. It seems that especially in the application of the principles of sensory integration we have at times been questioned and doubted and often placed in a defensive position about its merit.

As most of you know by now, we were publicly challenged by "An Open Letter to an Occupational Therapist" which appeared in the *Journal of Learning Disabilities*, January 1981. We were challenged to look at ourselves and to think about what we may be saying and doing in practice that raises concern about the need for occupational therapy services and the use of a sensory integrative approach. We were stimulated to think about the value of

the theoretical framework offered by sensory integration to our practice as occupational therapists and its importance to our clients. We were motivated to organize our ideas and to formulate some unified statements about our purpose in bringing this approach into practice.

As problem-solvers and facilitators of change, our intent has always been to assist in dealing with complicated problems. A letter to this effect was written by AOTA to the editor of the *Journal of Learning Disabilities* as a response representing the thinking of many occupational therapists who reacted to this issue through the SI Specialty Section.

The critical need or challenge which we must now deal with most directly is the documentation of change which could be attributed to occupational therapy intervention. Research is receiving greater emphasis in our profession because we realize that clinical practice alone is not enough to verify that we do offer valuable services. Both the medical and educational communities, especially under strained economic conditions, are asking for valid evidence of the need for related support

services. We recognize that to remain viable we must present written proof of our contribution to advanced practices in health and education.

Since the area of research presents a new horizon for exploration by occupational therapists, AOTA, the American Occupational Therapy Foundation and the specialty sections are offering information and services to assist us in this new effort. You will note that a recent issue of the *SISS Newsletter* focused on the case study method of research. This represents a very practical method which can be applied in our clinical settings as we consistently record responses to treatment and note improvements. Our current newsletter provides us with some additional information on computer searches and copyright laws which may be of value in preparing to conduct research. We must face this challenge with confidence and take pride in our ability to grow and adapt when the demand is apparent, gaining new skills and expanding our professional foundation in the process.

Sensory Integration
Special Interest Section Newsletter; Vol. 4, No. 2, 1981

Visual Function in Adults With Brain Damage

By Mary Jane Bouska, OTR

Mary Jane Bouska is an occupational therapist in a private practice limited to the adult with brain-damage. She has recently completed eight years of full-time research at Temple University. Prior to this she was engaged in clinical practice in the United States and Australia. She lectures at both Temple University and the University of Pennsylvania occupational therapy schools, presents workshops, and is currently writing a chapter on visuo-perceptual disorders to be included in a book on management of the patient with neurologic deficit.

Many adults with brain-damage exhibit deficits in one or more aspects of the visual system, i.e., primary visual input, oculomotor control, visuo-perceptual processing, visuo-motor function, higher cognitive processing and other functional and anatomical aspects of the visual-sensory-motor system. It is of great importance to clinically investigate the presence of pri-

mary and secondary visual manifestations of neurologic disease in brain-damaged individuals. Many texts are devoted to the study of this relationship.[1,2]

Unfortunately, members of the rehabilitation team are often unaware of the presence and/or functional significance of visual system disorders during the rehabilitation process. Historically, problems inherent in this population (i.e., language disorders, cognitive deficits, apraxia) have made evaluation of visual system disabilities difficult. In addition, ophthalmologists have not been trained to translate primary findings into functional terminology and management or treatment suggestions. We, as therapists, have likewise been unaware and unable to view visual system pathology in terms of functional meaning which can engender treatment programs. A critical awareness of the normal and abnormal visual system and its

role in skilled tasks such as reading a newspaper, picking up a penny, walking through an aisle or driving a car has been long overdue in the field of rehabilitation of the adult with brain-damage. As therapists, we have typically used the words "visuo-perceptual" and "visuo-motor" with too little regard for the "visual" component of the disorder.

It was in response to this need that Temple University's Rehabilitation Research and Training Center No. 8 began to conduct visual system dysfunction studies in 1973. The research team included a psychiatrist, optometrist, bioengineer, neuropsychologist and occupational therapist. One of the major goals of these studies was to develop a quantitative assessment of visual function in brain-damaged adults. Visual function was defined as encompass-

(continued)

Visual Function

ing the following abilities: a) to respond to stimuli incident on all parts of the retina and adjust focusing for near and far objects (anatomical and physiological integrity); b) to move the eye and head to gather information (oculomotor and vestibulo-ocular control); c) to meaningfully interpret this information (visuo-perceptual ability); d) to quickly and accurately move a limb in response to a visual cue (visuo-motor abililty); and e) to integrate all of the above abilities.

This assessment battery was given to 128 adults with brain-damage secondary to CVA, traumatic head injury, cerebral palsy, multiple sclerosis, tumor and cerebellar lesions. The most common primary visual deficits noted were; visual field losses, decreases in near or distance acuity, inadequate accommodation, double vision, inability to move the eyes in one or more directions, poor eye movements (i.e., slow, missing target), and poor integration of eye and head movements.

Common secondary visual deficits included visuo-spatial, visuo-constructive and visuo-memory difficulties, visual neglect or left or right space, slow and inaccurate motor responses to increasingly complex visual targets and general confusion during tasks requiring visual processing. Reading difficulties (unrelated to language) were directly related to decreases in acuity or accommodation, visuo-spatial problems, unilateral visual neglect, problems with oculomotor control and visual processing problems *per se*.

Unilateral visual neglect was seen more frequently in right than left hemisphere lesions and was noted both with and without homonymous hemianopsia. This finding is in agreement with others[3,4] who suggest that neglect represents an additional (and

separate) lesion to field defects. One of the most significant findings was that during perceptual testing, patients with neglect consistently or inconsistently neglected images on one-half of the test page contralateral to their lesion and, therefore, chose answers more frequently (or only) on the half of the "seen" page (ipsilateral to their lesion). Even though patients were given the option of selecting no answer, in almost all cases they chose a wrong answer in the "seen" space rather than not answer. This over-responsiveness to one-half of the test page, of course, resulted in many incorrect visuo-perceptual choices. A method was designed to measure responsiveness to left and right test space and, thereby, rule out the influence of neglect on raw perceptual score. This finding as well as Gianotti's work[5] suggests that results of conventional assessments given by occupational therapists, speech pathologists and psychologists may be invalid in some patients unless unilateral visual neglect is considered when interpreting results.[6]

Patients demonstrated all combinations of visual system disorders. Some had performance difficulties related to both primary and secondary visual deficits; others had normal visual input but were unable to carry out perceptual tasks; still others had only primary visual problems (i.e., field defects). Patients in this category compensated most efficiently. Visual symptomology did not always correlate with diagnosis, although some deficits were observed more frequently in certain diagnostic catagories.

After gathering comprehensive visual function evaluations on a number of patients, it became clear that the visual function battery could help define rather spe-

cific treatment programs. Twenty patients were given individualized treatment programs aimed at teaching compensation for visual deficits or alleviating visual deficits. Fourteen of these patients showed improvements in visual function, i.e., reading, eating, maneuvering a wheelchair, etc., which might not have been expected by chance. Although the treatment design did not include a control sample, preliminary results *suggest* that definition of primary and secondary visual deficits may help engender effective treatment designs, and, furthermore, that effective treatment programs can enhance visuo-perceptual and visuo-motor function in adults with brain-damage. Further research is needed to duplicate and augment this study.

The final report of this research is available from the author upon request at 6143 Wayne Ave., Philadelphia, PA 19144. Enclose $4.00 to cover expenses. In addition, the author also conducts three-day workshops on visual function assessment and treatment of the adult with brain-damage.

1. Walsh, F.B. and Hoyt, W.G. *Clinical Neuro-Ophthalmology*. Williams and Wilkins Company, Baltimore, 1969.
2. Critchley, M. *Parietal Lobes*. Hafner Publishing Company, Inc., New York, 256-325, 1953.
3. Friedland, R. and Weinstein, E. Hemi-Inattention and Hemisphere Specialization: Introduction and Historical Review. In: Weinstein, E. and Friedland, R. (eds.). *Advances in Neurology. Hemi-Inattention and Hemisphere Specialization*. Volume 18. Raven Press, New York, 12-26, 1977.
4. Heilman, K. Neglect and Related Disorders. In: Heilman, K. and Valenstein, E. (eds.). *Clinical Neuropsychology*. Oxford University Press, New York, 268-289, 1979.
5. Gianotti, G., and Tiacci, C. The Relationship Between Disorders of Visual Perception and Unilateral Spatial Neglect. *Neuropsychologia*. 9: 451-458, 1971.
6. Bouska, M. and Biddle, E. The Influence of Unilateral Visual Neglect on Diagnostic Testing. Presented at the American Speech and Hearing Association Annual Convention, Atlanta, Georgia, 1979.

Sensory Integration
Special Interest Section Newsletter; Vol. 4, No. 2, 1981

Computer Searches in Reviewing Literature

Medlars

Medlars, formally known as The Medical Literature Analysis and Retrieval System, is based on a computer system derived from journals indexed for *Index Medicus, Index to Dental Literature* and the *International Nursing Index*. This system has over 1,800,000 citations from approximately 3,000 medical and health related scientific journals dating back to 1964. A computer

print-out gives author, title and bibliographical notations under subject headings taken from medical description terms. The National Library of Medicine in Bethesda, Maryland houses the computer base for this system. Many medical schools and hospital libraries (over 400) in the U.S. have access to the Medlars system.

Medline

Medline is a shortened form of the Medlars

system. It has over 400,000 citations taken from 1,200 major journals indexed for *Index Medicus*. The Medline system has more current citations and is programmed to include journal citations for the last two years.

Reference: Stein, Franklin, *Anatomy of Research in Allied Health*, John Wiley & Sons, New York, 1976.

(continued)

Computer Searches

ERIC

The Educational Resources Information Center (ERIC) is a nationwide network, but decentralized. Sponsored by the National Institute of Education (NIE), it is tailored to gather educational documents and make them available to educators, researchers and other interested persons. The ERIC network publishes a monthly abstract journal entitled ''Resources in Education'' (RIE). The journal announces all documents that are acquired by ERIC and that pass its selection criteria. ERIC attempts to provide comprehensive coverage of recently completed significant documents relevant to education.

The research papers announced in RIE (except for some copyrighted materials) can be purchased in microfiche or reproduced paper copy from the ERIC Document Production Service (EDPS). EDPS forwards complete sets of ERIC documents and microfiche to over 650 customers nationwide and abroad. All documents announced in RIE must be made available to the public via EDPS or an alternate source.

The ERIC data base is accessible at many locations via computer searches of ERIC magnetic tapes. The retrieval service is one of the most popular and lowest cost data bases available.

ERIC has sixteen subject oriented clearinghouses (located at nonprofit institutions) and three contractors.

Information taken from ''Submitting Documents to ERIC, Educational Resources Information Center''. The National Institute of Education. U.S. Dept. of Health, Education and Welfare, Washington DC 20208.

Submitted by: Sandra Edwards, MA, OTR, Associate Professor, Western Michigan University, Kalamazoo, MI

Sensory Integration
Special Interest Section Newsletter; Vol. 4, No. 2, 1981

Protection of Intellectual Property: Copyrights, Patents, and Registrations

The following abstracts of articles on Protection of Intellectual Property from the AOTA Federal Reports, Volume 79, should be relevant to those Sensory Integration Specialty Section members interested in research, stimulated to publish, or reading related literature. The Information can be a useful guide to therapists in protecting their published material as well as becoming aware of the responsibilities related to publishing (giving recognition to others for their ideas by referencing their source of knowledge. This is true for both oral and written presentations).

PART I. COPYRIGHT

The hallmark of a profession is the development of theories, methodologies, instruments and processes and the application of these from a cohesive conceptual base. Knowledge and its application is protected as ''intellectual property'' by copyright.

The Nature of Copyright

Literary works, theses, graphics, audiovisual materials or sound recordings are examples of what can be copyrighted. However, the concepts described within become a part of the public domain.

If an occupational therapist writes a monograph describing an invention, the article can be copyrighted; the invention can not be. It needs a patent to be protected.

Copyright's Duration

Copyright laws were revised in January 1978. They now protect the authors during their lifetime and their heirs through an additional 50 years following the author's death. Other statutes cover works ''made for hire'' and for publications in force through copyright prior to January 1, 1978.

An owner has exclusive rights pertaining to reproducing, preparing derivative works and distributing copies of the copyrighted work for sale and transfer of ownership.

Fair Use Exceptions

Exceptions to using copyrighted material are criticisms, news-reporting, teaching (including multiple copies for classroom use), scholarship or research.) These are not considered copyright infringement.

Securing Copyright Protection

The published copy of a work bears a copyright notice with a symbol © enclosed in a circle, a ''copyright,'' ''copr,'' the year of first publication, the name of the copyright owner, an abbreviation of his name or a known designation.

The copyright applicant obtains forms from: *Copyright Office, Library of Congress, Washington, DC 20559.*

Remedies For Infringement

Registration of claim is made with a deposit of two copies of the work with the Registrar of Copyrights; remedy for infringement is sought by:

1. Impounding and disposition of the infringing articles;
2. Recovery of damages to the owner and illegal profits of the infringer;
3. Recovery of costs and attorney's fees. (Recovery in the form of an injunction is available)

Infringement is a criminal offense; fines are provided from 2,500 to 50,000 dollars with terms of imprisonment up to two years.

PART II. THE PATENT LAW

A Patent For An Invention

A patent is a symbol of the government's permission to the inventor to have the right to prevent others from making use of his invention for their profit in the United States. This grant or permission is received through the U.S. Patent and Trademark Office.

Duration Of The Patent

The patent law protects against use without permission for 17 years. The patent is not renewable; the invented item becomes public property when the patent expires. Nearly everything that can be invented and the process of the invention can be protected by a patent.

Granting A Patent

Granted a patent, the patentee is required to mark his articles with ''patent'' and the patent number. The patented item must be ''new'' and ''useful'' as defined by the patent law.

Patent Application

To apply for a patent, the following application components must be sent to the Com-

(continued)

Intellectual Property

mission of Patents and Trademarks in Washington, DC.

1. $65 application fee;
2. a petition for the patent;
3. specifications and claims describing the invention;
4. a declaration;
5. an illustration of the invention.

A patent attorney is useful to represent inventors and to conduct a search of patents and other records before applying for a patent. The patent and trademark office examiner may reject claims in an application on the basis of prior patent publications.

Pamphlet Or Attorney

The following pamphlets are available through the Superintendent of Documents, Washington, DC 20402 or through any U.S. Department of Commerce, District Office:

Pamphlet or Attorneys and Agents Registered to Practice,

General Information Concerning Patents,
Patents and Inventions,

An Information Aid to Inventors.

PART III. REGISTRATION

Trademark/The Professional Logo

Once a professional logo has been adopted, the logo will be registered with the US Patent and Trademark office as an official identifying mark. The mark will symbolize professional status and differ from the collective mark, a symbol of service.

The advantage of the trademark/ professional logo is that these qualify for the Federal Principal Register placement which confers nation-wide exclusive rights to use the registration symbol. After a five year period of registration, the mark becomes the Association's exclusive right to use as it sees best. The law provides for "remedies of injunction, recovery of profits and destruction of advertisement and infringing labels."

Information abstracted by Yvonne Norton,
MA, OTR
Hitchcock Rehabilitation, Center,
Aiken, SC

Sensory Integration
Special Interest Section Newsletter; Vol. 4, No. 1, 1981

The Case Study Method of Research—Introduction

By Richard Cox, PhD

Richard Cox, PhD, teaches measurement and evaluation at the University of Pittsburgh. The value of the case study method in clinical practice was demonstrated in his presentation at the AOTA National Conference in Detroit in 1979.

Using the case study approach can be an interesting way to conduct clinical research. There are some unique characteristics of this methodology that make it particularly suited for the clinician and especially attractive to the beginning researcher.

The case study is a detailed, in-depth description of a single subject, unit or event. Sometimes called $N = 1$ research, the case study is longitudinal by nature, with data being collected over a period of time extending anywhere from a few weeks to several years. Although a case study typically focuses on a person, other units which could be studied are a family, a community, a hospital ward, or a piece of equipment.

Comprehensive data collection is characteristic in case studies. Data are gathered from a variety of sources and at periodic intervals during the course of the study. Most often, the individual or unit is studied in a natural or clinical environment, rather than in a laboratory or some other artificial setting.

The case study is a descriptive research technique, the primary purpose of which is to describe, in detail, certain characteristics of the subject. Although there may be some experimental aspects in a particular study, case studies typically do not utilize randomization or control, two essential elements in experimental research design.

The replication of a case study can be a useful way for the novice to begin thinking about research. Replication is also important in and of itself if the results of a case study are to be generalized to a variety of situations. Researchers must be very cautious in making generalizations from a single case study since it may be difficult to decide which data are unique to one particular case and which are generalizable. A series of replications using different subjects in different locations may provide consistent evidence that will allow for generalization.

Unique Advantages of Case Studies

A case study can provide an in-depth look at the whole individual. Summaries of data collected from large groups often mask individual differences, and group statistics can be misleading. In a case study all data are related to the single subject being studied and can, therefore, be quite extensive and detailed.

In some instances it is not easy for researchers to quantify certain types of variables. It is difficult, for example, to assign a number to a specific type of emotion or to a particular child-play activity. The case study is particularly amenable to the study of variables difficult to quantify. In addition, the case study is well suited to the study of special situations, unique circumstances, or the unusual subject. For example, Goodenough studied a congenitally deaf-blind girl who had received no schooling or intervention and had no language. Erhardt reports data for a 15-month-old twin girl diagnosed as a spastic quadriplegic with questionable visual and auditory abilities. Obviously, group research is not very feasible in these instances where only a few cases exist (see references).

(continued)

Case Study Method of Research

The case study is quite appropriate as a research technique for the practicing clinician. Clinicians have access to patients, some of whom may present particular characteristics which could be related using the case study approach. A detailed description of an unusual case could be a valuable contribution to the existing body of knowledge, as well as being useful information for other clinicans.

The case study can also be useful in the early investigations in a particular area. The variety of data typically collected in a case study gives the researcher some latitude to explore the relationships among variables, to verify or generate speculations, and to uncover the unexpected.

Disadvantages of the Case Study Approach

The lack of generalizability may be a serious drawback to using the case study as a method for discovering systematic knowledge about human behavior. The particular subject may not be representative of a larger population and, in fact, may have been selected because of convenience or due to certain biases of the investigator. Any of these selection processes may mean that the results of the case study are not valid in other situations.

Maintaining objectivity in data collection can be difficult in case studies. Often the investigator becomes too involved with the subject and interprets the data subjectively. It is easy to fall into the trap of seeing something in a subject because you want to see it. This may be especially true of the clinician looking for improvement in a patient.

Since there may be a large amount of data collected in a case study, it can become difficult to decide what is relevant and what is not. It would be nice prior to the study to be able to decide which variables are the most important; however, this is difficult in an exploratory approach such as the case study.

It must be remembered that a case study is a descriptive technique and, as such, the research has little or no control of variables. "What" has happened can be described, but not "why" it has happened. Cause and effect statements should not be made.

Some Examples of the Case Study Approach

Axline, V.M. Dibs: *In seach of self*, Boston: Houghton Mifflin, 1964.

Ayres, A.J., & Heskett, W. Sensory integrative dysfunction in a young schizophrenic girl. *Journal of Autism and Childhood Schizophrenia*, 1972, 2(2), 174-181.

Erhardt, R.P. Sequential levels in development of prehension. *American Journal of Occupational Therapy*, 28(10), 592-596.

Goodenough, J.L. Expressions of the emotions in a blind-deaf child. *Journal of Abnormal Psychology & Social Psychology II*, 1932, 27(3), 328-333.

Norton, Y. Neuro development and sensory integration. *American Journal of Occupational Therapy*, 1975, 29(2), 93-100.

Piaget, J. The language and thought of the child. London: Kegan Paul, 1926.

Roemer, R.B., Culler, M.A., & Swartt, T. Automated upper extremity progressive resistive exercise system. *American Journal of Occupational Therapy*, 1978, 32(2), 105-108.

Wehman, P., & Marchant, J.A. Improving free play skills of severely retarded children. *American Journal of Occupational Therapy*, 1978, 32(2), 100-104.

Suggested Readings
For The Beginning Researcher

Single Case Experimental Designs: Strategies for Studying Behavior Change, Michael Herson & David Barlow, Pergamon Press, New York, Toronto, 1977.

Research: The Validation of Clinical Practice, Otto D. Payton, F.A. Davis Co., Philadelphia, 1979.

Quasi-Experimentation: Design & Analysis Issues for Field Settings, Thomas Cook and Donald Campbell, Rand McNally College Publishing Company, Chicago, 1979.

Experimental and Quasi-Experimental Designs for Research, Donald T. Campbell, Julian C. Stanley, Rand McNally College Publishing Co., Chicago, 1963.

Pitfalls in Human Research: Ten Pivotal Points, Theodore X. Barber, Pergamon General Psychology Series, Pergamon Press Inc., New York, 1976.

Sensory Integration
Special Interest Section Newsletter; Vol. 4, No. 1, 1981

Case Study Methodology

by Richard Cox, PhD

As with other approaches, the case study must include certain basic elements of the research process. The researcher should specifically identify the problem to be studied including a rationale, the significance of the study, and a theoretical base if appropriate. A statement of the problem together with operational definitions, limitations, and assumptions should be made explicit. A review of related research should be conducted in order to provide a knowledge base for the study. The researcher should be aware of what is known and what needs to be studied so that the results of the case study can contribute to existing knowledge. Even though the purpose of the case study may be exploratory, the researcher should specify which characteristics will be studied and which relationships among characteristics seem to be worthy of investigation. Up to this point in the research process, the case study is quite similar to other types of research.

Selecting the particular subject for the case study is an important first step in the procedure. While the selection of a subject will often be made with convenience and accessibility as primary concerns, it should be done keep-

(continued)

Case Study Methodology

ing in mind the problem to be studied. Remember that the case study is especially suited to providing information about special situations and uncommon or specific types of behavior.

Data Collection

There is a wide selection of data that may be useful in a case study. Although the majority of the data collected should relate to the variables of interest, the procedure is also nicely suited to exploratory data collection. Specific types of information sought can include (a) physical measures, such as height, weight, age, sex, disabilities; (b) psychological measures, such as general ability tests, personality profiles, interest inventories and attitude scales; and (c) socio-economic data, such as family composition, race, income, religion, work experience, level of education and social activities. Measures will vary depending on the focus of the study.

As in any good research, attention must be given to the reliability and validity of all measures used in data collection. Care should be taken to find the best types of measurement tools for obtaining the most relevant information. The advantages and disadvantages of using techniques such as direct observation, interviews, psychological tests, questionnaires and medical records should be carefully weighed.

Data Analysis

Although the analysis of data is often perceived as the most difficult part of the research process, it need not be. The analysis should follow logically from the questions the study is designed to investigate. Since the case study is primarily a descriptive technique, the data analysis should be designed to present the description of the case in as straightforward a manner as possible. There is no need to impose a complicated analysis on a simple descriptive study. In many instances, common descriptive statistics such as frequencies, percentages, averages and trend lines are sufficient. It can be quite helpful to examine other case studies to see how data are presented.

If the researcher has included a treatment variable in the study, there are several choices for data analysis. The baseline-treatment, (B T, or sometimes labled A B) model reports data collected prior to the introduction of the treatment contrasted with data collected following the treatment. The B T B T (or A B A B) design adds the collection of baseline data again, following the first treatment data, and subsequent data being collected following a repeat of the treatment. Other models, which are considered quasi-experimental, include time series or multiple time series analyses. A thorough discussion of data analysis models when a treatment variable is included in a case study is presented by Anton (see references).

It must be remembered that considerable caution should be used in the interpretation of data using these designs. None is an experimental design. Random selection and control of extraneous variables have not been adequately included; therefore, attributing observed changes in data to the treatment variable must be done cautiously if at all.

Findings

The remaining elements of the case study parallel those found in other types of research. The researcher should present the results and provide an interpretation and discussion which is consistent with the data analysis. Implications and conclusions of the study should be stated. As previously mentioned, caution should be exercised when suggesting any generalizability of the results. Replications to other situations most certainly should be suggested.

Some References About Conducting Case Studies

Anton, J.L. Studying individual change. In L. Goldman, *Research methods for counselors.* New York: John Wiley and Sons, 1978, 117-153.

Becker, H.S. Observation: Social observation and social case studies. In D.L. Sills (Ed.), *International encyclopedia of the social sciences* (Vol. 11). New York: Crowell-Collier and Macmillan, 1968, 232-238.

Dukes, W.F. $N = 1$. *Psychological Bulletin*, 1965, 64, 74-79.

Good, C.V. The individual and case study. *Essentials of educational research.* New York: Appleton-Century-Crofts, 1966, 310-344.

Kratochwill, T.R. *Single subject research: Strategies for evaluating change.* New York: Academic Press, 1978.

Llewellyn, L.N. Case method. In E.R.A. Seligman (Ed.), *Encyclopedia of the social sciences* (Vol. 3). New York: Macmillan, 1930, 251-254.

Miller, E., & Warner, R.W. Single subject research and evaluation. *Personnel and Guidance Journal*, 1975, 54, 130-133.

Selltiz, C., Jahoda, M., Deutsch, M. & Cook, S.W. *Research methods in social relations* (Rev. ed.). New York: Holt, 1960, 59-65.

Simon, J.L. *Basic research methods in social science.* New York: Random House, 1969, 277.

Sensory Integration
Special Interest Section Newsletter; Vol. 4, No. 1, 1981

Critical Analysis of Research

Listed below are questions to serve as guidelines for your critique of research articles.

I. Purpose, Problem, and Justification

A. To what extent is the purpose or problem clearly stated?
B. To what extent is the justification logical and convincing?
C. Is the problem significant?

II. Review of the Literature

A. To what extent is the literature discussed relevant to the problem?

(continued)

Critical Analysis

B. Are the citations recent enough to reflect current status of the problem?

C. Are the results of the studies in the literature review indicated and summarized?

D. Does the status of the research cited support the researcher's claim that he or she has a researchable problem?

III. Hypothesis

A. To what extent are they clear and precise?

B. Are they directional?

C. If there is only a problem statement rather than a hypothesis, is that problem statement sufficient? Is it clearly stated?

IV. Definitions

To what extent are the major terms clearly defined?

V. Sampling

A. To what extent is the sample clearly described?

B. Does the method of sampling seem appropriate?

C. To what extent is it adequate in size? Is rationale for sample size discussed?

D. To what extent are the limitations on generalizability presented?

VI. Instrumentation

A. To what extent are the instruments clearly described?

B. To what extent are the instruments reliable? Are they appropriate and valid for the study? Why or why not?

C. If the researcher developed the instrument, did he or she pilot it (try it out prior to the study being reported)?

VII. Procedures

A. To what extent are they clearly described? Could you replicate the study from the procedural information given?

B. To what extent were extraneous variables controlled?

C. Were the rights of human subjects protected? How?

VIII. Data Analysis

A. In what scale(s) were the data in the study?

B. Do the methods selected to analyze the data seem appropri-

ate? Were they applied correctly?

C. Are reasons given for decisions to tabulate and analyze data in the manner they were?

IX. Results

A. To what extent are they clearly presented?

B. If a hypothesis was directional, was the test of significance used appropriately?

C. To what extent is the written description consistent with the data?

D. To what extent are the tables, graphs or figures used helpful in understanding the data?

X. Discussion or Interpretation

A. To what extent is the interpretation of the data consistent with the results? Are the conclusions justified?

B. To what extent does the total report clearly distinguish between actual findings and the researcher's interpretation of the findings?

C. To what extent does the researcher place the findings in broader perspective by comparing the results to earlier research or theory?

D. To what extent does the research display any biases?

E. Are limitations of the study noted?

F. Are generalizations confined to the population from which the sample was drawn?

G. To what extent do the results or discussion closely relate to the original hypothesis?

XI. Problems With Internal Validity

A study has *internal validity* if the outcome of the study is a function of the program or approach being tested rather than the result of other causes not systematically dealt with in the study. There are several *threats to internal validity*. Evaluate the study according to each of the following (when relevant). Does the researcher recognize and appropriately discuss threats to validity?

A. *History:* did anything else happen between the time the treatment started and finished that could have affected the results?

B. *Maturation:* did the subjects become wiser, older, more tired, more or less alert with the passage of time as the study progressed?

C. *Testing:* did taking a pretest sensitize the subjects?

D. *Instrumentation:* did the measuring instrument, observer or scorer change as the study progressed?

E. *Selection Bias:* did the method of sample selection bias the results?

F. *Statistical Regression:* very high scores and very low scores tend to move toward the mean on retesting. If pretest scores were extremely low or high, could posttest scores be due to statistical regression?

G. *Experimental Mortality:* was there differential loss of respondents from the comparison groups? Was loss of subjects usually high? If a questionnaire needed to be returned, was the rate of return so low that bias was introduced?

H. *Other:* Were the experimental and control groups truly similar? Were extraneous variables controlled? Did the experimental treatment differ from the control treatment *only* in terms of the independent variable, or were other differences present? Did the *order* in which part of the treatment was administered inadvertently affect the next part of the treatment? Did the very presence of the researcher, observer or measurement instrument affect the study or results?

XII. Problems With External Validity

A study has external validity if the results obtained would apply in the real world to other similar programs and approaches. Threats to external validity would include poor sampling procedures, use of extremely restricted or artificial conditions, sensitization to the experimental variable, the researcher, the experimental setup, and so forth. Threats to external validity are threats to the generalizability of the study. Evaluate the study with respect to external validity.

XIII. Strengths

What are the good points of this research?

What are the strong features?

— *Jean A. Morse, PhD*
Medical College of Georgia

Sensory Integration
Special Interest Section Newsletter; Vol. 3, No. 4, 1980

Establishing a Private Practice By Kayleen R. Hall, OTR, and Lois E. Hickman, OTR

A private practice is a small business. If your motives are mainly financial, perhaps you should reconsider, since it takes two to three years for a business to become self-supporting and make a profit. (One solution is to work part time for another agency while "phasing in" your private practice—but be aware of conflict of interest!) Also, analyze your skill and readiness for working independently. It is best to have experience in a clinical setting, working with other therapists before taking primary responsibility for evaluation and treatment.

Some initial considerations before beginning your private practice are:

1. Establish the need for an SI practice. Do you have a product the community needs and will buy?
2. Survey the rates for comparable treatment. You should be competitive with other centers in the community without undercharging.
3. Consider taking a bookkeeping/accounting adult education course.
4. Know AOTA's standards of practice for private practice and for therapists in the public schools.

If you decide to take the big step, then:

1. Notify area agencies (we phoned first) that might send you referrals. (Examples are; Handicapped Children's Programs, social services, children's hospitals and diagnostic services, pediatricians, neurologists and pre-schools.) Follow up your phone contact with a letter of identification outlining your professional credentials, educational and work experience, service provided and charges for service.
2. Consider listing your practice, not only under your name but also in the yellow pages of the phone book under such headings as; Rehabilitation, Child Guidance and Development and Special Educational Services.

Now you are ready to tackle the specific challenges and growth that will come from working on your own!

Part I. Initial Expenses

When establishing a private practice, consider the initial expenditures carefully. It may be difficult to assess what is truly necessary to operate a business and what is a luxury treatment item.

Business expenses may be around $500, initially, if you already own a typewriter. If not, plan to purchase a typewriter or employ a reliable typing service. Business cards and/or letterhead stationery are highly recommended for professionalism as well as one source of advertisement. Keep the printing simple and avoid logos. Other initial business expenses may include; business statements, postage, printing and distribution of announcements, telephone advertising, ledgers and other items for bookkeeping. (Browse through an office supply store.)

Plan to spend between $200 to $300 a month for clinic rental, including utilities, cleaning services and supplies. This expense may be reduced if you develop a private practice in your home or utilize the client's home, but your transportation costs and travel time will increase. You will need to consider an answering service for your home and/or office. Phone installation is another initial expense. Monthly phone rates vary greatly between private and business usage. The phone company can assist you in deciding on what systems will fit your needs.

Liability insurance is recommended for all addresses where treatment is provided. For your protection consider obtaining malpractice insurance. (Maginnis and Associates can help you establish your insurance needs.)

Initially, you have to prioritize your equipment needs. Consider the space you have rented or the transportation of the equipment if you work out of the client's home. If you are at all handy, scooter boards, ramps, rocking boards, etc., can be made. (We contracted a retired carpenter to build the larger pieces of equipment as they could be afforded.) Some items may be picked up inexpensively at garage sales, such as barrels, innertubes, tactile activities and games.

Testing materials are another initial cost, ranging from $150 to $300 depending on the number of evaluations you will use in your assessment of the child.

The initial expenses of therapeutic equipment is the one area that you, alone, can make decisions on what you need. The business needs must be met initially to establish and maintain a viable practice in occupational therapy.

Part II. Insurance Coverage

Third-party reimbursement is a challenging aspect for a private practitioner. Each claim filed will be different, using different companies, physicians referrals and diagnoses.

Before filing a claim, work with the family to obtain a physician's referral. (We have yet to find an insurance company that does not require a physician's referral.) In addition, read through the family's policy booklet to become familiar with the items used and rehabilitative services included in their coverage. If outpatient occupational therapy is not directly addressed, it is advisable to call the regional or local claims office for clarification. Before calling, generally long distance, have the claim form or provider's statement (usually picked up at the policy holder's place of employment) partially filled out with the policy number and group number if applicable, the policy holder's full name and place of employment. (Occupational Therapy Provider's Statements are available from: OT Resources, 8000 East Girard, Suite 617, Denver, CO 80231. They are $6.00 for 100 forms and $.60 for postage and handling.) When you have reached the regional office be sure to note the claim's agent or clerk's name since this allows you to continue to direct future questions and communications regarding the claim to a specific person.

If the claim is denied ask the insurance company to issue you and/or the family a statement describing the grounds for the denial. This statement can be used to avoid future denials with that insurance company and occasionally, with clarification from you and the attending physician, the claim may be reviewed and accepted.

(continued)

Establishing a Private Practice

Part III. Frustrations of Private Practice

Your private practice will have its own frustrations and satisfactions. You will be dealing on a personal basis with insurance agents, medical and school-based professionals and parents. You need to maintain your professionalism and your patience when explaining for the millionth time: What OT is, what SI treatment is, why it is a legitimate form of treatment, why the child needs treatment, and why you should be reimbursed for your professional services.

You will have to organize your schedule around school hours, snow storms, childhood illnesses and your own problems. If the children are not seen, then you are not paid. In private practice there are no paid vacations. Your income will often fluctuate because of late payments and you will need to learn to deal with collections. (A phone call or letter is usually a sufficient reminder of a late payment.)

You will often provide informal consultation with parents, teachers and other professionals at no charge. It is impossible to charge for all the time spent for the client, so plan your treatment rate accordingly.

Satisfactions from a Private Practice.

A trust relationship develops between the therapist, the child and his or her family as a result of the personal attention the therapist can provide. There is more time to explain treatment goals and activities to the family. A home program to augment your therapeutic goals is often followed more faithfully by the family because of the trust relationship established.

Many times parents become enthusiastic co-workers, as they see the progress from home programs and scheduled therapy sessions. (Our parents are encouraged to observe and participate frequently in the therapy sessions.)

Educating the family about sensory integration does not jeopardize your professional role. It does in fact help parents become more aware of their child's needs. They seem more comfortable and less defensive about asking your advice regarding appropriate toys and activities as well as appropriate family interactions with the child. We recommend that you establish a library of resources and book lists for parent use.

The private practitioner is a 'free agent' and can therefore act as an advocate for the child and his or her family. You may be asked to defend the child's educational needs at a school staffing. You may also be requested to be the third party in justifying the child's special needs in a due process hearing. You may be freer to assume the advocate role than the agency-based therapist.

Be aware that there will be problems with which you may not be able to cope and children with dysfunctions that you are not qualified to treat. Families may become dependent upon you for advice in dealing with such problems as; marital problems, diets, medical and psychological needs. Don't hesitate to use the other resources in your community. Useful contacts to establish early in your practice would be; a dietician, a lawyer, a psychologist or psychiatrist, a social worker, a special educator, a speech pathologist, etc.

Lois Hickman and Kayleen Hall are currently practicing in the Denver, Colorado area.

Sensory Integration
Special Interest Section Newsletter; Vol. 3, No. 4, 1980

The Parent Component

By Winnie Dunn, MEd, OTR

When dealing with the young child in therapy, a major concern also involves parent relations. Parents of children with dysfunction need support from the professionals with whom they deal. This may be the first time they are faced with the problem.

They need ideas about many aspects of their (parents) life with this child:

1. What is wrong with him/her?

Why is this happening? (the parent wants to know if they are to blame, and usually need to be reassured that many factors affect development).

3. What should I expect from my child? What is unrealistic to expect?

4. What are some of the things we can do at home? (try to find activities that will fit into the daily routine, and life style of the family with which you are dealing. In your parent contacts find out what is available at home — i.e.; a swivel or rocking chair; carpeted floors; step stools; a place to climb or jump that's safe. Then fit some of these objects into appropriate activities, rather than asking the parent to purchase special equipment such as barrels, or scooter boards.

Learning Through Play, by J. Marzolla and J. Lloyd, is a good reference.

5. What is "normal" about him/her? (Emphasize the strengths or relative strengths, and give the parents realistic, but hopeful goals for which to strive.)

6. How do I manage my child's behavior? Many references on this topic are available (most in paperback)

Children the Challenge — R. Dreikers
Logical Consequences — R. Dreikers

(continued)

The Parent Component

Little People — E. Christopherson
Toddlers & Parents — T. Brazelton
Systematic Training for Effective Parenting — (a kit, by Am. Guidance Serv) (includes parent handbook that can be purchased separately) — D. Dinkmeyer and G. McKay
Parents and Teachers — W. Becker

7. What are *you* trying to accomplish?

The parent needs to know why sensory integration therapy is going to be beneficial. They need to hear how the things we do will affect the child's development and ability to cope with school demands as the child grows older.

Basically, parents need to be dealt with in an honest, compassionate manner, gaining some realistic answers and the support they need throughout the formative years.

A suggested source on interviewing parents is available in *Journal of Learning Disabilities*. Vol. II, No. 2 — February 1978. Five dimensions are discussed with respect to the parent interview:

1. the parent's evaluation of the child
2. autonomy with this child
3. affection
4. hostility
5. pressuring

This includes questions for addressing these areas that provide helpful insight.

Sensory Integration
Special Interest Section Newsletter; Vol. 3, No. 4, 1980

Benefits from Private Practice in Occupational Therapy

There are four reasons for occupational therapists to consider part-time, if not full-time participation in private practice. First, the occupational therapist involved in private practice can gain a greater appreciation of the business aspects of health care delivery. By doing so, an individual therapist can better understand the need for cost-efficiency. When one engages in private practice, there is no "buffer" institution (such as a school, hospital or charitable organization) between the therapist and those who are purchasing the service. The therapist must therefore deal directly with such issues as billing and monetary collection systems, rate setting, third-party payments, etc. In addition, the private practitioner must actively deal with professional accountability since the therapist is interacting directly with the person or organization purchasing the service. Certainly, professional accountability is an issue with which all therapists must cope. However, the private practitioner may confront the following questions (pertaining to accountability) almost daily. First:

1. Is my service really necessary? Upon what evidence is the decision for occupational therapy based?

2. What can the client (or third-party paying for the service) realistically expect to gain as a result of therapy?

3. How long will therapy be necessary? What are the criteria for discontinuation of service?

Second, just as private practice in occupational therapy increases a therapist's responsibility regarding fiscal matters, it also increases a therapist's responsibility regarding the implementation of the treatment plan. For it is the therapist acting as an independent health professional (who may or may not be working in collaboration with others) who determines the plan of action for any given client. Consequently, a therapist's self direction pertaining to case management is increased. Obviously, within any job setting there should be opportunity for an occupational therapist to have significant input regarding case management. But an occupational therapist in private practice has primary responsibility for determining case management.

Third, there is greater potential for involving parents and family members in the therapy program, especially if the services are being purchased directly by the parents or family. Direct and repeated contact with the consumers of occupational therapy services (parents of learning-disabled children, spouses of stroke victims, etc.) can enhance their understanding of the client and his other dysfunction. Increased understanding may, in turn, lead to better family relationships.

Fourth, an occupational therapist in private practice must develop a referral network. Community hospitals, schools and health care professionals such as psychologists and psychiatrists must be carefully "cultivated" for referrals. Thus, the private practitioner spends much time teaching others about the need for occupational therapy, whom to refer and what to expect from therapy. Indirectly, our profession benefits from private practice, for the private practitioners publicize occupational therapy in an important way.

In summary, if professionalism includes understanding of cost efficiency and accountability, self-direction as an independent health care professional, involvement with the family or parents of a client and interaction with other professionals, then private practice promotes professionalism among occupational therapists by fostering these behaviors.

Charlotte Brasic Royeen, MS, OTR
Special Center for Learning
Cincinnati, Ohio

Evaluation of Pre-Schoolers

By Winnie W. Dunn, MEd, OTR

One of the major concerns in working with the preschool population is that of appropriate evaluation techniques. Following is an example of areas to cover in a typical evaluation of a preschooler. The suggestions here are by no means exhaustive or all inclusive, but rather, an example of areas that may be included.

Clinical Observations (critical to any evaluation)

Flexion in Supine: Can the child move against gravity in supine? Normal preschoolers should be able to hold this position for a few seconds.

Prone Extension: Can the child lift upper trunk, head and arms up against gravity? Normal preschoolers should be able to maintain upper trunk extension for several seconds, but not the full body extension position. This may not be fully integrated until school age.

TNR Inhibition: Preschoolers may still exhibit the effects of a combination of tonic neck responses, and body and head-righting responses. This will show up in the all-fours position and in purposeful activity. TNR responses should not interfere with normal exploration; the child may show a lot of elbow flexion in the all-fours position, but should not show an entire body collapse.

Muscle Tone: Palpation of integrity and balanced muscle tone seems to yield the most helpful information.

Cocontraction: The usual method for testing this by having the child seated and grasping examiner's thumbs is not successful with preschoolers. They don't seem to understand the directions for pushing-pulling. Observe the child in a free play situation for tone and cocontraction information to identify whether they can stabilize joints for purposeful activity. Activities such as tug of war, catching a Tumble Forms ball, or picking up and throwing different sizes and weights of objects can help to determine integrity of stability mechanisms.

Protective Extension Equilibrium: Observing the child on an insecure surface, such as a tilting board, in several positions (i.e., prone, supine, sitting, kneeling, all-fours, standing) is a good way to gather basic information about the child's level of postural control with motion. Preschoolers will still show a predominance of protective responses even with the presence of head, spinal, and trunk

changes to compensate for the movement. The child should also be observed in activities to determine the integrity of this system with purposeful movement. (An example would be "save the people." (Child is on the 'boat' (tilt board), and reaches down on one side for the 'people' (large pegs), then carries them to the other side to place them on the 'raft' (large pegboard).)

Rolling Pattern: While engaged in activity, does the child separate head, trunk and limb motion? Some separation should be present.

Standing up Pattern: How does the child get from supine to standing? Preschoolers should be able to rise to standing without using all-fours as an intermediary step.

Developmental Information: To determine the extent that the child's sensory integrative difficulties are affecting milestones, some sort of developmental information should be gathered. Both present and past information can be helpful. Possible sources:

Denver Developmental Screening Test

Denver Prescreening Checklist—filled out by parent

Portage Guide

Learning Staircase

Santa Clara Inventory

Gesell or other developmental inventories

Brigance Diagnostic Inventory of Early Development

Gross Motor Areas: Jumping from floor and platform; hopping; skipping; walking alike—forward and backward; running; one foot balance; stairs—up and down; marching; rolling; somersaulting; ball skills—catching, throwing, and kicking; and bilateral/reciprocal movements.

Fine Motor Areas: Beery Test of Visual Motor Integration; use of blocks—stacking, making a train and making a bridge; coloring, cutting; drawing—objects and scribbles; tracing; manipulation skills, such as use of nuts and bolts, pegs or clothspins; stringing beads; paper folding; grasp/release patterns; and use of nonpreferred hand to stabilize on bilateral tasks.

Language: Understanding directions; naming objects, actions, use of concepts receptively and expressively; ability to use abstract ideas.

Personal Skills: In addition to the checklist type of information from above, I add information from the parent included on the *Functional Status Rating Scale,* (which is being developed by Carol McEnulty and Brendan Smith). This rating scale goes into detail on the sensory integrative aspects of the child's behavior in all family settings, i.e.; postural changes the child uses to get into and out of the tub; and the tactile responses to the bathtime as well as behavior manifestations in different settings. Ratings are written in lay terms, and are categorized 1, 2, 3, 4.

Behavior: Therapist observations in conjunction with the parent's observations are considered here.

Sensory Processing: In addition to clinical observations, child should be observed for reactions to different types of sensory input.

Does the child tolerate/enjoy activities with a high degree of: tactile/proprioceptive/vestibular input?

What are his/her responses?

Is the child interpreting this information correctly to execute an adaptive response in play?

Include a sensory history from the parent, which will include the child's reactions as an infant to these types of stimulation, and the types of activities the child chooses at home.

Pre-Readiness: Visual and auditory perceptual skills are also a consideration. This should include basic awareness of the visual and auditory world, skills developed, and presence or absence of distractibility to this type of input.

The Cognitive Skills Assessment Battery, The Developmental Indicators for Assessment of Learning Kit, and the *Learning Staircase* include many skills that will be necessary for school readiness, and both are easy to administer.

An informal check can be done with blocks, pegs, beads, and puzzles. Sequencing, matching memory, discrimination and figure ground should be included.

Areas described above may be more or less emphasized, depending on the child's presenting behaviors. The life situation of the child needs to be considered when planning the emphasis of evaluation and treatment planning; some children may

(continued)

Evaluation of Pre-Schoolers

not need the emphasis upon pre-readiness evaluation at the initial visit, but will need this at the end of your treatment, as they approach school age.

Evaluation of preschoolers will be more streamlined when the *Miller Assessment for Preschoolers* is complete because it includes many of the areas described, and will have standardization data available.

Winnie Dunn is employed at St. Luke's Hospital, Kansas City, MO. She has had extensive experience with preschoolers.

Sensory Integration
Special Interest Section Newsletter; Vol. 3, No. 3, 1980

The Transdisciplinary Approach for the Pre-School Child

By Ruth R. Lyddy, OTR

As OTs, most of us have worked within a multidisciplinary team approach, where each professional individually evaluates a child, determines appropriate intervention strategies in the professional's own area, and then carries them out. Formal communication between members occurs at regularly scheduled team meetings, to which members bring their independently and previously determined impressions, recommendations, and progress reports.

Recently, an alternative framework for evaluation and service has been developed that seems particularly useful in a preschool setting: the transdisciplinary model. This is a brief introduction to some aspects of this approach. More complete information on the transdisciplinary model can be found by consulting the suggested readings listed at the end of this article.

Underlying the transdisciplinary approach is the belief that the areas of a child's function cannot be compartmentalized, but rather, that all areas—sensory, motor, cognitive, language, social/emotional—should be considered in light of their shared interaction. In order to implement this belief, the model makes use of two concepts: the "arena" assessment and the primary care provider. Both of these require coordinating the varied skills and knowledge of the team members— including parents—to form a single multidimensional intervention plan for the child.

During an arena assessment, only one member, designated the facilitator, interacts with the child throughout the session. All other team members are present to observe the child perform activities that range across the entire developmental spectrum. At the conclusion of the observation period, the team and parents

share their perceptions and begin the process of developing a unified plan of action. Their success depends on having team members with specialized skills in assessment, ability to readily apply theory to observed behavior, ability to integrate their knowledge with that of other disciplines, and ability to communicate effectively across disciplinary boundaries.

When goals and a treatment plan have been established, one member is chosen as the primary care provider (PCP). The PCP will then provide all the direct service to the child and instruction to the parents, except where specifically decided otherwise. This eliminates the need for the child and family to cope with multiple individuals, environments, and transitions, and thus fosters development of a single, more effective working relationship. This service model requires frequent, regular communication among the entire transdisciplinary team to ensure appropriate program implementation and optimal progress for the child.

The frame of reference that the occupational therapist brings to the transdisciplinary team is an extremely valuable one. The OTs understanding of how dysfunction in sensory integrative processes affects a child's performance in all developmental areas is itself often an integrating framework for the diagnostic impressions of the other team members. Since the formulation of an integrated therapy plan is central to this model, the OTs application of sensory integrative developmental theory and treatment principles is an important component. Specific techniques to increase attentional mechanisms, enhance learning readiness, and facilitate normal sensorimotor experiences can be given to the PCP, who then applies them as she/he works with the child in all the therapeutic areas.

It appears that time efficiency, cost effectiveness, increased learning between team members, and increased parent involvement are all benefits of the transdisciplinary approach. But most importantly, its use in a preschool setting can result in more effective assessment, planning, and service implementation for the young child with special needs.

Suggested Readings:

Connor, F.P. et.al. (eds.), *Program Guide for Infants and Toddlers with Neuromotor and Other Developmental Disabilities*; Teachers College Press, Columbia Univ., NY, 1978.

Hart, V., "The Use of Many Disciplines with the Severely and Profoundly Handicapped" in E. Sontag (ed.), *Educational Programming for the Severely and Profoundly Handicapped*, CEC-MR Division, Reston, VA, 1977.

Maxwell, S.E., "A Transdisciplinary Model for Diagnosis and Remediation in Early Childhood", Paper given at 18th Congress of the International Ass'n of Logopedics, Washington, DC, August 1980, (Proceedings to be published).

Servis, B., "Developing IEP's for Physically Handicapped Children: A Transdisciplinary Viewpoint", *Teaching Exceptional Children*, 10: 78-82, 1978.

United Cerebral Palsy—*Staff Development Handbook: A Resource for the Transdisciplinary Process*, Nationally Organized Collaborative Project to Provide Comprehensive Services for Atypical Infants and Their Families, NY, 1976.

Ruth is presently working in the Walpole, Massachusetts Public Schools providing evaluation, treatment and consultation services. She has worked with preschoolers during the past 5 years and is certified to administer and interpret the SCSIT.

Sensory Integration
Special Interest Section Newsletter; Vol. 3, No. 1, 1980

Treatment of the Autistic Child—A Demanding Challenge

By Karen Pettit, MEd, OTR, Assistant Director, Occupational Therapy, Warren State Hospital

The evaluation and treatment of the autistic child is filled with more questions than answers. Therapists involved with these children are constantly faced with many dilemmas that require much thought, exploration, sensitivity and astute observation in order to solve them. As I reviewed the literature on autism with respect to treatment, it becomes apparent that we currently have three basic approaches from which to formulate a treatment rationale; a biochemical, behavioral and/or a sensory motor frame of reference.

One of the most significant implications from Isaacson (1974) and Pribram and McGinness (1975) is the fundamental and diffuse nature of the autistic's problem. It is more basic and complex than any sensory integrative deficit. What could be more primary than the organization of sensory input to engage in purposeful motor activity? .. the registration, modulation and response to sensory input! Without orienting and modulating sensory input it's very difficult to make meaningful, productive responses to the incoming sensory input. Thus, we see the disturbances of motility, attention, perception, the ritualistic and compulsive behaviors, the language and visual disturbances, as well as the failure to develop normal social relationships that Demasio and Maurer (1978) and others describe.

Consequently, this proposed imbalance that Isaacson, Pribram and McGinness discuss as being between the amygdala, basal ganglia and the hippocampus circuitry is thought to be responsible for the inability of the autistic child to be aroused in order to respond to the sensory input; his inability to have the physiological readiness to respond to the input; and his inability to make the effort to coordinate the arousal and activation processes required to respond. This concept plays a considerable role in the theoretical basis of the treatment of autism.

In this paper we will be discussing evaluation and treatment implications of autistic patients, and identifying a variety of issues that we must become competent with in order to evaluate, treat and organize priorities that will help us to keep the treatment process and our own expectations for the austistic patient's growth in perspective. The frame of reference will be the precursors to the process of sensory integration that is to say sensory processing and their difficulty with the registration, modulation and response to sensory input.

Evaluation and treatment go hand in hand. One without the other often creates meaningless effort and little help to the patient. It is the evaluation, the process of reviewing, categorizing and processing our pre, during and post-treatment observations that increases our understanding of the patient, thus strengthening our body of knowledge to grow as a profession. The field of psychiatric occupational therapy has long experienced the agony and frustration of dealing with the psychotic child as well as the adult. Dr. A. Jean Ayres' profound exploration into the neurological basis for autism has indeed provided us with the structure to continue to make sense out of our clinical observations, our formal and informal test results and our treatment.

Evaluation of the autistic is difficult. Many are unable to participate in such formal testing, the SCSIT, the Carrow Language Comprehension Test, the Bruininks-Oseretsky Test of Motor Proficiency and the Peabody Picture Vocabulary Test. Thus, the need for a test that was not dependent upon cooperation but would provide information about the autistic individual's ability to respond to sensory input, assess his ability to orient and register sensory input as well as whether he could modulate the input. As a result, Dr. A Jean Ayres has been devising and refining such a test, and conducting research regarding the autistic children and their relationship to sensory integration procedures. It will suffice to say that Dr. Ayres' (1979) study and results soon to be published suggest "children who registered sensory input but failed to modulate it responded better to therapy than those who were hypo-responsive or failed to orient to sensory input." This study will close the holes that occur between this description and Ginny Scardina's discussion that appeared in the Spring Issue 1979 of the *Sensory Integration Specialty Section Newsletter*. This concept of hyper-responsivity versus hyporesponsivity as a predictor of a responder to sensory integration procedures is of significant importance both in determining priorities for treatment, criteria for admission into programming and in having a deeper understanding of the area and its depth that we must explore to transcend the autistic's world of psychosis.

After assessment with Ayres' adaptation of the Ornitz Scale evaluating the child's response to 14 different sensory input (auditory, visual, olfactory, touch, vestibular, joint traction, vibration, pain, gravity, and his hyperresponsivity-hyporesponsivity) is determined and are combined with clinical observations of the child relating to this environment, the therapist will have a starting point.

The therapist's ability to be sensitive to the autistic child's non-verbal cues and their need for control, understanding and respect, as well as the therapist's ability to place very simple, achievable demands is always on the line. It is with these qualities that the therapist is able to provide the environment and the initial stimulation to enable the autistic child to produce simple adaptive responses to his environment ... consequently a change in the way he has related to his environment. As Joan Erikson (1976) states, "activity-action is the vital component of all change and without change recovery is an illusion. Without activity and change which is life itself, there is no growth."

As with any field dealing with people there are only some general guidelines that can be shared regarding the treatment of the autistic child. As no two human beings are alike so it is with the autistic patient. There seems to be three basic areas directly related to the initial phase of treatment: (1) the intensity of the need for appropriate kind of stimulation; this seem to be so great you almost get the idea they could lie on the oscillator, or spin in an axial plane inside an inner tube, or ride down a ramp on the scooter board, hour after hour or session after session; (2) the most progress seems to be made with autistic children (as with other sensory integrative deficits) when they are involved with producing an adaptive response; and (3) the therapist must be able to recognize when the child needs to be "pushed" or is able to self-direct his treatment sessions.

The three primary skills the therapist must have to recognize those guidelines and aid in treatment are (1) the ability to be in touch with the patient . . . read the non-verbal cues sent through gestures, moves toward equipment or away from equipment; (2) trust the patients and respect their communications; they know how the stimuli feels to them; and (3) the ability to have a positive attitude toward patients and the patients' treatment.

Ashley Montagu (1979) states

... for through what other avenues than our senses are we able to enter into the dimension of human existence? It is our senses that frame the body of reality. The Western man has increasingly relied for the purposes of communication on the 'distance senses'—sight and hearing. The 'proximity senses'—touch, taste, smell, the vestibular and joint-muscle sense have either been tabooed, or ignored.

Have we as therapists ignored or been afraid of using our 'proximity senses' to experience in treatment the kind of stimulation that our patients seek? Could that mutual participation in the treatment session aid

(continued)

our understanding of the non-verbal messages our patients send us? For most autistic children the therapist's dependence on the distant senses of sight and hearing to establish a relationship and a process of communication would make it virtually impossible to understand or have any idea of how or what the patient is feeling. The therapist must be committed to exploring, processing and reviewing each encounter with the patient within a sensory and psychodynamic frame of reference. Although we theorize the autistic child has a disordered registration, modulation and response to sensory input, that does not mean he cannot feel your respect or lack of respect, your understanding or lack of understanding for him! He may not be able to register and respond to our often fast, complex verbal messages but he can, through those unidentified extra senses, feel our warmth, sincerity and concern through our touch and approach.

The art of therapy is dependent upon the therapist having the three primary skills of "getting into the patient's spaces," trust and respect for the patient, and the therapist's positive attitude toward the patient and the patient's treatment, in addition to the therapist's proficiency in guiding the patient, designing the environment and often manipulating the environment toward the goal of the patient self-directing the treatment session and producing adaptive responses.

The issue of self-direction with the autistic child is not as clearcut as it is with the learning-disabled child. On the continuum for the autistic child is self stimulation versus self-direction. For the learning-disabled child it is disorganization versus self-direction.

What is the process of moving from self-stimulation to self-direction? It is of utmost importance to have a basic neurological understanding of the autistic child's difficulty in the irregularity of the registration function of the amygdala hippocampus circuitry as well as the limbic system components that regulate emotional tone. Many autistic children have too much or too little emotional tone. If it is this imbalance in the function of the amygdala-hippocampus mechanisms that causes the autistic child's under or over registration of input then we must under-

stand as much of the neural pathways, projections and sensory convergence involved in order to provide the appropriate stimulation. There are connections with the vestibular, stretch of the muscle, touch pressure and olfaction. The visual and the auditory connections and projections at this point in our knowledge do not seem to be as significant. This is not to say that if we provide vestibular, proprioceptive and olfactory stimuli that the problem of autism would be solved. The complexity is great.

The process then of moving from self-stimulation to self-direction is slow, tedious and often filled with much frustration and puzzlement because of the lack of answers. Simple expectations and instructions are critical in the outcome of treatment. The first several sessions may be spent on separating the child from the family or living unit in order to begin individual treatment. It is also most important that the child's "6th sense" picks up your warmth, understanding and acceptance. After these phases are past, one then can begin to focus on the non-verbal communication to begin to understand the child. In other words we have to begin to analyze what the behavior tells us about how their brain is working. Each child is different and his preferred type of stimulation is dependent upon his sensory integrative deficits combined with his degree of difficulty in registering sensory input. In general, vestibular stimulation seems to have the greatest effect. For some the proprioceptive system needs to be stimulated first in order to help them begin to modulate the vestibular input. Most autistic children seem to enjoy the vestibular input and it often serves as a motivating force in treatment. At various stages in the treatment linear, axial, and orbital vestibular inputs play significant roles at other times tactile input is meaningful, still at other times proprioceptive input is the most meaningful. We therefore must be as "in touch" with our patient's needs as possible.

As I mentioned earlier, the adaptive response is very important in the treatment process. An adaptive response occurs when the individual self-initiates, a subcortical, generalized, self-reinforcing, purposeful, goal directed, functionally meaningful response to his environment in order that he

might become master of his needs and wants. In other words, an adaptive response is the behavior act that causes excitement, pleasure, the desire to go further into a task or the desire to repeat the task because it was right, it was successful, if felt good; it is that behavior act that one performs that makes him feel proud and is that extra push necessary to take on a more complex task that had been too difficult and was avoided. It is that task that has meaning and purpose.

Recognizing and promoting adaptive responses has many implications for treatment and is the art of therapy. Since planning and executing movement provides one of the most basic means through which the brain produces and organizes stimuli, our ability to analyze movement is critical to the treatment process. If the movement for the individual has zest, satisfaction, excitement and often is repeated again and again one has probably reached and appropriate level for the individual's maturation. If his nervous system was able to modulate the stimuli and the activity was growth promoting, fulfilling, organizing and integrating, he will receive fulfillment with the right combination of challenge and success.

Thus, during treatment, the therapist must have as the major goal the patient's self-fulfillment, not cooperation. The session must have a task with the possibility of success in order to be motivating, thus, a challenge. Our patient's brains hold the answers to the question "Of what should therapy consist?" We must learn to watch the brain through behavior.

Opportunity and freedom to explore is a necessary element so that we can determine the complexity, accuracy, appropriateness, and effectiveness of the behavioral response. It is only with the patient in control that we as therapists know how to better design the environment to promote more mature adaptive responses and thus help him to grow. Joan Erikson states "the fundamental purpose of (the hospital) treatment is to permit the patient to regress to a stage of dependence in which he can "nurse" his weakness and relearn strength and hope, and it must unremittingly encourage him to regain autonomy and the will to help himself."

Sensory Integration
Special Interest Section Newsletter; Vol. 3, No. 1, 1980

Autism—A Neurological Model

By Mary Becker, OTR

This brief article will explore some information relevant to the role of the occpuational therapist in the assessment and treatment of autistic children. Although there are many ways to approach the problem of autism, this article is written primarily in the sensory motor frame of reference. At present, we actually know relatively little about this complex dysfunction. It is therefore important to take a broad-based approach to the problem. As occpuational therapists working with autistic children, we must be informed about the various modes of treatment and understand the importance of an interdisciplinary approach. As the knowledge base expands, so must our mode of assessment and treatment.

We tend to interpret problems in light of the times. In the psychoanalytic era, we interpreted problems in psychoanalytic terms. Today, with increased neurological data, we interpret problems in terms of central nervous system dysfunction. Our hypothesis today will probably not hold true in years to come. We must, therefore, hold these hypotheses lightly, move ahead with flexibility, and strive for increased knowledge and understanding.

Definition:

Kanner first described autism in 1943. He was quite accurate in his observations of behavioral manifestations and many of his descriptions still hold true today. Autistic children, according to Kanner, have an inability to relate to other people, a delay in speech, abnormalities of language (particularly reversals of pronouns and echoing), and excellent rote memory and an obsessive desire for maintaining sameness.

Rutter expanded on the description in his review of 30 years of research on autism. He described the abnormalities in interpersonal relationships by a relative lack of eye-to-eye gaze, limited emotional attachment to parents, little variation in facial expressions, and a lack of interest in people. Autistic children often fail to cuddle and do not usually seek comfort from their parents when they are hurt or upset. Their speech and language delay is often accompanied by some reduction in response to sounds. When language does develop it is usually abnormal (i.e. pronoun reversals and echolalia). Deficits are evident in all forms of non-verbal communication such as gestures and facial expressions. The child provides examples of ritualistic and compulsive behavior in which there is often a morbid attachment to unusual objects, peculiar preoccupations and a resistance to change.

Rutter explored the relationship of mental retardation in the autistic syndrome. He found that features characterizing autism were present in autistic children of both high and low intelligence. The mentally retarded autistic children did show a more severe autistic picture. Mentally retarded autistic children were more apt to exhibit self-injury, hand-finger stereotypes and deviant social responses. A wide range of perceptual deficits and neurodevelopmental abnormalities was evident. They were more likely to develop epileptic seizures during adolescence. Mentally retarded autistic children were found to have poorer prognosis than autistic children with normal intelligence.

Several writers have described aberrant responses to sensory stimuli. This observation has particular significance within the sensory motor frame of reference. Autistic children have a shorter and less sustained orientation toward visual stimuli than do normal or retarded controls. They use peripheral vision more than central vision. According to Rimland although they may not respond to a very loud sound, they may respond excessively to a barely audible siren. There are also documented reports of decreased response to pain, with excessive response to tactual, gustatory or olfactory stimuli. Ayres has explored this facet in a research study which will be published in the near future. Children exhibiting hyporesponsivity to sensory stimuli were found to have a poorer prognosis with regard to sensory integrative therapy. Those autistic children in her study that demonstrated signs of hyperresponsivity to sensory input such as gravitational insecurity and tactile defensiveness were found to respond to sensory integrative therapy.

The above-mentioned lack of responsiveness to stimuli, or perhaps inappropriate response seems to suggest a deficit in that system which allows us to analyze and integrate incoming information. According to Gold and Gold, autistic children appear to perceive the incoming input as non-novel and insignificant.

Neurological Considerations:

The following is a brief examination of that part of the nervous system which evaluates the importance of incoming stimuli. The limbic system plays an important role in this process. It helps the individual know what stimulus is important and which is not important and allows the appropriate attention and orientation to these stimuli. This takes place at different levels of limbic processing according to the nature and complexity of the stimuli involved.

Isaacson defines "orienting" as preparation for assocation of a new stimuli with memories from the past and expectation for the future. The hippocampus and the amygdala, structures of the limbic system, serve opposite functions in terms of orienting. We need both responses well modulated in order to pay the right amount of attention for the given situation.

There is some evidence linking the behavioral manifestations of autism to defects in limbic structures and functions. Hauser, DeLong and Rosman describe pheumoencephalographic (PEG) findings in a group of chidren exhibiting the austic syndrome. The PEG demonstrated an enlargement of the left temporal horns in 15 of 17 cases of autism indicating a deficiency of brain substance or atrophy. The widened left temporal horn was attributable, at least in part, to a distinct flattening of the normal hippocampal contour. They speculate that these children may fail to profit from experience because they lack the hippocampal mechanisms necessary to store and integrate new information. They add that the hippocampus and surrounding structures flavor all experience with a personal, appropriate, emotional meaning. It is precisely in these areas that the autistic child is most deficient, according to these authors.

What other data to we have to support a hypothesis linking autism to limbic systems dysfunction? Damasio and Mauer attribute autism to dysfunction in a system of "bilateral neural structures that includes the ring of mesolimbic cortex located in the mesial frontal and temporal lobes, the neostriatum and the anterior and medial nuclear groups of the thalamus. The mesocortex is a relay point for information coming from the perceptual neocortex on its way to structures such as the hippocampus, or to subcortical limbic system structures such as the amygdala according to these authors' experimental work. Their speculations, in addition to those of Hauser, etc., do suggest limbic system dysfunction. This hypothesis is certainly in the embryo stage. The picture is quite complex and there is much need for further research. This information does, however, provide some exciting data for beginning exploration of this most perplexing syndrome.

Etiology:

To what possible causes do researchers attribute these deficits?

Kanner (1943) felt that it was an inborn disturbance of affective contact. He wrote that "these children have come into the

(continued)

Autism—A Neurological Model

world with an innate inability to form the usual biologically provided affective contact with people, just as other children who come into the world with innate physical or intellectual handicaps." Kanner later focused on the traits of the parents of autistic children, writing that they were cold, aloof, and unusually intellectual. Bettleheim (1967) and Lotter (1967) were proponents of this view.

At present, most researchers agree that autism is a neurobiologically based dysfunction. Evidence comes from neurological data and EEG abnormalities. Small (1975) found autistic children to have a high incidence of abnormal EEGs and positive neurological data. Rutter (1967) found the presence of seizures in adolescence in 1/6 of cases of autism.

As one of the possible causes of autism, Damasio and Mauer include perinatal infection. Autism is postulated to be associated

with viral disease, as it is associated with patients with congenital rubella, measles encephalitis and cytomegalovirus infection. Hypoxia is another possibility, causing damage to parts of the brain. A genetic disturbance could be responsible for deficient maturation of neurons in specific areas concerned with the production of neuromediators. According to Rutter (1968), the rate of autism in siblings is considerably above that in the general population.

As one can see, there are many possibilities. Not all have been listed. At present, we can only postulate. The varied clinical picture associated with autism suggests that there is not one simple etiology. Perhaps factors interact in a very complex manner, varying in nature and intensity and contributing to the variety in the clinical picture.

This article attempted to define the syndrome of autism with an emphasis on the apparent hyporesponsivity, or aberrant

responsiveness to sensory stimuli seen in autistic children. Some neurological considerations were also explored that emphasize the relationship of the apparent hyporesponsivity to sensory stimuli to limbic functions, or more specifically, to the amygdala, basal ganglia and the hippocampus circuitry. Etiological factors were also touched upon. The intent was to introduce the occupational therapist to this frame of reference. If we are to make progress with autistic children we need an in-depth understanding of the nervous system, with an emphasis on the functions of the limbic system. We need to develop assessment tools and collect data on children in treatment to evaluate responsiveness to treatment. As occupational therapists working within the sensory-motor frame of reference, the challenge of working with the autistic child is great. Let's meet this challenge with vigor, and contribute to this ever expanding body of knowledge.

Sensory Integration
Special Interest Section Newsletter; Vol. 3, No. 1, 1980

Calm—A Therapeutic Device

By Mary Silberzahn, MA, OTR

The strong drive for linear movement such as bouncing, jumping, body rocking evidenced by autistic children prompted further investigation of the importance of linear movement to this population of children. An electric device, which provided controlled alternating linear stimulation, named CALM was constructed and has been used in the treatment of autistic children as well as with children with a variety of diagnostic categories of sensory integrative dysfunction since 1975. Observations of behavioral changes, especially when used as a major treatment modality over a period of time include a decrease in muscle tension and an increase in environmental awareness. Alerting reactions developed in the nonresponsive child and became more selective in the hyperresponsive child. Eye contact gradually developed and increased. While all of the children treated showed an increase in receptive language and in vocalization, verbal communication was enhanced in those children who had previously acquired some verbal communication but not in nonvebal children. Postural insecurity decreased and children began to tolerate experiences in various planes and to initiate more purposeful motor action. Children no longer displayed a defensive reaction to touch but

began to seek hugging and comfort from the parent.

Premature and infant stimulation studies have reported similar results from continuous rhythmical stimulation, i.e., more rapid neurodevelopment, cessation of crying, more and longer periods of quiet sleep, calming and alerting, decrease in heart rate and irregular respiration, greater visual, auditory and motor maturity. Studies of infant rocking which used controlled electrical devices reported that frequencies of 60 to 90 cycles per minute were more effective than lower frequencies. Pederson and Ter Vrugt (1973) found that an amplitude of 5 inches was more effective in calming and alerting than was 2 inches and that rocking in a vertical direction (head to toe) was more effective than rocking in a horizontal direction.

It may be that autistic children, as well as other types of neurologically dysfunctioning children, have not been able to benefit appreciably from the early passive movement experiences which prepare the developing nervous system for adaptive responses. It appears as though many of these children require a great deal more rhythmic, repetitive stimulation in the linear plane for primitive organization of movement experiences than was previously provided or than can be pro-

vided through self-initiation or therapist-assisted activities. Therefore, an electric device which can be controlled for speed and amplitude was made available to these children both during therapy sessions and for home use. The length of time spent on the device varied from 5 to 10 minutes to 1 hour per treatment session with the more hyperresponsive or hyporesponsive children using the device the longer periods of time. If the child initally rejected this type of movement experience, linear stimulation was introduced through other activities such as prone swinging or bouncing on a bolster or platform swing suspended from coils. As tolerance increased the child then selected the more constant movement provided by CALM. Although children generally began to use the device while prone or supine, they would later initiate motor action in all positions.

An initial concern was whether the amount of time some children spend on CALM was promoting perseveration rather than integration or delaying the development of self-initiated motor action. However, observations over a period of 4 years have alleviated this concern. Children vol-

(continued)

Calm—A Therapeutic Device

untarily leave the device, apparently when sufficient input has been received as well as voluntarily return to the device when additional stimulation is needed. Such perseverative behaviors as body rocking, bed rocking, and head banging have been extinguished and no substitute behaviors have been reported. The observation that children return to CALM during a treatment session may be similar to the rocking of normal children while in transition between motor stages such as between sitting and crawling. In addition, the integrative of passive movement appears to be essential for the development of active movement.

The effectiveness of CALM may lie, not only in the multisensory stimulation but in the repetition of movement for an extended period of time. Input of the same frequency and amplitude may build up a constancy and consistency of sensory patterns fundamental for the perception of changing patterns of sensory input. Goody (1958) has suggested that the repetitive rhythmical action of the nervous system is important to internal sequencing of external events. The personal concept of time, the timing of motor movements for the coordinated use of body parts, and thus for body scheme development and motor skill, as well as of perception and memory may be in some way related to the constant flow of energy throughout the nervous system.

The neurophysiological rationale for the use of controlled alternating linear movement continues to be developed and publications are being prepared. CALM, as an electric device to provide controlled alternating linear movement, is being perfected as a marketable device available from this author.

References:

Goody, W.: Time and the nervous system. *The Lancet*, 31 May, 1958, *i*, 1139-1144.
Pederson, D.R., & Ter Vrugt, D.: The influence of amplitude and frequency of vestibular stimulation on the activity of two-month-old infants. *Child Development*, 1973, *44*, 122-128.

Sensory Integration
Special Interest Section Newsletter; Vol. 2, No. 4, 1979

Sensory Integration and Infants

Introduction

The numbers of hospital neonatal units employing occupational therapists as part of the team is routine care, evaluation and follow-up care are increasing at a rapid rate.

While 0-3 programs have been in existence for several years, they are becoming far more efficient at identifying risk factors and instituting specific therapeutic programs to help remediate or lessen the effects of those factors. Because we are no longer in a passive phase of watch and wait, but rather in an active phase of diagnosing and remediating, our role with the 0-3 population has changed radically.

This change brings challenge and excitement but primarily it carries enormous responsibility. Responsibility for acquiring in-depth knowledge of the developing nervous system and the normal and abnormal neurophysiological reactions to touch, pressure, movement, position, feeding and sleep and wake states, as well as a skilled working knowledge of normal growth and development concepts as they relate to the acquisition of gross and fine motor skills, auditory/speech/language skills, visual form and space skills and social-emotional growth and development. The concepts of convergence, divergence and interdependence have led us to a team approach for adequate diagnosis and program planning for our patients. My own experience is that these principles applied to team members have facilitated enormous professional growth which results in increased competency of care and programs.

This issue illustrates untold hours of multidisciplinary involvement. Several articles represent the combined efforts of the following therapists (Dottie Ecker, MA, OTR; Carolyn Fiterman, RPT; Patricia Montgomery, MA, RPT; Eileen Richter, OTR; Kathy Swenson-Miller, MS, OTR; Patricia Wilbarger, MEd, OTR). I appreciate their contributions and hope my writing reflects their expertise.

Now is the time to submit articles for the next summer's issue on adult psychiatry and to begin thinking about your contribution to the preceding issue on Geriatrics. Please send your comments, long or short articles and the names of people who may be encouraged to contribute their expertise.— *Patti Oetter, OTR, editor*

Our thanks to Kathy Swenson-Miller, MS, OTR for the feature articles on SI and the Infant. Kathy received her BS in OT from the University of Minnesota and her MS in health sciences from Boston University (focus on developmental disabilities and neuropsychology). She is CSSID faculty and is currently director of OT, as well as research assistant, Division for Disorders of Development and Learning, Biological Sciences Research Center of the Child Development Institute, University of North Carolina at Chapel Hill. She is also clinical assistant professor, Department of Allied Health Sciences, University of North Carolina at Chapel Hill. Kathy has presented numerous lectures and papers. She has a published training videotape entitled "Feeding Evaluations", DDDL, 1979, and has contributed to a chapter by H.R. Chamberlin, "The role of other disciplines and the interdisciplinary team" in the forthcoming Child Development and Developmental Disabilities. Also to be published are articles, "Tactile defensiveness—neurological and cultural aspects", and "Sensory responsiveness of hypotonic infants."

Sensory Integration Theory Applied to Infant Intervention During the First Three Years of Life

Since sensory integration is an inherent part of every individual's spectrum of abilities and disabilities, it seems appropriate to apply sensory integration theory to the infant population. It can help in understanding normal infant development more comprehensively. It can also help in understanding, assessing and intervening effectively with the handicapped infant. Through a progression of operational definitions of sensory integration (see Glossary), the following questions can be answered in an organized way:

1. What are the sensory integration abilities in the normal infant? That is, what is the defined developmental progression of the following abilities for the infant 0-3 years: tactile discrimination, kinesthetic awareness, ocular-vestibular and postural-vestibular responses, auditory discrimination, postural reflex expectation, motor planning, prehension skills as part of bilateral hand useage? Currently we have only gross developmental principles to guide our observations until therapists systematically develop ways to measure these aspects and thereby gain normative data.

2. Can sensory integrative dysfunction be validly identified in infants? That question is difficult to answer, because sensory integrative dysfunction may be: (a) an adjunct problem as part of a definable diagnosis, e.g., mental retardation, autism; or (b) the primary diagnosis. My own experience leads me to believe that we are not yet sophisticated enough to identify infants with primary sensory integrative dysfunction such as ideomotor dyspraxia. Probably we will eventually be able to identify, then treat, entities such as moderate to severe ideomotor dyspraxia in infants (especially those with accompanying oral and verbal dyspraxia) by concentrating our observations on *how* an infant feeds, manipulates toys, and approaches new mobility patterns.

3. How can sensory integration be assessed in handicapped infants? (See Assessment Tools section in this newsletter for names and sources of infant assessment tools.) First, good baseline developmental data is needed (i.e., social, fine motor/adaptive, gross motor, speech, expressive and receptive language) to give us information about "end products"—*what* an infant can do. To appreciate *how* an infant approaches tasks, careful sensory and motor expression analysis is done of the following: observation of the developmental testing; infant temperament by observation and parent interview; and observation and parent interview regarding the infant's play, interactional and self help (especially feeding) patterns. Now our normative data is limited so we must rely upon a tremendous amount of clinical judgement to determine sensory integrative patterns, decide if the patterns are significantly atypical or delayed, label the patterns for reporting and parent education purposes, decide most appropriate form of intervention, and find ways to measure progress. As occupational therapists become increasingly zealous in applying sensory integration theory to the handicapped infant population, it is important for us to keep a good perspective of all factors, intra-child as well as environmental, influencing the infant. For example, what may appear to be biological tactile defensiveness in a given infant may actually be a behavior which reflects child abuse. In this case, the intervention needs to be directed to the environment as well as to the infant.

4. How can sensory integration theory be translated into intervention for handicapped infants? The sensory and motor qualities of activities can be analyzed in terms of what best promotes a functional attending/arousal level, what position is best for an activity, how can functional play interactions be facilitated through controlled sensory input, etc. Adaptation of the neurophysiological approaches to treatment (Ayres, Bobath, Rood) can be effective with infants. When using any neurophysiological treatment technique, one must assume responsibility for having the necessary theoretical background, have an understanding of the limitations as well as potential of the technique, constantly reassess effectiveness, and know precautions of the approaches. For instance, sensory integration theory and techniques were effective when applied in combination with a developmental intervention and parent education program to an 18-month-old, moderately mental and motor retarded little boy who demonstrated low muscle tone and flat affect (primary diagnosis was not sensory integrative dysfunction). "Jazzing up" facilitatory experiences (primarily play experiences incorporating angular and linear vestibular stimulation and generalized vibration) to enhance general alerting and arousal level were found useful during each intervention session prior to incorporating self-initiated mobility and Piagetian cognitive-play experiences. — *Kathy Swenson-Miller*

Addendum A: Operational Definitions Of Sensory Integration

Sensory integration is the ability to organize sensory information for adaptive use.

Sensory integration theory uses neural function/dysfunction principles in assessing/intervening an individual's sensory integration constellation of abilities/disabilities.

Sensory integration dysfunction implies aberrant processing of sensory information resulting in maladaptive responses, as reflected in the infant's play, interactional and self-help behaviors.

Sensory integration therapy uses controlled sensory input (facilitation or inhibition) to organize sensory information for adaptive use.

Sensory integration therapy techniques are: creatively derived from natural play/leisure time activities that provide opportunities for controlling sensory input resulting in an adaptive response; are age appropriate for the client; and are goal directed as well as self directed.

Criteria for Referral to Occupational Therapy

The numbers of identified risk factors are many and all may or may not be appropriate OT referrals. Few hospital nursery departments have the financial luxury of following every infant. As a result adequate referral criteria is needed from the units gathering long-term data. Therapists working in hospital units have tentatively identified the following criteria.

(continued)

Criteria for Referral

A. Newborn
1. Small prematures and others requiring prolonged hospitalization see risk factors
2. Any abnormal neurological exam (EMI scan, seizures, increased or decreased muscle tone, peripheral nerve injuries, drugs/alcohol)
3. Any infant who has been on a ventilator (oral motor development and possible small blood vessel leakage within brain due to increased pressure.
4. Orthopedic problems
5. Sensory deficits including vision and hearing
6. Congenital anomalies and chromosome anomalies
7. High risk social
8. Feeding problems

B. Developmental
1. High risk social
2. Parental concern—parents appear to be 80% efficient in "gut feelings" about developmental discrepancies and they need to be encouraged to seek evaluation and intervention.
3. 2 weeks—hyper-irritable, increased or decreased muscle tone
4. 4 months—inability to get hands to midline in supine position, weak neck flexion or weak total flexion posture, inability or delay in following or turning to sound, tactile defensiveness, postural insecurity, is not cuddly, dislikes bath or clothes changed.
5. 7 months and up—child should be competent with hands. At this age, development is multifaceted and requires standardized assessment tools. (See list compiled by K. Swenson-Miller)

Sensory Integration
Special Interest Section Newsletter; Vol. 2, No. 4, 1979

Affective Development and Sensory Responsiveness

By Kathy Swenson-Miller

Recent research[1,2] demonstrates correlation between infant affective and cognitive development. Four aspects of affective development have been emphasized in the research: smiling, laughter, fear and surprise. (Affective development scales are now being developed.) An interesting study deals with correlation of affective and cognitive development in normal and infants with Down's Syndrome[3], using a "smile scale," the Uzgiris-Hunt and the Bailey Tests. Research results indicate that Down's Syndrome infants' cognitive and affective development to progress at one-half the rate of normal infants as one would anticipate.

The authors do not analyze the sensory parameters of the smile scale items. But their data do indicate that the infants with Down's Syndrome were more highly responsive to near receptor stimuli (tactile, vestibular, vibration) than to auditory stimuli in the first stage of affective development. This trend supports sensory integrative thinking that low muscle tone infants, in order to be responsive to their environment, require experiences that have a primitive stimuli base. Also, the infants with Down's Syndrome rarely laugh, but rather smile, in the first 18 months of life. Hypothetically, this observation might be related to limited muscle tone tension sufficient for a laugh.

Such research may eventually help us to organize documentation of comments frequently made about results of sensory integrative treatment: a happier child, laughs more often, knows danger (development of fear) for the first time, etc. Further research of affective development promises interesting avenues for documenting changes effected at a spontaneous, automatic level.

1. Johnson N, Jens K, et al. Affect and cognition in infancy: Implications for the handicapped. In *New Directions in Special Education*, J. Gallagher (Ed.), New York: Jossey-Blass. (Book in preparation)
2. Stroufe LA, Waters E. The ontogenesis of smiling and laughter: a perspective on the organization of development in infancy. Psychological Review, 1976, 83, 173-189.
3. Cicchetti D, Stroufe LA. The relationship between affective and cognitive development in Down's Syndrome Infants. Child Development, 1976, 47, 920-929.

Useful general references regarding infant evaluation and intervention:

Erickson, Marcene: *Assessment and management of developmental changes in children*, CV Mosby Company, Saint Louis, 1976. (One chapter covers infant temperament assessment.)

Gross L, Goin K (Eds.): *Identifying handicapped children, a guide to casefinding, screening, diagnosis, assessment and evaluation*, Walker and Company, 720 Fifth Avenue, NY 10019, 1977. (Includes an extensive bibliography of assessment tools.)

Caldwell B, Stedman D (Eds.): *Infant education, a guide for helping handicapped children in the first three years*, Walker and Company, 720 Fifth Avenue, NY 10019, 1977.

Connor FP, Williamson GG, Siepp JM; *Program guides for infants and toddlers with neuromotor and other developmental disabilities*, Teachers College Press, Columbia Univ., NY, 1978.

Nystagmus in Infancy

By Patricia Montgomery, MA, PT

A review of the literature in the area of infant nystagmus can be very confusing. This is due to the wide variety of procedures used in testing for the response.

Two recent studies, however, have indicated that the nystagmus response may serve as an index of central nervous system maturation. Eviatar (et. al, 1974) studied the nystagmus response of 11 premature and 110 term infants categorized as small, large or appropriate for gestational age (SGA, LGA, AGA) to movement in a torsion swing and caloric stimulation. Results showed that all but one of the LGA term infants and 83% of the AGA infants had prerotary vestibular responses within 10-75 days of birth compared to only 24% of the SGA infants. All of the LGA term infants, 69% of the AGA and 26% of the SGA responded to cold caloric between 10-75 days. None of the pre-term infants showed a response to either test within 10-75 days of birth, but all demonstrated a response at four to nine months of age.

Rossi (et. al, 1979) studied the nystagmus response (presence or absence) of 91 full-term and 10 pre-term infants to rotary stimulation. Eighty-six of the 101 children (15 not followed) showed a nystagmus response by the 49th post-conceptual week. The majority of full-term AGA infants demonstrated the response by the 45th week. The full-term SGA infants demonstrated a significant delay in nystagmus response compared to the AGA infants, supporting the view that delayed vestibular responsivity is related to delayed maturation of the CNS.

It is important for the therapist who is evaluating nystagmus in infants to understand the neurophysiologic basis of the response. The slow component of nystagmus is attributed to stimulation of the peripheral vestibular apparatus, whereas the quick component is thought to be due to central connections between the vestibular nuclei and the reticular formation. There may be a lack of a quick component in young or premature infants (eye deviation only), especially during sleep, or in conditions which would affect the level of consiousness (i.e., medications, following feeding, etc.). This would be explained by immaturity or depression of central reticular pathways. Indeed, caloric testing of comatose adults results in a nystagmus with a slow component only and reflects depressed reticular system function.

Eviatar, L., Eviator, A. & Naray I. Maturation of neurovestibular responses in infants. *Developmental Medicine and Child Neurology*, 1974, 16, 435-446.
Rossi, L., Pignataro, O., Nino, L., Gaini, R., Sambatro, G., & Oldini, C. Maturation of vestibular responses: preliminary report. *Developmental Medicine and Child Neurology*, 1979, *21*, 217-224.

Identification of the High-Risk Infant

The concept of the high risk infant is an infant who is at significantly increased risk of dying or of suffering morbidity, including physical and/or developmental abnormalities. Such an infant may be born to a mother who demonstrated risk factors during her pregnancy or labor and delivery or to a mother without previously identified risk factors. —Dr. A. Orgill, Children's Hospital, St. Paul, MN.

Labor, Delivery, and Neonate
High Risk Factors

1. Prolonged duration of active labor
2. Ruptured membranes at 24 or more hours
3. Infant too large or too small for period of gestation
4. Placenta previa or abruptio placenta
5. Any difficult delivery or Apgar score of 5 or less at 1 minute of life.
6. High or midforceps delivery
7. Caesarean section (at least for brief observation)
8. Breech delivery (at least for brief observation)
9. Birth weight under 5½ lbs. (2.5 kg.) or over 9 lbs. (over 4 kg.)
10. Meconium-stained amniotic fluid
11. Multiple pregnancies
12. Any infant requiring resuscitation
13. Prolapsed cord
14. Respiratory distress syndrome or other respiratory distress
15. Malformation or other significant abnormality in newborn infant
16. Evidence of birth injury
17. Drug or other depression at birth
18. Evidence of infection in infant
19. Candidates for surgery, preoperatively and postoperatively

Maternal High Risk Factors

1. Age
   Under 16 or over 40
   Current first pregnancy in a mother age 35 or more
2. Prior pregnancy history
   Complications in previous pregnancies
   History of infertility (involuntary sterility)
   RH sensitization
   Previous multiple pregnancies
   Previous premature births
   Previous births with malformations
   Previous births of infants 9 or more lbs. (even if previous studies for diabetes mellitus were negative)
3. Multiple pregnancy
4. User of drugs/alcohol
5. RH negative or maternal antibody sensitization
6. Bleeding after 20 weeks of gestation
7. Maternal medical problems
   Toxemia, hypertension, chronic renal disease, etc.
   Cardiac disease
   Persistent albuminuria
   Diabetes mellitus
   Obesity
   Chronic urinary tract infection
   Infectious disease (tuberculosis, syphilis, etc.)
   Viral (and protozoan) diseases: rubella, herpes simplex (especially cervicitis), cytomegalovirus (CMV), toxoplasmosis
   Anemia
   Surgery during pregnancy
   Metabolic disease (e.g., hyperthyroidism)
   Drugs prescribed by physicians (e.g., iodides, propylthiouracil, rauwolfia, sulfas, etc.)
   Premature labor or threatened labor
   Postmature labor (two or more weeks beyond expected date of confinement)

Sensory Integration
Special Interest Section Newsletter; Vol. 2, No. 4, 1979

Purpose of Occupational Therapy in Infant Programs

A. Normalize the sensory environment. Balance facilitation and inhibition, as well as balance stimulation and relaxation. Our responsibility is to protect the immature nervous system as much as possible and to provide as close to normal a sensory environment as medically possible. Skill and knowledge are required, especially for the pre-term infant.

B. Provide a variety of appropriate sensory experiences. Caution and knowledge are key issues. New literature is becoming increasingly available which reviews normal neurophysiological development.

C. Encourage active motor responses. This can be done through positioning and in increasing or decreasing the effects of specific types of sensory input. Skill, knowledge and constant assessment of adaptive responses are critical during therapy. Another critical issue is the design of a home program within the level of the parents' cooperativeness and ability.

D. Plan an effective home program within the level of the parents' cooperativeness and ability.

Sensory Integration
Special Interest Section Newsletter; Vol. 2, No. 4, 1979

Oral-Motor Factors

One of the major at risk factors appears to be oral-motor deficits and/or feeding problems. The ability to organize neuromotor mechanisms for adequate nutritional intake has many implications. Most obvious and primal is for support of life-normal growth and maturation of all systems. A hungry or insufficiently nutritioned baby has neither the energy nor the motivation to explore or learn about himself or his environment. The bonding process becomes altered as the stress bounces from mother to baby and back again with the desperate need to provide and get food. Feeding normally provides both parent and baby with a warm loving time to interact. The oral motor reflexes (rooting and suck-swallow) facilitate the baby's first real interaction with his environment in contrast to other newborn reflex patterns which elicit protective or withdrawal responses. Feeding invites environmental interaction patterns to develop.

The suck, swallow, breathe synchrony is critical not only for intake of food but also for early motor planning skills which allow the infant opportunities for exploring himself and his environment. The larynx is high and in back of the tongue of the newborn, which allows the semi-supine position for feeding, and is the reason for the high pitched, hypernasal, and little variation in voice quality. By 5-6 months the larynx has dropped into position. Babbling begins as a result of this and upper chest expansion is facilitated in the prone extension position and the baby requires a near vertical position to keep from choking.

The pressure of the tongue on the palate flattens and widens the palate for later use in phonation. Breathing patterns and rib cage alignment change from belly breathing and obligate nose breathing in the newborn (the upper chest is almost flat) to upper thorax breathing patterns and alternating nose or mouth breathing as situations require. The rib cage is tilted down and out by 18 months of age as a result of well-established feeding patterns and the prone on elbows position which in turn promotes adequate postural responses, chest expansion, rhythmical breathing, and fluency in speech production.

There are many competency levels required for various types of sucking (nipple, breast, pacifier, finger). Assessing or offering practice on one area may not reflect competency in another area. In truth, we may be overtiring the infant and reducing his efficiency during feeding.

This progression of events may give us some clues to assessment and treatment goals for the 0-3 population. It may also help identify problem areas in the older child. How many of our children (of any diagnostic category) display one or more of the following? 1) oral defensiveness, 2) oral sensory seeking behaviors, 3) high arched palates, 4) poor suck swallow synchrony, 5) arrhythmical breathing patterns, 6) inadequate mouth closure, 7) drooling (constant, intermittent or under stress), 8) pot bellies and relatively flat upper chest configuration. And how many of those children have significant histories of early feeding problems?

In reviewing only a fraction of the available literature related to oral motor development, it becomes apparent that the influences of the cranial nerves, V, VII, VIII, IX & X tactile, proprioceptive and vestibular sensory input via position, movement and muscle activity before, during and after feeding are enormous. Please refer to the bibliography for references. Knowledge of these influences is critical for responsible and accurate diagnosis and remediation of oral-motor problems and their subsequent effects on sensorimotor integration.

Role of Occupational Therapy With Infants During the First Three Years of Life

A. Assess the child's ability to problem solve. In the neonate or pre-term infant, begin by assessing the autonomic nervous system's ability to close down or become excited by incoming stimuli. As the nervous system matures this ability becomes more subtle, discreet and less variable. Special training is required for this type of assessment (i.e, Brazleton).

B. Assess infant's muscle tone, reflexes, sensations and movement patterns. While this training is inherent in OT training, it requires much experience with normal newborn infants to become skilled in detecting abnormalities. Special training and experience are necessary to detect discrepancies in the pre-term infant or the infant in an intensive care unit.

C. Help plan programs for individual infants in cooperation with hospital staff and parents. The therapist can become a vital link between hospital staff and parents if well prepared.

D. Implement parent and staff education programs, and provide models for both parents and staff offering the best possible environment to promote normal growth and development.

E. Refer child to community agencies if long-term programming is appropriate.

F. Complete follow-up evaluation of developmental programs.

G. Gather data to begin providing information on risk factors appropriate for follow up and criteria and effect of intervention.

Sensory Integration and Mental Retardation

by Jeanetta D. Burpee MEd, OTR

Our thanks to Jeannetta Burpee, MEd, OTR, for the featured articles on SI and MR. Jeannetta received her BA in OT from Colorado State University and a master's degree in educational psychology from Temple university. She is CSSID faculty and is currently working as supervisor of the psychosocial clinic (serving 1500 MR individuals) at Pennhurst Center, Spring City, PA. She is also currently involved in the development of a theoretical framework detailing the interdynamics of cognition neuromotor, and psychosocial development.

Using sensory integrative theory and therapy with mentally retarded individuals opens doors in all parameters of development, the neurodevelopmental, psychosocial, and the cognitive. It remains for each of us as a therapist to be ready for and have the skill to accept and nurture growth risks in those other spheres along with the neuromotor. When developmental problems are as diffuse and severe as we find them in the severely and profoundly retarded, every developmental process seems disabled and in need of support for the most rapid and complete gains toward individualization.

Sensory integrative theory examines the interdynamics between neural systems. Deficits in primal systems, the vestibular and tactile, can readily cause subsequent deficits at higher levels of neural integration and their resultant behavioral skills, such as visual perception and motor planning. However, the ladders of support are not only vertical, rather also horizontal. If a person is so defensive of movement input that the most direct path of treatment through the vestibular system is precluded, the therapist can and does treat through the tactile and proprioceptive systems and can effectively alleviate certain vestibular hypersensitivities. If a therapist should be so lucky as to have all forms and manner of sensory input available in the treatment session and a nonthreatened patient, then the gains during treatment are most likely going to be even more rapid due to interactive support between neural systems. The lines of support, communication, and organization are highly interactive within our central nervous system and if used will more effectively remediate problem areas. Similarly, when working with the mentally retarded, where deficits are pervasive and well beyond the neuromotor developmental parameter, we need to sustain and support integration by treating all behavioral parameters involved.

Lois is a profoundly retarded lady who shows many classic signs of severe vestibular system deficit (hypotonus, inability to co-contract, inability to assume a pivot prone position, very weak extensors, refusal to be moved or positioned, postural insecurity, refusal to be tested for postrotary nystagmus, constant body rocking, and head rotating) but also active withdrawal from all social-emotional and interpersonal interaction, a flat affect, and few if any cognitive schemes for exploration and controlled manipulation of her surroundings. There is little doubt that she needs more in her therapy sessions than sensory integration and little doubt that before hands-on treatment can begin, Lois will need to trust enough or want enough from another to allow space sharing and eventually contact with another individual. She will need to establish some apparent control within her environment and be allowed to maintain some control to assuage her fear of being in turn controlled by others, out of control herself, and physically as well as emotionally threatened in the process, if not actually hurt. Lois refuses contact but without further evidence it remains to be seen whether this is an extreme end result of postural insecurity or in fact a tactile system deficit resulting in tactile defensiveness. At this point in evaluation and treatment I have decided to leave it at as such and call it spatial defensiveness, a place where the therapist cannot reach to provide sensory integrative hands-on treatment anyway. The initial effort begins not with hands-on but rather by identifying the complex of behavioral parameters in deficit (sensory integrative-neuromotor, an emotional-social problem, and a cognitive deficit).

(continued)

Sensory Integration and Mental Retardation

This complex is predominated by withdrawal and total resistance in all three developmental spheres. Neurodevelopmentally, there is insecurity with an emotional response of threat and a total coping schematic response of active resistance to any form of interaction. Being spatially defensive, Lois is not even secure in her own body self and the space around her which is empty of objects and other persons. She is as yet without the ability to even accept spatial changes, other than those simple movements she imposes on herself and in total control by herself. She is unable to control basic reflexes and assert her position against gravity. She controls the imposition of these reflexes by avoiding movements or positions which might elicit a reflexive response (namely prone positions where a residual tonic labyrinthine and lack of extensor tonus disallows any resistance of gravity's pull downward). She is also further inhibited by the environment and its surrounding people who insist upon changing her already insecure status quo, and imposing more threats of change and more loss of self-control. By acknowledging that Lois must initially take control of the space around her, learn to be able to expect and anticipate what is happening, where the therapist is in relation to her own body self and what the therapist will and will not do to that space surrounding her, Lois comes to trust her body self in its space. She initially becomes less spatially defensive and more spatially secure. Once this sense of space and position is secured, Lois and therapist can proceed to ever closer interactions in space and eventually interactions involving contact.

To jump forward in the treatment process a bit and glimpse gains at a higher level of integration and interaction, it is possible to watch how neuromotor, emotional-social, and cognitive schemes evolve concomitantly. As Lois gains control of her extensor muscles, she is able to assume pivot prone and resist gravity's pull. She shows real resistance in muscle tone and a resistance that allows her to assert a degree of control over her body position. She is no longer without the means to help herself, no longer defenseless and without choices or alternatives in movement patterns. At the same time Lois begins to assert herself emotionally and no longer resists with anger all that is offered to her. She now pulls the therapist to her, smiles, or frowns and pushes the contact away. Her choices for feelings have expanded as have her reasons for expressing them. She sits and watches the therapist who is with another peer, begins to cry, scoots closer, pushes her peer away and stretches out her own arm for a rub and closeness. Now she laughs excitedly. With greater control of herself, knowing she herself can manipulate the environment to get what she wants, there is greater demand for more involvement, greater needs to be met and more assertion in order to get it from those who give. The emotions and their demands do not always seem immediately positive as they come out and are tried in their newness and need for expression but the therapist must somehow accept them and move on. When someone gets hit in jealousy and it is the first time an overt gesture is given that shows there is a need for being recognized and a need to get closer, then it behooves the therapist to find a way to accept and in no way to reject that reaching out. It is just as when Lois first walks over to the swivel chair and gives it a good shove to show her control of it despite her refusal to sit in it that is the beginning of a trust situation. She is now showing the most secure gesture in her interaction but it is the place where she must begin. Equally apparent are those cognitive schemes developing in interaction with the total process. From simple withdrawal, Lois learned to push or pull people and objects around her, to smell, taste, feel, watch as she processed information.

She begins to pick objects up and turn them over, throw them away, pull the swivel chair to her, sit in it and push with her feet or sit beside it and turn the seat around watching it. To get into the therapy room she learned how to rotate the door knob or to get out when she'd had enough she learned to turn the lock on the door, open it, and walk out. Schemes of exploration and schemes for play expanded as she gained neuromotor control, decreased defensive responses, gained emotional and social expression, wants, assertiveness, and generally found more pleasureful alternatives in risking and reaching out.

Unless a therapist is ready for and can assist by accepting and nurturing all those risk-taking ventures embarked on when an individual begins to integrate and cope with this world, the learning process will not be as complete nor nearly as rapid. Where the etiology is often diffuse and the results severe, multiple problems result. Treating one without the constant regard for the other is much like disregarding the obvious facts that a pyramid needs all sides and a base for support where each resists the others' fall, and assists in the others' climb. When one needs to rebuild, all angles are considered and interposed concomitantly. It is a problem of interparameter support in conjunction with interneural support.

Self-Abuse And Self-Stimulation

Along similar lines, it seems that when there is a problem such as self-stimulation or self-abuse, the individual shows root problems in several behavioral parameters of development, not just the neurological, or just the social, or just the cognitive. Meg is a blind, profoundly retarded lady who spent much time sitting upside down in a chair, feet up against the chair back and head dangling over the edge, for long periods of time alone and seemingly content. Other time was spent literally shoving furniture and people around, pulling or pushing, and then hanging on very tightly to staff. With sensory integrative therapy stressing vestibular, proprioceptive, and tactile input, together with consistent tactile, verbal, and tonal acknowledgment of her presence during therapy whether in contact or spatially separated from others, Meg's needs reached less intensive levels and "bizarre" activities decreased. The problem was seen as one with two primal need deficits—sensory integrative (specifically vestibular and proprioceptive) and emotional dependencies unmet.

Dean was a head banger, particularly when upset and apparently threatened by another's presence and/or demands on him, or when he was sitting alone. He hid his hands inside his shirt cuffs or pants and often pulled his shirt over his head, rocked and bounced on the sofa. His only interactions with the external environment were simple repetitive object schemes, spinning and twirling balls or pieces of paper or shoelaces. On the other hand, he might come and sit in an aide's or therapist's lap cuddling and clinging. If staff persons were farther than one or two feet distant, there was no eye contact, no acknowledgment of their presence, and Dean would not come if called unless a direct contactual and manual signal was given. Dean's needs were seen as a triad of interacting and intensifying root systems. He was in need of sensory stimulation provided by those he trusted, by those who would respond to his nonverbal signals to let go or accept him when he came for contact. He needed to be in "control," while simultaneously participating in a dependent all-accepting relationship with another. This relationship provided a dynamic which contained elements of an adualistic infant's existence where subject is not separate from object and infant is not separate from the rest of the world and the ever-present parent. Within this structure the individual is not dependent or independent but rather simply in complete harmony where needs are known to others without their being stated and met without the need to reach out to take. It is quite a passive existence but a very accepting existence as well. It seemed that Dean thrived with just such a consistent relationship where he had no doubt of getting the warmth, contact, sustenance his central nervous system and psyche needed, where he would receive without even reaching out or having to ask. His sim-

(continued)

Sensory Integration and Mental Retardation

ple intellectual schemes were entirely wrapped up in accepting, as an infant suckles the readily available nipple and molds into its mother's body.

Head banging was understood as a behavioral alternative which in some way attempted to fulfill several needs. The first was neurological and seen as a need for sustaining sensory integrative levels. It tapped or provided vestibular, tactile, and proprioceptive input. It was also seen as a psychological defense and also a means for immediate cathexis. Where the environment and those surrounding Dean threatened demands and painful or frightening interaction, self-stimulation seemed calculated as a means of inner distraction. By evading or distracting oneself with self-involving activities, activities which diffuse and redirect energy, there is less to attend to which is external to the body self. It is also possible that when the situation peaks with painful ambivalence, and Dean is caught between

wanting to be with others and yet too threatened to reach out, he head bangs as a means of diminishing or desensitizing that painful psychic ambivalence. We rub away a painful itch or we kick a stone when faced with an angry situation, so that Dean butts his head in a similar scheme. His third need was for cognitive schemes which would allow for and offer viable alternatives in dealing with his situation with other persons and his environment. Spinning and twirling were not enough and just seemed to fulfill the purpose of taking him farther away by enacting a point of focus not respondent to environmental activity around him.

Treatment in all three developmental parameters, with techniques which merge and interact allowed Dean not only to decrease headbanging but to release his hands from his pockets, uncover his head and begin to reach out and take hold of himself and his ever-present situation. He eventually opened his mouth and said, "More!,"

while laughing and spinning around the room with the therapist in an old bicycle inner tube.

Thus far I've attempted to discuss how parameters of development interact to exacerbate and create a pervasive holistic system of dysfunction. The individual who is mentally retarded finds him/herself in need of many types of support and facilitation in the process of individualization. But this is only the beginning of the therapeutic experience. The real challenge comes as the therapist watches and permits these interdynamics to continue as ever higher levels of adaptation are reached. The sensory integrative process continues to expand with the process of ego differentiation in the personal-social sphere and both processes intertwine with expanding cognitive adaptations. For our purposes they are easier studied separately but for the individual in process they are certainly one.

Sensory Integration
Special Interest Section Newsletter; Vol. 2, No. 3, 1979

How Long Do You Spin?

"How long do you spin a child with nonobservable nystagmus?"

"Should I tell the parents to spin their child five or ten minutes?"

Child spinning in net, stopwatch ticking: "Six minutes already! Isn't that great?!"

"This boy has depressed nystagmus but can't tolerate any spinning. That rules out SI therapy, doesn't it?"

"We have some learning-disabled children and I've heard that spinning is supposed to be good for them. Will you tell me how to do it?"

The answer to all these questions is the same: a resounding, unequivocal "NO."

The last therapist went on to ask, "You're an SI therapist but you don't believe in spinning? Don't tell me you don't use it?" Again, the answer is "No," but further, "I understand the effect of spinning as one form of vestibular input, and I apply it in therapy where appropriate, according to my trained clinical judgment, but I'm not advising you to use it and I can't tell you how."

At least these therapists asked and could

be answered. It has come to our attention that many others, having heard about the therapeutic use of vestibular stimulation but not sufficiently understanding it, believe that spinning is the only or the best method for all, that anybody can try it, and that the more spinning the better.

Spinning can, in carefully selected instances, be an effective, appropriate therapeutic tool. It is by no means the only or always the most desirable type of vestibular stimulation, but SI-certified therapists, using it advisedly, find some limited application for it. It can be employed responsibly only by those who understand the neural mechanisms involved, the appropriate techniques and positions, the expected effects, both positive and negative, and the subtle clinical signs that are indicators of these effects; they know why, how, what happens and how you know, as well as who and when. As in all therapeutics, dosage is an important factor and must be understood and controlled; one or two units of medication may be effective, but ten or twenty are not necessarily better

or even safe. Duration of spinning depends entirely on the patient's reaction, not the clock, and is a matter of seconds, not minutes. And there is an important distinction, actual and semantic: *you* don't spin, the patient does.

Arbitrarily applied, excessive spinning can and has harmed patients, and such irresponsible use has reflected not only on the practitioner in question, but on all SI therapy, and has jeopardized the status of occupational therapy programs in some communities. SISS has gone on record with a statement that OTs are expected to apply neurotherapy responsibly. Follow this simple rule: if you are interested in using SI therapy, including spinning, but don't know much about it, don't dabble. Get serious. There are many learning opportunities available. For your clients' sake, your own and your profession's, become competent first.

How long do you spin? There is only one answer: If you have to ask that question, don't spin your client. — *Antje Price, OTR, SISS Standing Committee Member.*

Individual Differences in Autistic Children

At the annual CSSID Faculty Meeting held at Denver, Feb. 23-25, Dr. A. Jean Ayres presented a significant paper which had previously been prepared for and presented at the Piagetian Conference, Feb. 2, sponsored by the University Affiliated Program and the University of Southern California.

In this study, she compared the reactions of 11 autistic children with 11 aphasic dyspraxic children to 14 different stimuli. Their reactions were scored most frequently on a contiuum from under-reaction to over-reaction using four gradations. Exploring presentation of these carefully selected stimuli allows the therapist concerned with dysfunction in sensory integration to observe the differences in one child's ability to process various types of sensory input.

In this very brief overview, it seemed ap-propriate to report that all of the autistic children demonstrated hyporeactive or no clinically observable nystagmus following rotation; 5 were hyposensitive and 5 were hypersensitive to movement; 5 were posturally insecure and 4 demonstrated tactile defensiveness. Five sought vibratory stimuli. None were over-reactive to a puff of air, firm pressure, pain or distasteful food. Their regard for a specific visual stimuli seemed most significant.

These findings can serve as a guide to assist in observing the autistic child's behavior and not necessarily as a guide for therapy.

Ayres' complete report will be published by the University of Southern California within the next six months. In this interim, therapists should continue to thoroughly review functional neurology. Ayers identified that the amygdala, hippocampus, hypothalamus and basal ganglia may be related to dysfunction. The limbic system circuitry with the frontal lobe and mesocortex needs thorough investigation with relation to attention.

Studies that scientifically measure a client's reactions to sensory stimuli are to be developed and reported by the therapists working with multiply involved children and adults, as one proceeds with full professional responsibility. Professional competency is based on knowledge of the nuerosciences, theories of sensory integration and processing, normal development, and clinical experience.—*Ginny Scardina, CSSID Faculty Member.*

Therapy Suggestions

The Bay Area Association for Sensory Integration shares with other SISS members the following summary of guidelines for sensory integration therapy as suggested by Dr. Ayres:

There are two determinants for therapy: age and nature of the problem. Under five years, any diagnosis can benefit from a few months to a year in therapy. By four years of age, two years of therapy is recommended, and if the child continues to show improvement, a further year would be suggested. From five to seven years, not more than two years of therapy is recommended. At eight years and beyond, not more than a year of therapy is recommended. If the child is making progress, no matter what the age, therapy should be continued until a plateau of behavior of six months duration is reached.

Types of disorders that respond to SI therapy are: delayed speech with a postrotary nystagmus of short (Dr. Ayres uses the word attenuated) duration responds best; vestibular and bilateral integration syndrome with attenuated nystagmus are candidates below age eighteen; dyspraxic children with attenuated nystagmus, or somatosensory dysfunction, or postural ("gravitational" is the word used by Dr. Ayers) insecurity, or high IQ are good candidates; they often are emotionally disturbed.

Delayed speech with normal or prolonged nystagmus and evidence suggestive of left hemisphere dysfunction are poor candidates. Autistic diagnosis is still under study and good predictors are still tentative. Those that seem to do best have gravitational insecurity and tactile defensiveness, will orient to a strong odor or air puff, or are considered high level autistics. Least appropriate for therapy are Down's syndrome, and trainable developmentally delayed.

Any child with tactile defensiveness and gravitational insecurity can benefit. Children with chromosomal abnormalities have not been assessed for their response to SI, but if it is possible to identify dysfunction in tactile or vestibular processing, they can possibly benefit.

Sincere thanks to the Bay Area Association for sharing this valuable information with SISS members!!

Sensory Integration
Special Interest Section Newsletter; Vol. 2, No. 1, 1979

Suggestions for Adolescents

1 — A version of "King of the Mountain" utilizing two rather shakey balance beams joined with a hinge (can be done on one extra long balance beam but its not as much fun). Players approach from opposite ends and beat each other with laundry bags filled with cotton (or dacron) stuffing until one falls off. This was extremely popular with both staff and patients.

2 — An "Exercise" program that was done self-placed in groups of 2 or 3 to earn points. A daily program to complete was posted and recorded on a separate posted chart. This included traditional situps etc. plus jump rope, barrel rolls, use of other equipment including a body flexor from Sears (great for vestibular). The boys did surprisingly well with this and after supervised sessions they would go in sensory integrative room and do it well without constant supervision.

3 — Bicycling. We had old bicycles donated, and parts were donated by local bike manufacturers, the patients repaired bikes and then went on short trips around the grounds (good for top-bottom integration, reciprocal patterns and vestibular especially). We did the same with a couple of go carts.

4 — Soccer. Very popular—this was organized to provide sensory motor experience as well as social skills. They would play in the mud and got very skillful. This is great for all sorts of SI experience.—*Beth Moyer*

Cookie Factory is a game that can include many forms of input to the skin. Some ideas follow—use your imagination to adapt these to each child's needs.
  1. Add ingredients—chocolate chips—apply deep pressure with finger tips; sugar—light touch, etc.
  2. Mix ingredients—use vibrator (pretend electric mixer).
  3. Roll out dough—use a rolling pin covered with material (held in place with rubber bands).
  4. Cut out cookies—use dull cookie cutters or geometric forms, pressing on body. Ask child to identify shape being "cut".
  5. Bake the cookies—wrap child in blanket—ask to lie still—dim lights use hair dryer—(warm air). —*Wendy Eichstaedt, OTR.*

Going Swimming—a game for tactile involvement. Child swims prone (crawl) or supine (backstroke) on top of an outstretched parachute. Then gets out of (water) parachute and rubs dry body with terry towels. I used scented lotions, i.e., coconut, honey for suntain lotion which they rub on after they have dried off.

Bubble Balance—a game to increase balance and equilibrium response and assist with body identification. Child stands on balance disc, balance beam etc.; therapist blows bubbles through wand and asks child to pop bubble with a specific body part.—*Debby Sprenger*

Yoga In Therapy—Several yoga positions have been used to facilitate prone extension, supine flexion, and trunk rotation in high-functioning children; e.g.—the "cobra" and "bow" to facilitate prone extension, the "plough" for supine flexion, and "spinalk twist" for rotation. The children responded well and enjoyed the yoga, especially if their parents were involved in yoga also. The use of animal imagery helped but the positions on a more subcortical level.—*Jo Teachman*

Lynn Andrews, OTR with professional photography assistance has developed a slide/tape presentation introducing the role of occupational therapy in the public schools, "OT: A Complement to Special Education." It is available on a loan basis only from Katherine Moore, Division for Exceptional Children, State Department of Public Instruction, Raleigh, NC.

The demand will be great. You may want to write early and be placed on the waiting list.—*Ginny Scardina*

Sensory Integration
Special Interest Section Newsletter; Vol. 1, No. 2, 1978

Sensory Integration Library

Since the formation of the specialty sections the membership has expressed various areas of concern. Some examples include:

A. Evaluation
  —of adults, adolescents, etc.
  —screening tools (e.g. as predictors of children needing services; early infancy, etc.)
  —Re-evaluation tools
  —etc.

B. Treatment
  —Precautions
  —Record Keeping
  —Sharing of techniques and ideas

C. Interpretations of Sensor Integration
  —To teachers, parents
  —To administrators
  —To physicians (etc.)

D. Sensory Integration as it applies to
  —Adolescents
  —Adults
  —Emotionally disturbed
  —Geriatrics
  —Infancy
  —Learning disabilities
  —Mental Health
  —Mental Retardation
  —Multiply Handicapped
  —Special sensory losses

E. Theory and Neurophysiology

F. Etc., Etc.

Many therapists across the country have met some of these obstacles and dealt with them effectively. Other therapists are still struggling and searching for assistance.

In order to expedite more effective communication, a central "library" of sensory integration information is being developed. All therapists are asked to share their experiences and knowledge, as the library depends entirely on membership contributions. **No piece of information is too insignificant to share!** Some examples of pertinent contributions might include:

• Graduate and undergraduate papers (e.g. information not necessarily prepared for publication, but that the author has found interesting and helpful in some phase of SI study).

• Papers or outlines found helpful in communication with individuals not familiar with SI (e.g. Physicians, parents, educators administrators, Speech Therapists, Physical Therapists, etc. etc.)

(continued)

Sensory Integration Library

- Compiled (and/or annotated) bibliographies
- Critiques of current literature
- Tapes and Videotapes (Although tapes of workshops may not be acceptable without the consent of the instructor, many SI therapists have lectured to parent groups, students, etc. Could these not be taped for sharing?

- General information (e.g. liability and legal concerns, private practice, 3rd party payer, consultation etc.)

Please send all contributions to: Michelle Catellier, Coordinator of Continuing Education, SISS, 312 S. Downey Ave., Indianapolis, IN 46219, (317) 359-7349)

The status of contributions and procedure for borrowing will be announced in a future newsletter. —*Submitted by the Committee for Coordination of Continuing Education for SISS, Michelle Catallier, OTR, Kathy Claussen, OTR, Debi Ludeman, OTR, Becky Sanders, OTR, Karen Szatalowicz, OTR, Diane Zaitz, OTR.*

Sensory Integration
Special Interest Section Newsletter; Vol. 1, No. 2, 1978

Results of Research Survey

Many thanks to all those people who returned the research survey sent out in the last *Newsletter.* I was staggered at the amount of people who are willing to do independent research in the area of Sensory Integration. All people submitting the research survey results will receive a letter giving them the names and addresses of a) people involved in similar research and b) the name of a resource person, if the need for assistance had been indicated.

For interest to other readers the following is a list of research topics which was submitted. The names and addresses of principle investigators will not appear publicly however, if you desire to get in contact with a particular resource, you may write to me for the name and address.

Effects of Time of Day Southern California Postrotary Nystagmus Test

Tactile Stimulation for Geriatric Patients

Influencing the Development of a Developmentally Delayed Child Through Vestibular and Tactile Stimulation

Effects of a Program of Tactile Stimulation on Weight Gain in Premature Infants

Improving Visual Motor Skill Through Sensory Integration

Determining Biofeedback as a Means to Quantify Hyperactivity

Effects of Sensory Integration Treatment on the Low Achieving College Student

Haptic Perception in the Hyperactive Emotionally Impaired Child

Validation of a Simple Method to Identify Children with Vestibular Dysfunction

Establishment of some Norms for Kindergarten Children on the Clinical Observations

Relationships Between Sensory Integrative Function and Emotional Distrubance in Children

Pilot Study to Determine Trends of Mean Scores on Clinical Observations on Children 4 to 10 Years

Vestibular Input: Its effect on feeding and sleeping behavior of premature infants

Visual Tracking of Normal Children

Effects of Tactile Stimulation on Normal Preschool Children

Determination of the Reliability of Certain Observation Criteria of Motor Abilities as Predictors of Future Sensory Integrative and Cognitive Abilities

Provide a Program that can be run by local schools under the direction of Sensory Integrative OTR

Breaking up an ATNR in a 13 Year Old Spastic Quadriplegic CP: Case Studies

Effectiveness of Sensory Integrative Treatment in Comparison to Operant Conditioning on Mentally Retarded Children

Development of a Screening and Diagnostic Tool for Preschool Children

Sensory Integrative Treatment Effects on Unsocialized Aggressive Children

Verification of Normative Data: Postrotary Nystagmus

Refinement of the Proposed Linkage between the Depressed Postrotary Nustagmus and Language Disorders

The Incidence of Sensory Integrative Dysfunction in Children with Orofacial Cleft

Autonomic Effects of Vestibular Stimulation in Autistic Children

Identification of Sensory Integrative Dysfunction in an Autistic Population

Measuring the Effects of Sensory Integration Therapy in Chronic Schizophrenic Adult Males

A Program Evaluation of Sensory Integrative Therapy in the Treatment of Adult Schizophrenics

Preliminary Normative Data for the Tactile-Kinesthetic Tests on the SCSIT

The Effects of Vibratory Tactile Stimulation on Tactile Defensiveness in Hyperactive Children

The Effects of Perceptual Motor Programs on the Perceptual Motor Development with Developmentally Disabled Adults

Vestibular Function in Mildly Mentally Retarded Adults

Prediction of Ritalin Effectiveness through Sensory Integrative Diagnostics

Correlations Between Selected Skills and Academic Readiness at the Kindergarten Level.

Relationship of Vestibular Function to Academic Readiness

Patterns of Sensory Integrative Dysfunction in Adult Hemiplegia

Survey Sheets are still being sent to me. An updated list will appear in the next issue of this newsletter.

Thanks again for your response. For those of you interested, there *may* be a research workshop held in the future specifically designed to help those of you who are working on a project and do not have good resources. If you would be interested in such a workshop, maybe you could write—I will keep the names and contact you specifically when the workshop is planned. —*Chris Chapparo, OTR*

Sensory Integration
Special Interest Section Newsletter; Vol. 1, No. 1, 1978

Why Is Sensory Integration a Separate Specialty Section?

Recently there has been much questioning of the need for a separate sensory Integration Speicalty Section. Since sensory integration and sensory integration disorders are common to so many diagnostic categories, why is it not included in all specialty sections — why is it treated differently?

Sensory integration is a unique body of knowledge within the Occupational Therapy field. It arose from within the field and its development has primarily been nurtured by occupational therapists. More research is necessary at this time to further solidify its position as a viable neurobiologically based treatment approach. Occupational therapists must continue to nurture sensory integration theory, to assure its acceptance by persons outside the field. That nurturance and the "power" needed to further research will be fragmented if sensory integration were distilled into the other specialty sections. Sensory integration must be firmly identified as an area of practice for occupational therapists and its development must be encouraged.

In the field of medicine there has been a phenomenon similar to that which the Occupational Therapy profession is facing. The original concept of general paractice gave way to increasing specialization, ad infinitum, as medical knowledge expanded. Within the medical field there is now a swing back to that concept of the G.P. — the difference being that the knowledge accumulated through specialization is now available to the G.P. The G.P.'s own knowledge is expanded by exposure to the bodies of knowledge acquired through specialization. In addition, acknowledging that no one person can accumulate or retain all that knowledge, specialists continue to be available to the G.P.

AOTA seems in the beginning stages of specialization. We are rapidly expanding our theoretical bases and refining our evaluation and treatment procedures in all specialty areas. More textbooks and research articles are being published; the university curricula are stuffed to the bursting point! These benefits of increasing specialization are becoming available to the generalist. The specialists are developing coherent bodies of knowledge which can be used by the generalist; and the generalist can refer to the specialist if appropriate.

The concept of a separate sensory integration specialty section is not intended to exclude persons without "expertise." It is envisioned that there will be several levels within the specialty section. A resource network of experienced persons has been developed to pass on the benefits of their experience and knowledge to those members of the Sensory Integration Specialty Section seeking to expand their knowledge of sensory integration. One need not be a sensory integration "specialist" to belong to the S.I.S.S. — one needs only to desire more knowledge in this area.

Many therapists have opted to join more than one specialty section, reflecting the many desirable areas of overlap between the specialty sections. The specialty section chairs will determine how that overlap is dealt with — already, communication between chairs is occurring to share knowledge, goals, common interests, etc. Last fall a grass roots meeting of persons interested in sensory integration was held at Good Samaritan Hospital in Cincinnati. Possible objectives for the Sensory Integration Specialty Section identified at the meeting included developing a resource network, generating research, developing more continuing education, and increasing public relations efforts.

These objectives were adopted by the S.I.S.S. steering committee. It would appear that these objectives can best be carried out at this time by a separate Sensory Integration Specialty Section.

Jo Teachman
Eastern Kentucky University

Index